Medicode's 1999 Publications & Software For Coders

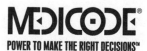
POWER TO MAKE THE RIGHT DECISIONS™

Medicode, Inc. 5225 Wiley Post Way, Suite 500, Salt Lake City, UT 84116 • 801-536-1000 • FAX 801-536-1011

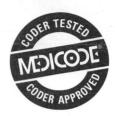
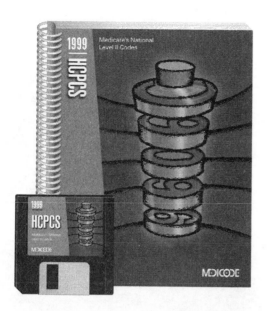
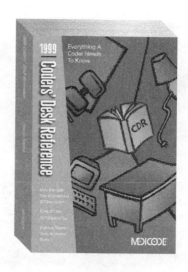
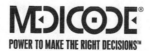

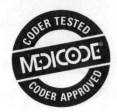
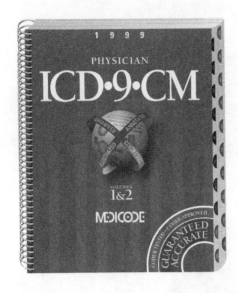
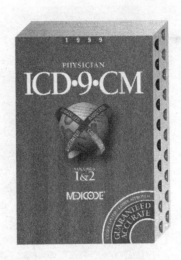
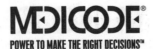

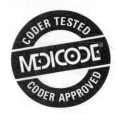
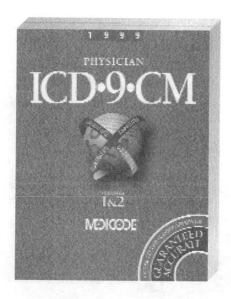
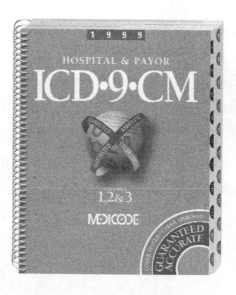
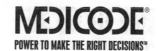

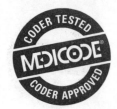
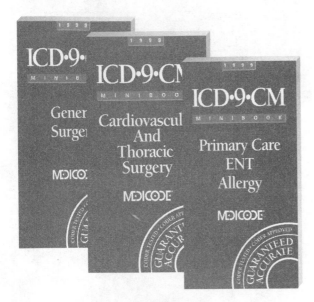
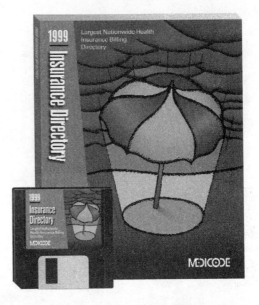
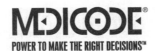

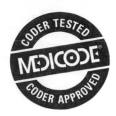
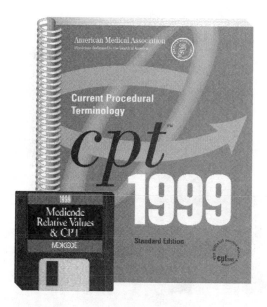

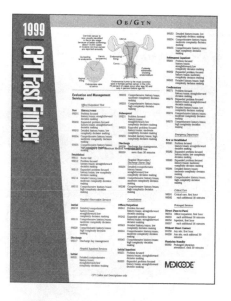

Stay Current With 1999 CPT Codes

Cheat Sheets For CPT

Choose from two versions of CPT in 1999: *Professional Edition* or *Standard Edition*. Both come with all the 1999 code information you need, but the *Professional Edition* also includes color keys, anatomical illustrations, medical terminology, thumb tabs and your choice of spiral binding or a 3-ring binder.

1999 CPT, Professional Edition	**$64**⁹⁵	(No. 2612)
1999 CPT, Professional Edition Binder	**$72**⁹⁵	(No. 2623)
1999 CPT, Spiral	**$49**⁹⁵	(No. 2611)
1999 CPT, Softbound	**$47**⁹⁵	(No. 2610)
1999 ASCII File*	**$229**⁹⁵	(No. 2724)

*For single-user license only. Call for multi-user pricing.

New for 1999. Our double-sided, laminated *CPT Fast Finder* provides a quick reference list of the most common codes for that specialty. Choose from 21 different specialties

- **1999 Codes.** Includes updated codes.

- **Saves Time.** Each sheet includes surgery, E/M, lab radiology and the most commonly used codes for that specialty to save you time.

- **Illustrated.** Each sheet contains anatomical illustrations to orient you to physiology.

- **Slightly Undersized.** Fits easily into your coding book.

1999 CPT Specialty Fast Finder   **$24**⁹⁵   **per sheet**

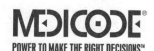

Medicode, Inc. 5225 Wiley Post Way, Suite 500, Salt Lake City, UT 84116 • 801-536-1000 • FAX 801-536-1011

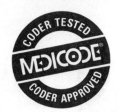
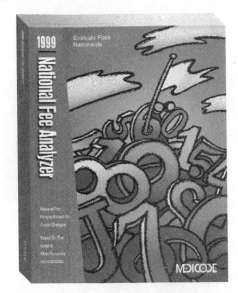
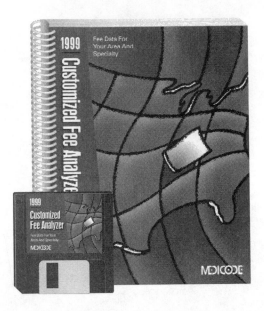
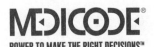

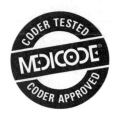
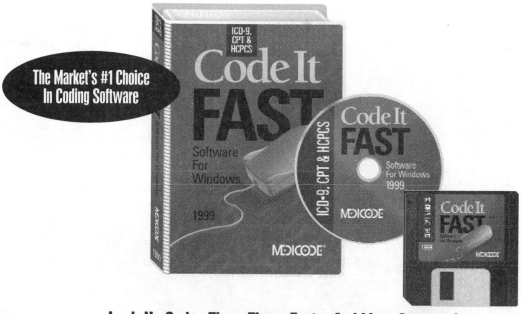
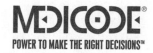

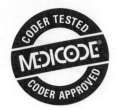
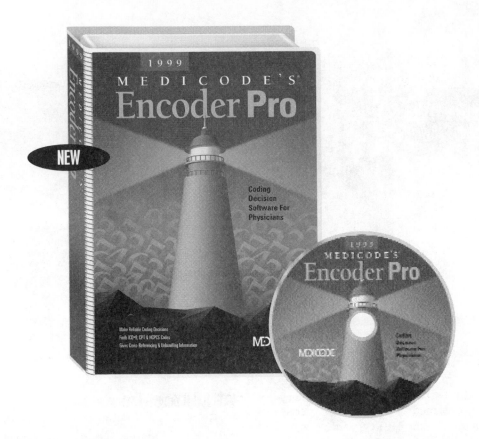

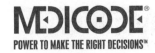

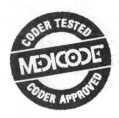
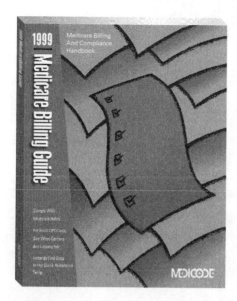
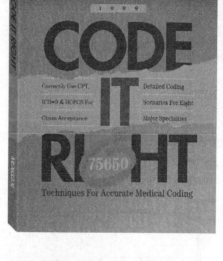
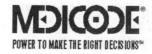

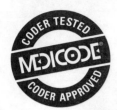
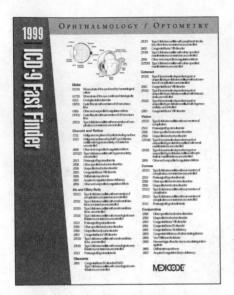
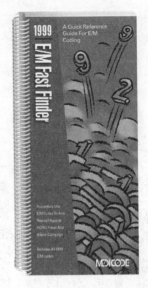
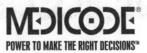

Code It Right

MEDICODE®

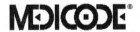

5225 Wiley Post Way, Suite 500
Salt Lake City, UT 84116-2889

Publishing Staff

Publisher	*Susan P. Seare*
Associate Medical Director	*Thomas G. Darr, M.D., F.A.C.E.P.*
Editorial Director	*Lynn Speirs*
Product Managers	*Anne Petrie, M.B.A.*
	Ralph S. Wankier, M.B.A.
Project Editor	*Christine B. Fraizer, M.A.*
Editor	*Kimberli Turner*
Clinical Editors	*Lauri Gray, A.R.T., C.P.C.*
	Charlene Neeshan, L.P.N., C.C.S., C.P.C., C.P.C.-H.
Designer/Typesetter	*Kerrie Hornsby*
Editorial Assistant	*Lisa Singley*

PLEASE NOTE

This book does not replace the CPT, ICD•9•CM, HCPCS Level II, or other coding system books. It serves only as a guide.

Attention Educators

Enhance your students' learning with curriculum developed especially for *Code It Right*. The curriculum includes a student workbook and an instructor's manual that provides workbook answers and a test bank.

This curriculum was developed by health careers educator Kay Cox, R.N., M.A. Ms. Cox is founder of Achiever's Development Enterprises and program coordinator of the medical assistant program at Saddleback College in Mission Viejo, California. A nationally known author and editor of clinical and administrative medical textbooks, Ms. Cox worked for the California Department of Education as a contract consultant for 10 years and was formerly chairperson of the California Health Careers Advisory Committee.

For more information or to order your curriculum call:

949-364-0540

or write:

Code It Right Curriculum
Achiever's Development Enterprises
PO Box 4122
Mission Viejo, CA 92690

Contents

Introduction

As simple as it sounds, if you want to get paid for what you do, you have to speak the language. Physicians use a common language of names and terms (nomenclature) to communicate with other physicians and with the organizations that reimburse them for the services they perform. Specific codes serve as a shorthand for this nomenclature and are recognized and accepted by most insurance payors. These codes represent diagnoses, physician services and procedures, and medical services and supplies. To be fairly and adequately reimbursed in a timely fashion by third-party payors, physicians and their reimbursement specialists must understand and use these codes correctly.

Code It Right is a comprehensive introduction to medical coding. This newest edition, published by Medicode, is easy to use. Its textbook format lists objectives at the beginning and discussion questions at the end of the chapter sections so coders can test themselves. Coding tips, definitions, and rules are highlighted in a brief, concise manner in the margins. It includes a description of the three coding references with the directions to use them accurately, as well as chapters on inpatient and Medicare coding. Eight specialty-specific coding scenarios illustrate appropriate coding in every chapter.

The first primary coding system to be discussed in *Code It Right* is the diagnostic reference, *International Classification of Diseases, 9th Revision, Clinical Modification*, referred to as ICD-9-CM. Within this system, the code for acute appendicitis with generalized peritonitis is 540.0, and a closed shaft fracture of the ulna is coded as 813.22. Chapter 1 of *Code It Right* establishes a fundamental understanding of ICD-9-CM conventions and applications.

The second reference, *Physicians' Current Procedural Terminology*, known as CPT, is published annually by the American Medical Association (AMA) and contains codes for services provided by physicians and other health professionals. Correlating the diagnostic examples above, the appendectomy is coded as 44960, and closed treatment of a closed ulnar shaft fracture without manipulation is 25530. The bulk of the information contained in *Code It Right* is about CPT and is broken out with a chapter for each of its sections. Chapters 2 through 8 detail specific information on anesthesia, modifiers, evaluation and management, surgery, radiology, pathology and laboratory, and medicine services. The specialty-specific coding scenarios presented at the end of each chapter apply the coding rules to physician practices and inpatient reporting.

The third reference is the *Health Care Financing Administration (HCFA) Common Procedure Coding System*, commonly called HCPCS (pronounced "hick-picks"). These codes report medical services and supplies not specifically identified in CPT, including drugs administered by injection and durable medical equipment. Codes in this system are not as widely accepted as an industry standard as are CPT and ICD-9-CM codes, though their use is growing. HCPCS information is presented in Chapter 10.

No coding reference would be complete without an overview of the complex system underpinning today's government and third party reimbursement to hospitals, exemplified by Diagnosis Related Groups (DRGs). Inpatient coding, the critical hospital coding system often overlooked in coding manuals, is presented in Chapter 9.

After ICD-9-CM, CPT, and HCPCS coding systems are explained, the foundation is laid for an introduction to Medicare coding in Chapter 11. This chapter in *Code It Right* reviews the Medicare policies and procedures to follow when filing claims for services to Medicare patients.

All examples and clinical scenarios offered in *Code It Right* are drawn from many years of medical coding experience by the authors and do not represent actual clinical cases. The coding schemes presented should not be substituted for similar coding tasks without first consulting proper references.

1 Diagnostic Coding

Historical Perspective

The *International Classification of Diseases, Ninth Revision, Clinical Modification, Fifth Edition,* more commonly referred to as ICD-9-CM is the classification system used by physician offices as well as inpatient and outpatient facilities for the purpose of coding and indexing disease data. ICD-9-CM Volumes 1 and 2 are used in coding diagnosis information and are the focus of this chapter. Volume 3 is used in coding inpatient procedures which will be explained in chapter 9. The medical coder's role in this process is to translate written diagnoses into numeric and alphanumeric codes. This coded information is used by physician offices primarily as means of communicating the reason for the medical services to commercial and government payors, though that was not the original purpose of diagnosis coding. As a communication tool, ICD-9-CM diagnosis codes relate the disease, condition, complaint, sign, symptom or other reason for the medical services provided. In addition to being a means of communication between provider and payor, these diagnosis codes are used as a means to gather statistics for purposes such as: research, grants, financial analysis, compliance with standards set by the National Committee on Quality Assurance (NCQA), and Healthplan Employer Data and Information Set (HEDIS) reporting.

ICD-9

Interestingly, ICD coding was not developed as a diagnostic-reporting tool, but as a statistics-gathering tool. After centuries of disease tracking localized by country or continent, the World Health Organization (WHO) began in 1948 to track sickness (morbidity) and death (mortality) worldwide. Many revisions have occurred, but today's *International Classification of Diseases* (ICD) is still primarily a tool for statisticians. In 1978, WHO published its ninth revision of this list (ICD-9).

ICD-9-CM

Once ICD-9 was internationally recognized, the United States National Center for Health Statistics (NCHS) moved to create a more precise clinical picture of the patient than was needed for statistical groupings and trend analyses. NCHS modified ICD-9 with clinical information that allows a more thorough indexing of medical records, medical case reviews, and ambulatory and other medical care programs. The current *International Classification of Diseases, Ninth Revision, Clinical Modification* reflects these changes. In the United States, ICD-9-CM codes are often referred to as simply ICD-9.

ICD-10

ICD-10 is the tenth revision to the International Classification of Diseases created by the World Health Organization for tracking disease and deaths worldwide. WHO adopted this

OBJECTIVES

Differentiate the origin and objectives of ICD-9, ICD-9-CM, and ICD-10, ICD-10-CM, ICD-10-PCS

Understand the increasing importance of diagnostic coding to quality of care, medical necessity issues, and reimbursement

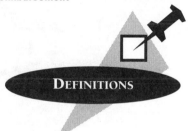

DEFINITIONS

WHO: World Health Organization. This international agency with advice from participating countries developed ICD-9 to track morbidity and mortality statistics worldwide. It recently updated its coding system with ICD-10. WHO can be contacted at: 525 23rd St. NW, Washington, D.C. 20037.

NCHS: National Center for Health Statistics. This U.S. government agency with HCFA jointly refines the diagnostic portion of ICD-9-CM every year to reflect advances in medical diagnostics. NCHS holds several hearings a year to consider changes or additions in ICD-9-CM. NCHS can be contacted at: Room 036, 6525 Belcrest Rd., Hyattsville, MD 20783.

AHA: American Hospital Association. This private agency acts as a clearinghouse for ICD-9-CM coding rules developed by HCFA, NCHS, and AHIMA (American Health Information Management Association). AHA publishes *Coding Clinic* quarterly. AHA can be contacted at: One N Franklin, Chicago, IL 60606.

new system in 1993, and it is currently used in dozens of countries. This new system greatly expands the number of codes available, an essential task, as ICD-9 is running out of room for new designations. ICD-10 was accomplished by changing the entire coding system from predominantly numeric to alphanumeric.

ICD-10-CM

Don't confuse ICD-10-CM with ICD-10. In the United States, ICD-10 is being clinically modified (CM) by the National Center for Health Statistics (NCHS) prior to code adoption. The clinical modification provides the specificity the United States needs for collecting data on our health status. ICD-10 codes contain three or four characters. ICD-10-CM codes may contain up to six characters. The first character is always a letter; the others are numbers. ICD-10-CM is expected to be implemented Oct. 1, 2001. The current draft of the tabular section, released late in 1997, is undergoing revision based on 1,200 public comments received by NCHS earlier this year. A new draft of the tabular section, and the first draft of the index, are expected to be released by mid-1999.

ICD-10-CM represents the most significant revision of the International Classification of Disease (ICD) since ICD's inception. The codes have more characters. They are alphanumeric. The organization of the codes has changed, and their number has jumped by more than 50 percent.

This greater coding detail is called "granularity" and is useful in healthcare policy and also in outcomes research. Naturally, this means a lot more detail will be required from the medical record for ICD-10-CM code selection. Because of the increased granularity, documentation becomes more critical than ever before. Even physicians who are providing documentation sufficient for current coding requirements will need to be educated as to the more detailed requirements of ICD-10-CM.

ICD-10-PCS

ICD-10-CM is an easy transition compared to ICD-10-Procedural Coding System (PCS). This procedural coding system was developed three years ago by 3M HIS under contract with the Health Care Financing Administration (HCFA). HCFA requested development of a single, comprehensive procedural system to supercede other procedural coding systems now in use. HCFA contracted with 3M to design a system that solves problems of specificity, redundancy, and data quality. This new procedural coding system revolutionizes the way we look at procedural coding, stripping it of Latin terms, eponyms, and acronyms, and distilling all of surgery into 30 simple procedures, differentiated by the anatomy upon which the procedure is performed, and the approach used.

Granularity is also a goal of ICD-10-PCS and this is reflected in the greater number of code choices in PCS when compared with both ICD-9-CM Volume 3 and CPT. However, there are other motives at work in the proposed procedural coding system. The government seeks a procedural coding system that is devoid of diagnoses (e.g., aneurysm, hernia, cleft lip, enterocele) and that uses standardized terminology. This standardization of terminology means that while the physician records a "laparoscopic cholecystectomy," the coder must find a code that reports the "endoscopic" "excision" of a "gallbladder."

If adopted, ICD-10-PCS would replace Volume 3 of ICD-9-CM and CPT-4 for procedural coding in the United States.

DEFINITIONS

HCFA: Health Care Financing Administration

HEDIS: Healthplan Employer Data and Information Set. This is a core of performance standards designed by participating managed health plans offered under the sponsorship of the National Committee for Quality Assurance (NCQA).

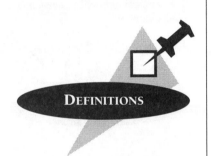

DEFINITIONS

ICD-9-CM: *International Classification of Diseases, Ninth Revision, Clinical Modification* is a hierarchal listing of codes describing medical conditions. Volumes 1 and 2 cover diagnostic codes and Volume 3 covers procedural codes.

CPT-5

To complicate matters further, the American Medical Association (AMA), which developed and maintains the CPT-4 coding system, this year formed a committee to develop CPT-5, a direct competitor to ICD-10-PCS. As a latecomer in the development process, the AMA has clouded the issues of when, how, and if, ICD-10-PCS would be implemented.

SUMMARY

Nearly everyone in the healthcare industry or in government healthcare policy will be affected by the new coding systems, slated for implementation in the United States in October, 2001. While it is important to remain current on proposed coding system changes, ICD-9-CM is the current system used in the United States for reporting diagnoses. Two systems are used for reporting procedures. ICD-9-CM Volume 3 is used to report inpatient procedures and CPT-4 is used to report physician and outpatient facility services. These current coding systems are the focus of this book.

In order to avoid confusing current coding systems and coding conventions with proposed coding systems, examples of these new coding systems are not provided here but can be found in Appendix 9.

DISCUSSION QUESTIONS

1. How do ICD-9 and ICD-9-CM differ?

_____

_____

_____

2. How does ICD-10 differ from ICD-9 and ICD-9-CM?

_____

_____

_____

3. What are the varied uses of ICD-9-CM codes?

_____

_____

_____

ICD-9-CM Diagnostic Coding

GOVERNMENT MANDATES

The advent of computerized claims processing has forced the medical community to learn a common language, and ICD-9-CM Volumes 1 and 2 provide the diagnostic half of that language. Care must be taken to select the correct code. Computer software applications can link diagnoses to the services provided and automatically reject claims when ICD-9-CM codes do not justify the service performed. Furthermore, for government claims, the correct use of ICD-9-CM codes is required by law. In 1988, Congress passed the Medicare Catastrophic Coverage Act. Although the act itself was later repealed, the mandate was

OBJECTIVES

Understand how to code to the highest level of specificity and why this is important

Understand the multiple uses of ICD-9-CM codes

Differentiate among Volumes 1, 2, and 3, how they are organized and what information each presents maintained to require ICD-9-CM codes on all physician-submitted Part B claims. Medicare's rules tightened in 1996 when it began to reject any claim that did not assign the most specific ICD-9-CM code available.

The ICD-9-CM diagnostic coding system translates written medical terminology into numeric and alphanumeric codes. Diagnostic codes from 001.0–V82.9 are used to:

- Identify symptoms, conditions, problems, complaints, or other reasons for the medical service or procedure being billed

- Report medical necessity by indicating the severity and emergent nature of the condition or complaint

- Translate written information into a numeric/alphanumeric system that can be stored and retrieved for use in medical education, research, reimbursement, and statistics

- Translate written information in the patient's chart into a form that can be submitted electronically for reimbursement

Another section reports external causes of injury and poisoning which are referred to as E-codes.

ICD-9-CM is published in three volumes. Volumes 1 and 2 contain diagnostic information used by physicians, outpatient facilities and inpatient hospitals, free standing surgical centers, and others. Volume 3 contains procedural information generally reserved for inpatient facility coding. See Chapter 9 for more information on Volume 3, procedure coding.

The Alphabetic Index to Diseases (Volume 2) is presented first. ICD-9-CM volume 2 is an alphabetical index to diseases and the corresponding codes. The Tabular List of Diseases (Volume 1) is presented second, listing information from Volume 2 in numeric order along with other pertinent coding conventions. This logical placement of the Alphabetic Index allows for quick location of terms for verification in the Tabular List.

ICD-9-CM Volume 2

The Alphabetic Index (Volume 2) is presented first in most publications because it is referenced first in selecting a diagnosis code. Volume 2 is divided into three sections: Section 1, Alphabetic Index to Diseases; Section 2, Table of Drugs and Chemicals; and Section 3, Index to External Causes.

ALPHABETIC INDEX TO DISEASE

Section 1 Alphabetic Index to Diseases lists conditions alphabetically by commonly used medical terms called main terms or main entries. Main terms are shown in bold type. Main terms are medical conditions not anatomical sites. Main terms may have a specific code assigned to them or may be modified by one or more terms which are indented and listed alphabetically below the main term.

To find the correct ICD-9 code it is necessary to correctly identify the main term in a diagnostic phrase. For example, the main term in the diagnostic phrase "closed fracture of femoral shaft" is fracture. Therefore, "fracture" is the term referenced in Section 1 of

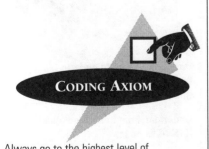

CODING AXIOM

Always go to the highest level of specificity when selecting a code from ICD-9-CM.

Volume 2. Next the modifying terms should be identified. In this case three modifying terms can be found: femur, shaft, and closed. If the main term had been incorrectly identified as "femoral," Volume 2 provides instructions on selecting the correct code, in this case a note to "see condition."

Section 2 Table of Drugs and Chemicals is one of three tables in Volume 2. The other two tables are presented alphabetically under the main terms "hypertension" and "neoplasm."

TABLES

Three main terms are presented in Volume 2 as tables. The *Hypertension* and *Neoplasm* tables are found in their proper alphabetical place in the index, but the *Table of Drugs and Chemicals* follows the alphabetical listing. Knowing how to use these tables correctly is essential to determine proper codes.

Hypertension Table

The complications, etiology, and clinical manifestations of hypertension are listed alphabetically under the bold heading Hypertension, hypertensive.

	Malignant	Benign	Unspecified
Hypertension, hypertensive (arterial) (arteriolar) (degeneration) (disease) (essential) (fluctuating) (idiopathic) (intermittent) (labile) (low renin) (orthostatic) (paroxysmal) (primary) (systemic) (vascular)	401.0	401.1	401.9
with			
heart involvement (conditions classifiable to 428, 429.0-429.3, 429.8, 429.9 due to hypertension) (see also Hypertension, heart)	402.00	402.10	402.90
with kidney involvement–see Hypertension, cardiorenal			
renal involvement	403.00	403.10	403.90
renal sclerosis or failure	403.00	403.10	403.90
with heart involvement–see Hypertension, cardiorenal			
failure (and sclerosis) (see also Hypertension, kidney)	403.01	403.11	403.91
sclerosis without failure (see also Hypertension, kidney)	403.00	403.10	403.90
accelerated–(see also Hypertension, by type, malignant)	401.0	—	—
antepartum–see Hypertension, complicating pregnancy, childbirth, or the puerperium			
cardiorenal (disease)	404.00	404.10	404.90
with			
heart failure (congestive)	404.01	404.11	404.91

There are three subcategories for each listing in this category: *Malignant, Benign* and *Unspecified.*

The table includes categories 401–405 plus additional codes, such as hypertension, that may complicate pregnancy, childbirth, or the puerperium. Read the diagnostic statement carefully, watching for the words "due to" and "with." These terms supply information necessary for accurate coding. Remember, the index table is only the beginning. Verify your code by looking it up in the tabular section. Also note that categories 402–405 require fifth digits.

Neoplasm Table

The *Neoplasm Table* lists neoplasms alphabetically by location and further identifies them by behavior as either Malignant, Benign, Uncertain Behavior, or Unspecified.

	Malignant			Benign	Uncertain Behavior	Unspecified
	Primary	Secondary	Ca in situ			
Neoplasm, neoplastic – continued						
marrow (bone) NEC	202.9	198.5	—	—	—	238.7
mastectomy site (secondary) (skin)	173.5	198.2	—	—	—	—
specified as breast tissue	174.8	198.81	—	—	—	—
mastoid (air cells) (antrum) (cavity)	160.1	197.3	231.8	212.0	235.9	239.1
bone or process	170.0	198.5	—	213.0	238.0	239.2
maxilla, maxillary (superior)	170.0	198.5	—	213.0	238.0	239.2
alveolar						
mucosa	143.0	198.89	230.0	210.4	235.1	239.0

DEFINITIONS

HYPERTENSION

Hypertension is persistently high arterial blood pressure ranging from 140 mm Hg to 200 mm Hg systolic and 90 mm Hg to 110 mm Hg diastolic.

Benign hypertension is a form of hypertension that responds to treatment and is favorable for recovery.

Malignant hypertension is a severe hypertensive state with poor prognosis, characterized by papilledema of the ocular fundus, thickening of the small arteries, and left ventricular hypertrophy.

Unspecified hypertension indicates that the type of hypertension has not been determined by the physician.

NEOPLASM

A neoplasm is any new and abnormal growth.

Malignant identifies neoplasms that show a greater degree of anaplasia and have properties of invasion and metastasis.

A **primary malignant neoplasm** is the original neoplasm which may metastasize to other sites.

A **secondary malignant neoplasm** is a neoplasm that has metastasized (spread) to an additional body site.

Ca in situ is a malignant neoplasm confined to the site of origin.

Benign identifies neoplasms that are not recurrent, not malignant, and are favorable for recovery.

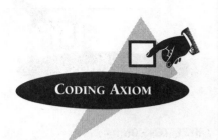

CODING AXIOM

More than one code is required to report poisoning. The first code indicates the substance that **caused the poisoning, and a second code should identify the patient's symptoms. A third code** should indicate the cause (e.g., assault, accident, suicide).

Malignant indicates a tumor has the potential to spread. Malignant neoplasms must be further defined as primary, secondary, or carcinoma in situ. When a neoplasm has metastasized (meaning the neoplasm has spread to a new location) the new growth is secondary to the primary (original) site.

Benign identifies neoplasms that are noncancerous but have neoplastic characteristics (e.g., fibromas and lipomas).

Uncertain Behavior identifies tissue that is beginning to exhibit neoplastic behavior but cannot yet be categorized as benign or malignant. Further testing by the physician is required. Watch pathology reports for information such as "further examination is necessary." If unsure about choosing the uncertain behavior category, query the physician.

To ensure correct representation to the insurance payor, make it a policy to code neoplasms after receiving pathology reports. Pathology report information should also be documented by the physician in the medical record.

Unspecified identifies neoplasms of unspecified morphology and behavior, based on documentation in the medical record.

Table of Drugs and Chemicals

The *Table of Drugs and Chemicals* appears after the alphabetical listing. It contains an extensive list of drugs, industrial solvents, corrosives, gases, noxious plants, pesticides, and other toxic agents in a six-column format. The first column identifies the substance. The second column identifies the corresponding poisoning code. The next five columns, grouped under the heading External Cause (E code), identify the circumstances of the poisoning or adverse effect.

| | | External Cause (E-Code) | | | | |
Substance	Poisoning	Accident	Therapeutic Use	Suicide Attempt	Assault	Undetermined
Carbromal (derivatives)	967.3	E852.2	E937.3	E950.2	E962.0	E980.2
Cardiac						
depressants	972.0	E858.3	E942.0	E950.4	E962.0	E980.4
rhythm regulators	972.0	E858.3	E942.0	E950.4	E962.0	E980.4
Cardiografin	977.8	E858.8	E947.8	E950.4	E962.0	E980.4
Cardio-green	977.8	E858.8	E947.8	E950.4	E962.0	E980.4
Cardiotonic glycosides	972.1	E858.3	E942.1	E950.4	E962.0	E980.4
Cardiovascular agents NEC	972.9	E858.3	E942.9	E950.4	E962.0	E980.4
Cardrase	974.2	E858.5	E944.2	E950.4	E962.0	E980.4
Carfusin	976.0	E858.7	E946.0	E950.4	E962.0	E980.4
Carisoprodol	968.0	E855.1	E938.0	E950.4	E962.0	E980.4
Carmustine	963.1	E858.1	E933.1	E950.4	E962.0	E980.4
Carotene	963.5	E858.1	E933.5	E950.4	E962.0	E980.4
Carphenazine (maleate)	969.1	E853.0	E939.1	E950.3	E962.0	E980.3
Carter's Little Pills	973.1	E858.4	E943.1	E950.4	E962.0	E980.4
Cascara (sagrada)	973.1	E858.4	E943.1	E950.4	E962.0	E980.4

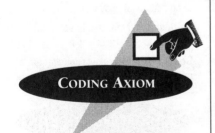

CODING AXIOM

Report 796.2 *Elevated blood pressure reading without diagnosis of hypertension* when elevated blood pressure is documented as having possibly been caused by stress or other problems occurring only during the visit or procedure.

The E codes in this table are defined as follows:

Accident codes identify accidental overdose of a drug, a wrong substance given or taken, a drug taken inadvertently, accidents in the usage of drugs and biologicals in medical and surgical procedures.

Therapeutic Use codes indicate an adverse effect or reaction to a drug that was administered correctly, either therapeutically or prophylactically.

Suicide Attempt codes identify the effects of drugs or substances taken to cause self-inflicted injury or to attempt suicide.

Assault codes indicate situations where drugs or substances are "purposely inflicted" by another person with the intent to cause bodily harm, injure, or kill.

Undetermined codes apply when the intent of the poisoning or injury cannot be determined as intentional or accidental.

Coding conventions and sequencing rules for poisonings and adverse effects are described later in the chapter.

INDEX TO EXTERNAL CAUSES

Section 3, Index to External Causes (E codes) is an alphabetic list of terms which classify the causes of injury and other adverse effects. It is organized by main terms which describe the accident, circumstance, event, or specific agent causing the injury or other adverse effect. This index identifies codes that are supplemental and should never be listed as the primary reason for medical care.

DISCUSSION QUESTIONS

1. Why is the alphabetic index (Volume 2) presented first? What are the three sections contained in Volume 2?

   _____
   _____
   _____

2. What information is needed to select the appropriate neoplasm code?

   _____
   _____
   _____

3. How is hypertension further defined in ICD-9-CM?

   _____
   _____
   _____

ICD-9-CM Volume 1

ICD-9-CM Volume 1, also referred to as the Tabular list, is a numerical list of the same diseases and conditions found in Volume 2. It is divided into three sections: Classification of Diseases and Injuries (Chapters 1-17), Supplementary Classification (V codes and E codes), and Appendices.

The main section, Classification of Diseases and Injuries, groups code numbers primarily by body system and secondarily by etiology.

KEY POINT

Presentation of ICD•9
Volume 2 – Alphabetic Index to Diseases

Volume 1 – Tabular List of Diseases

Volume 3 – Procedural Index & Tabular Sections

OBJECTIVES

Understand how diseases are indexed in ICD-9-CM

Learn how to use the Table of Drugs and Chemicals

Be proficient in the use of the hypertension and neoplasm tables

Chapter 1	Infectious and Parasitic Diseases (001–139)
Chapter 2	Neoplasms (140–239)
Chapter 3	Endocrine, Nutritional and Metabolic Diseases, and Immunity Disorders (240–279)
Chapter 4	Diseases of the Blood and Blood-forming Organs (280–289)
Chapter 5	Mental Disorders (290–319)
Chapter 6	Diseases of the Nervous System and Sense Organs (320–389)
Chapter 7	Diseases of the Circulatory System (390–459)
Chapter 8	Diseases of the Respiratory System (460–519)
Chapter 9	Diseases of the Digestive System (520–579)
Chapter 10	Diseases of the Genitourinary System (580–629)
Chapter 11	Complications of Pregnancy, Childbirth, and the Puerperium (630–677)
Chapter 12	Diseases of the Skin and Subcutaneous Tissue (680–709)
Chapter 13	Diseases of the Musculoskeletal System and Connective Tissue (710–739)
Chapter 14	Congenital Anomalies (740–759)
Chapter 15	Certain Conditions Originating in the Perinatal Period (760–779)
Chapter 16	Symptoms, Signs, and Ill-Defined Conditions (780–799)
Chapter 17	Injury and Poisoning (800–999)

Codes are arranged in numerical order in both this section and in the Supplementary Classification. Three-digit category codes are generally subdivided by adding a fourth and/or fifth digit after the decimal point to further specify the nature of the disease or condition. Codes with fourth digits are called subcategory codes, and those with fifth digits are referred to as subclassifications.

Knowing the three-digit category usually is not enough for accurate ICD-9-CM coding. In fact, there are only approximately 100 three-digit codes that are considered valid. The rest require the addition of further digits. See the appendix of *Code It Right* for a list of valid three-digit ICD-9-CM codes.

Numerical hierarchy plays a key role in ICD-9-CM coding. Each digit beyond three adds more detail. For example, the three-digit category code 802 identifies a fracture of a face bone. Add a decimal point and a fourth digit for the subcategory code, 802.2, and a closed fracture of the mandible is specified. A fifth digit, subclassification, 802.23 further clarifies that the fracture is the coronoid process of the mandible. Code to the highest level of specificity. Some payors will not accept generalized three- or four-digit codes if more specific ones are available, and Medicare in July 1996 began rejecting claims with incomplete ICD-9-CM codes. Incomplete codes are considered invalid, and may result in additional correspondence and delays.

Fifth digits are not always presented following a four-digit code in the hierarchical listing in ICD-9-CM. Sometimes, the fifth digit is presented in information at the beginning of the category or subsection. For instance, instructions for use of a fifth digit are presented under the three-digit category, 404 *Hypertensive heart and renal disease*, rather than repeated under each four-digit entry. The fifth digit describes the disease classification in relation to congestive heart failure or renal failure. Pertinent codes are then listed with fourth digits, but a fifth digit from the list at the beginning of the code category must be selected for the diagnosis to be coded to the highest level of specificity.

Medicode has developed icons for its ICD-9-CM publication that indicate when a code is incomplete and the reader should look further. Examples of these icons are given later in this chapter.

DEFINITION

ICD-9-CM Volume 1, also referred to as the Tabular List, is a numerical list of the same diseases and conditions found in Volume 2.

DISCUSSION QUESTIONS

1. Are three-digit and four-digit codes always invalid as diagnoses on claims forms? Why or why not?

   _____

   _____

   _____

2. How can you be sure that the code you selected is at the highest degree of specificity?

   _____

   _____

   _____

3. What appears in Volumes 1, 2, and 3 of ICD-9-CM?

   _____

   _____

   _____

Supplemental Classification: V Codes

The *Supplementary Classification of Factors Influencing Health Status and Contact with Health Services* (V01–V82), also known as V codes, describes circumstances that influence a patient's health status and identifies reasons for medical encounters resulting from circumstances other than a disease or injury classified in the main part of ICD-9-CM. The V codes immediately follow the injury and poisoning codes of Chapter 17. These alphanumerical codes are only listed as a principal diagnosis for inpatient coding or as a primary diagnosis for outpatient coding in very specific circumstances based on coding guidelines.

The main terms used with V codes reflect the nature of the medical service provided, such as:

Admission	Observation
Aftercare	Problem (with)
Attention (to)	Screening
Examination	Status
History (of)	Supervision (of)

V codes are divided into three main classifications:

Problem-oriented V codes identify circumstances that could affect the patient in the future but are neither a current illness nor injury. Use these codes to describe an existing circumstance or problem that may influence future medical care. Usually, problem-oriented V codes are not listed first on the medical claim form because they represent supplemental information.

V10.04	**Personal history of malignant neoplasm of stomach**
V15.3	**Personal history of exposure to radiation**
V17.3	**Family history of ischemic heart disease**

OBJECTIVES

Be familiar with the tabular listing of Volume 1 and its classifications

Understand when to use E codes and V codes

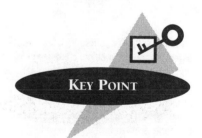

KEY POINT

V codes are generally used in three instances:

- When a physician identifies a circumstance or problem in a person who is not currently ill but has nonetheless come in contact with health services (e.g., organ donor, vaccination)

- When an ill or injured patient requires specific treatment (e.g., chemotherapy or removal of orthopedic pins or rods)

- When the circumstance is not itself a current illness but may affect future medical treatment (e.g., personal history of breast cancer or family history of heart disease)

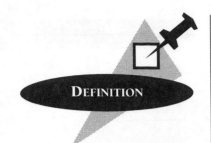

DEFINITION

E codes describe circumstances of an injury or illness. Their use can be pivotal in determining liability among payors such as medical insurance plans, car insurers, home insurers, or workers' compensation programs.

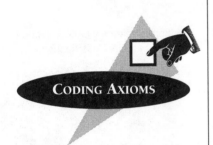

CODING AXIOMS

Usually, problem-oriented V codes are not listed first on the medical claim form because they represent supplemental information. Claims may be rejected if a problem-oriented V code is listed first rather than the actual diagnosis. However, a V code is listed first when no other service is performed. News of how V code usage may change can be found in *Coding Clinic*.

Information from the Appendices should not be listed on the claim form. For example, M codes for morphology of neoplasms are not listed on the claim form.

E codes are never listed as the primary or principal diagnosis on a claim form, because they provide adjunct information describing the circumstances surrounding an illness, but not the illness itself.

Service-oriented V codes identify or define examinations, aftercare, ancillary services, or therapy. Use these V codes to describe when a person with a known disease or injury, whether it is current or resolving, encounters the healthcare system for a specific treatment of that disease or injury. Follow the outpatient coding guidelines carefully to determine if these codes can be used as the primary diagnosis.

V54.8	Other orthopedic aftercare
V65.5	Person with feared complaint in whom no diagnosis was made
V67.2	Follow-up examination following chemotherapy
V76.2	Special screening for malignant neoplasm of cervix (Pap smear)

Fact-oriented V codes do not describe a problem or a service; they simply state a fact. These generally do not serve as an outpatient primary or inpatient principal diagnosis. Again it is important to check whether the code is listed as an acceptable inpatient principal diagnosis.

V21.1	Constitutional state in development: puberty
V27.2	Outcome of delivery: twins, both liveborn
V61.41	Alcoholism within family

SUPPLEMENTAL CLASSIFICATION: E CODES

The second set of supplemental codes in Volume 1 is the *Supplementary Classification of External Causes of Injury and Poisoning* (E800–E999), also known as E codes. The E codes are never listed as the primary or principal diagnosis; they are adjunctive. More than one E code may be necessary to describe fully the circumstances of an accident. Use E codes to establish medical necessity, identify causes of injury and poisoning, and identify the substance. The index for the E codes is found in Volume 2, following the *Table of Drugs and Chemicals*.

E884.0	Fall from playground equipment
E917.0	Struck accidentally by object or persons in sports
E922.0	Accident caused by handgun

Including E codes on a claim does not affect the amount of reimbursement. However, E codes add clarity and may speed up the claims process. For instance, in an industrial accident, workers' compensation could become the primary payor instead of the patient's private insurer. Or, two different plans may coordinate benefits depending on the circumstances of the injury. Knowing the circumstances prevents confusion and helps determine which agency or payors are responsible for payment.

Furthermore, E codes are an important statistic-gathering device for the federal government. Consistent use of E codes contributes to the compilation of valuable data on the frequency and cause of injuries in America. This data is used by federal agencies in public education campaigns and government safety regulations, aiding in the development of focused prevention plans.

APPENDICES TO VOLUME 1

Appendices to Volume 1 are provided for reference purposes only.

Appendix A	Morphology of Neoplasms
Appendix B	Glossary of Mental Disorders
Appendix C	Classification of Drugs by American Hospital Formulary Service List Number and Their ICD-9-CM Equivalents
Appendix D	Classification of Industrial Accidents According to Agency
Appendix E	List of Three-Digit Categories

DISCUSSION QUESTIONS

1. In what cases are V codes acceptable as primary or principal diagnosis codes?

   _____

   _____

   _____

2. What are the three main classifications of V-codes? Give an example of each.

   _____

   _____

   _____

3. Why should coders include E codes in their claim forms when these codes usually do not affect the amount of reimbursement?

   _____

   _____

   _____

Conventions

Just as customs direct how people behave, each space, type face, indentation, and punctuation mark determines how you must interpret ICD-9-CM codes. These "conventions" were developed to help you match correct codes to the diagnoses you encounter.

FORMAT

ICD-9-CM has an indented format. Subterms are indented two spaces to the right of the term to which they are linked. Continuations of lines that are too long to fit the column are indented four spaces.

> **Volume 1**
> **250.0** **Diabetes mellitus without mention of complication**
> Diabetes mellitus without mention of complication or manifestation classifiable to 250.1-250.9
>
> **Volume 2**
> **Pleurodynia** 786.52
> epidemic 074.1
> viral 074.1

TYPE FACE

Bold type identifies all codes and main terms in the Tabular List (Volume 1), separating it from subordinate information or notes.

> **Volume 1**
> **237.3** **Paraganglia**
> Aortic body   Coccygeal body
> Carotid body   Glomus jugulare

OBJECTIVES

Recognize and use various conventions of ICD-9-CM

Understand coding to highest specificity

Appropriately interpret notes and guidelines to ICD-9-CM

Italicized type identifies those categories that cannot be reported as a primary diagnosis and also for all exclusion notes. The italicized words in the following entry indicate that 580.81 *Acute glomerulonephritis* is not a primary diagnosis:

> **Volume 1**
>
> ***580.81***   ***Acute glomerulonephritis in diseases classified elsewhere***
>   *Code first underlying disease, as:*
>   infectious hepatitis (070.0-070.9)
>   mumps (072.79)
>   subacute bacterial endocarditis (421.0)
>   typhoid fever (002.0)

PUNCTUATION

Brackets enclose synonyms, alternative wordings, or explanatory phrases. The brackets may be regular type [ ] or italicized *[ ]*.

> **Volume 1**
>
> **460**   **Acute nasopharyngitis [common cold]**

Parentheses enclose supplementary (nonessential) modifiers that do not affect the code number. Modifying terms enclosed in parentheses need not be present in the diagnostic statement. Parentheses also enclose many *see also* references.

> **Volume 2**
>
> **Diarrhea, diarrheal** (acute) (autumn) (bilious) (bloody) (catarrhal) (choleraic) (chronic) (gravis) (green) (infantile) (lienteric) (noninfectious) (presumed noninfectious) (putrefactive) (secondary) (sporadic) (summer) (symptomatic) (thermic) 787.91

> **Volume 1**
>
> **568.81**   **Hemoperitoneum (nontraumatic)**

A **colon** indicates a term that is incomplete without one or more of the modifiers following it. They are used in Volume 1 to help assign a given category.

> **Volume 1**
>
> **695.4**   **Lupus erythematosus**
>   Lupus:
>   erythematodes (discoid)

A **brace** encloses a series of terms modified by the statement appearing to the right of the brace.

> **Volume 1**
>
> **685**   **Pilonidal cyst**
>   [INCLUDES]   fistula   } coccygeal or pilonidal
>   sinus

SYMBOLS

●   Medicode's red stop sign in ICD-9-CM identifies codes requiring an additional fourth or fifth digit.

> **Volume 1**
>
> ●   **671.4**   **Deep phlebothrombosis, postpartum**
>   [0,2,4]   Deep-vein thrombosis, postpartum

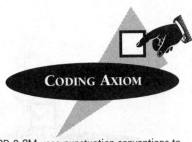

CODING AXIOM

ICD-9-CM uses punctuation conventions to save space and present information in a consistent manner.

Information enclosed in parentheses is supplemental to the diagnosis, and may not apply to every case for which a code is valid.

◆ In ICD-9-CM, Volumes 1 and 2, Medicode's yellow diamond indicates a code is not specific. These codes capture conditions that are not specified in other codes, and are sometimes the best option available. Other times, however, these codes don't give payors enough information and reimbursement may be delayed while queries are made. This symbol has a different meaning in Medicode's hospital ICD-9-CM.

Volume 1

◆ **255.3   Other corticoadrenal overactivity**

■ In ICD-9-CM, Volumes 1 and 2, Medicode's blue rectangle indicates that a code is not to to be used as a primary diagnosis. These codes should always be presented secondarily to the primary diagnosis. The symbol has a different meaning in Medicode's hospital ICD-9-CM.

Volume 1

■ *601.4   Prostatitis in diseases classified elsewhere*

NOTES

Notes are found in ICD-9-CM Volumes 1 and 2 and have no fixed length. They give coding instructions.

Volume 1

344 Other paralytic syndromes

Note: This category is to be used when the listed conditions are reported without further specification or are stated to be old or long-standing but of unspecified cause. The category is also for use in multiple coding to identify these conditions resulting from any cause.

Notes also list five-digit choices or define terms to give additional information.

574 Cholelithiasis

The following fifth-digit subclassification is for use with category 574:

0   without mention of obstruction
1   with obstruction

Volume 2

Cyst (mucus) (retention) (serous) (simple)

> *Note — In general, cysts are not neoplastic and are classified to the appropriate category for disease of the specified anatomical site. This generalization does not apply to certain types of cysts which are neoplastic in nature, for example, dermoid, nor does it apply to cysts of certain structures, for example, branchial cleft, which are classified as developmental anomalies.*
>
> *The following listing includes some of the most frequently reported sites of cysts as well as qualifiers which indicate the type of cyst. The latter qualifiers usually are not repeated under the anatomical sites. Since the code assignment for a given site may vary depending upon the type of cyst, the coder should refer to the listings under the specified type of cyst before consideration is given to the site.*

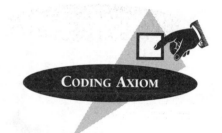

CODING AXIOM

Notes at the beginning of a section apply to all codes within that section.

Notes in Volume 1 are indented and printed in plain type, while those in Volume 2 are boxed and printed in italics. The placement of these notes is as important as their content. Notes at the beginning of a chapter apply to all categories within the chapter. Those at the beginning of a subchapter apply to all categories within the subchapter. Likewise, notes preceding three-digit categories apply to all four- and five-digit codes within that category.

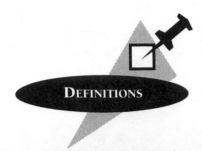

DEFINITIONS

Invalid ICD-9-CM code is a diagnostic code that is not as specific as it should be because digit(s) are missing. Claims will be rejected by Medicare and many private payors if invalid codes are used.

Nonspecific code: A catch-all code that specifies the diagnosis as "ill-defined," "other," or "unspecified." A nonspecific code may be a valid choice if no other code closely describes the diagnosis.

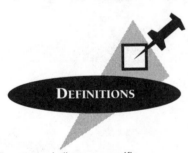

DEFINITIONS

Three terms indicate nonspecific diagnoses:

NEC: (not elsewhere classifiable) indicates that the condition specified does not have a separate more specific listing. This term is used only in Volume 2.

NOS: (not otherwise specified) is used only in Volume 1. It is used to designate diagnoses when the available information does not allow assignment of a more specific or "other specified" code.

Unspecified: indicates that more information is necessary to code the term to further specificity. In these cases, the fourth digit of the code is always 9. Fourth digits 0 through 7 identify more specific information of the main term or condition. The fourth-digit number 8 is reserved for identifying other information.

INSTRUCTIONAL NOTES

To assign diagnostic codes at the highest level of specificity, you must follow four additional kinds of notes:

Includes appears immediately under a three-digit code title to provide further definition or to give an example of the category contents.

> **Volume 1**
>
> **633 Ectopic pregnancy**
>   **INCLUDES**   ruptured ectopic pregnancy

Excludes indicates terms that are not to be coded under the referenced term, as they are listed elsewhere. A code reference directing the reader to the term or area is listed in parentheses.

> **711 Arthropathy associated with infections**
>   **EXCLUDES**   *rheumatic fever (390)*

Code first underlying disease identifies diagnoses that are not primary and are incomplete when used alone. In such cases the code, its title, and instructions appear in italics. This type of instructional note appears only in Volume 1. A code with this instructional note is referred to as the manifestation code and should be recorded second, with the underlying cause recorded first. Italicized brackets identify this situation in Volume 2.

> **Volume 1**
>
> **595.4**   *Cystitis in diseases classified elsewhere*
>   *Code first underlying disease, as:*
>   actinomycosis (039.8)
>   amebiasis (006.8)
>   bilharziasis (120.0-120.9)
>   Echinococcus infestation (122.3, 122.6)

Use additional code appears in Volume 1 in those categories where an additional code is available to provide further information and to give a more complete picture of the diagnosis or procedure. The additional code should identify other aspects of the disease, including manifestation, cause, associated condition, and nature of the condition itself.

> **Volume 1**
>
> **358.2**   **Toxic myoneural disorders**
>   Use additional E code to identify toxic agent

ABBREVIATIONS

NEC is an abbreviation for Not Elsewhere Classifiable. NEC is found only in Volume 2. Codes followed by "NEC" should only be used when the available information specifies a condition, but no separate code for that condition is provided. "NEC" codes report "other specified" diagnoses which do not have a more specific code.

> **Volume 2**
>
> **Infestation**
>   cestodes 123.9
>   specified type NEC 123.8

NOS is an abbreviation for Not Otherwise Specified. NOS is found only in Volume 1. Codes designated as "NOS" are to be used only when the information available is not sufficient to allow assignment of a more specific code.

> **Volume 1**
> **420.90   Acute pericarditis, unspecified**
> Pericarditis (acute):
>   NOS
>   infective NOS
>   sicca

DISCUSSION QUESTIONS

1. Which punctuation convention in ICD-9-CM encloses a series of terms modified by the statement appearing to the right of it?

    _____

    _____

    _____

2. What does the phrase, *Code first underlying disease, as* alert you to?

    _____

    _____

    _____

3. An *includes* notation provides what type of information about a code?

    _____

    _____

    _____

Assigning Diagnostic Codes

OBJECTIVES

STEP 1: DETERMINE THE MAIN TERMS
Analyze encounter forms, operative reports, and diagnostic statements for those words or main terms that identify the patient's condition or symptoms. Think of the main term as a common denominator — a total disease classification. Once you've located this general term, follow the alphabetic lists to the specific condition. The main terms in the following diagnoses are printed in bold type.

> Acute **otitis** media   **Fracture** of the leg
> Upper respiratory **infection**   Abdominal **pain**
> Infectious **mononucleosis**

Develop methods for swift and accurate code selection

Learn to correctly sequence ICD-9-CM codes when more than one code is necessary to describe the patient's condition

STEP 2: LOOK UP THE MAIN TERM IN VOLUME 2
Main terms in Volume 2 appear in bold type. Some conditions have more than one listing. If the term describing a condition can be expressed in more than one form, all forms appear in the main entry.

> **Volume 2**
> **Obstruction, obstructed, obstructive**
>   intestine (mechanical) (neurogenic) (paroxysmal) (postinfectional) (reflex) 560.9

There are exceptions to this guideline. For example, complications of medical and surgical procedures are listed under the main term *Complications* and under the main terms that identify specific complications such as *Infection and Dehiscence*. Late effects of certain conditions are found under the terms *Late* and *Status (post)*.

> **Volume 2**
> **Complications**
>   surgical procedures 998.9
>   burst stitches or sutures 998.3
> **Late**
>   effect(s) (of)
>   wound, open
>   head, neck, and trunk (injury classifiable to 870-879) 906.0

STEP 3: FOLLOW CROSS-REFERENCES

Volume 2 uses cross-references to possible modifiers for a term or its synonyms. Follow the cross-references to the correct code when the diagnosis is not located under the first term you find. There are three types of cross-references:

See indicates that you should reference the condition listed instead of the term you've found. You must follow the instruction to assign the correct diagnostic code.

> **Volume 2**
> **Glomerulonephritis**
>   desquamative — *see* Nephrosis
> **Elbow** — *see* condition

See also indicates that additional information is available. This cross-reference provides you with an additional diagnosis and code when the main term or subterm is insufficient. The additional information helps select the correct code. Always follow this instruction to ensure appropriate coding.

> **Volume 2**
> **Tuberculoma** — *see also* Tuberculosis
>   brain (any part) 013.2

When a single code does not fully describe a given condition, use multiple codes to identify all components of the diagnosis. However, medical record documentation must mention the presence of all the elements for each code to be used. If uncertain, query the physician.

See category directs you to an additional three-digit category in Volume 1, Tabular List. You cannot assign an appropriate code unless you follow this instruction and read the applicable notes in Volume 1.

> **Volume 2**
> **Laceration**
>   vagina
>   with
>   molar pregnancy (*see also* categories 630–632) 639.2

General adjectives such as *acute* and *hereditary*, and references to anatomic sites such as *arm* and *face*, appear as main terms, usually with a cross-reference to *see* condition or *see also* condition.

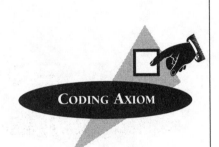

CODING AXIOM

Use multiple codes to identify all components of the diagnosis when a single code does not fully describe a given condition.

STEP 4: REVIEW SUBTERMS OR MODIFIERS

A main term may be followed by one or more subterms that further describe the patient's condition. These supplemental words, called modifiers, may describe the severity, location, or symptoms of the condition. There are two types of modifiers, essential and nonessential.

Nonessential Modifiers

These subterms are listed immediately to the right of the main term and are enclosed in parentheses. They serve as examples to help you translate written terminology into numeric codes and do not affect the selection of the diagnostic code.

Volume 2

Goiter (adolescent) (colloid) (diffuse) (dipping) (due to iodine insufficiency) (endemic) (euthyroid) (heart) (hyperplastic) (internal) (intrathoracic) (juvenile) (mixed type) (nonendemic) (parenchymatous) (plunging) (sporadic) (subclavicular) (substernal) 240.9

Essential Modifiers

These subterms are listed below the main terms and are indented two spaces. They are generally presented in alphabetical order, with the exceptions of *with* and *without*, which appear before the alphabetized modifiers. Each additional essential modifier clarifies the previous one and is indented two additional spaces to the right. These descriptive terms affect your code selection and describe essential differences in site, etiology, and symptoms.

Volume 2

Goiter
  simple 240.0
  toxic 242.0
    adenomatous 242.3
      multinodular 242.2

When a main term in Volume 1 has only one essential modifier, it appears on the same line as the main term, separated by a comma.

Volume 1

240.9   **Goiter, unspecified**

STEP 5: VERIFY CODE SELECTION IN VOLUME 1

Although it may be tempting to code strictly from the Volume 2 index, Volume 1 is the authoritative ICD-9-CM coding reference. It contains diagnostic codes, full descriptions, additional instructional notes, and examples of terms assigned to each code. These are intended to enhance the verification process and ensure proper code selection. There are times, however, when a descriptive term listed in Volume 2 is not found in Volume 1. In these instances trust the index as the volume most often updated to reflect current usage, check to verify the tabular entry is not contradictory to the term, and use the index code.

When choosing diagnostic codes, you must code to the highest level of specificity; in other words, use four- and five-digit codes when they are available. The first three digits comprise the category and identify the main condition or disease. Fourth and fifth digits further specify the diagnosis and are required when available. Based on the information found in the following example, an initial episode of care for acute myocardial infarction of the anterolateral wall is coded 410.01.

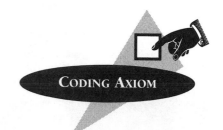

CODING AXIOM

Never code strictly from the Volume 2 index. Volume 1 is the authoritative ICD-9-CM coding reference.

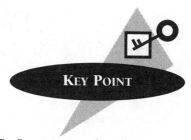

KEY POINT

The five-step process for assigning diagnostic codes can be summarized as follows:

1. Determine the main terms that describe the patient's condition or symptoms

2. Look up the main term in Volume 2 where the condition is alphabetized as a noun or an adjective

3. If indicated, follow cross-references such as *see, see also*, and *see category* to find the correct code

4. Review subterms and modifying words. Refer to any indented terms under the main term to clarify further the code selection

5. Verify the code listed in Volume 2, the alphabetic index, by checking its listing in Volume 1

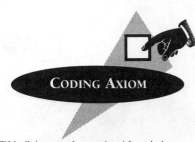

CODING AXIOM

Fifth digits are often omitted from index entries in ICD-9. Always confirm the code you find in the index by looking it up in the tabular section. To depend on the index for code selection is to invite error.

Volume 1

410	Acute myocardial infarction

The following fifth-digit subclassification is for use with category 410:

0	episode of care unspecified
1	initial episode of care
2	subsequent episode of care

410.0	Of anterolateral wall
410.1	Of other anterior wall
410.2	Of inferolateral wall
410.3	Of inferoposterior wall
410.4	Of other inferior wall
410.5	Of other lateral wall
410.6	True posterior wall infarction
410.7	Subendocardial infarction
410.8	Of other specified sites

If no five-digit code exists, code to the fourth digit if one is available. The following category includes only four digits:

Volume 1

413	Angina pectoris
413.0	Angina decubitus
413.1	Prinzmetal angina
413.9	Other and unspecified angina pectoris

Three-Digit Diagnostic Codes

Three-digit diagnostic codes are used only when no fourth or fifth digit is available. There are only about 100 codes at the highest level of specificity in the three-digit form. See the appendix of *Code It Right* for a list of these three-digit codes. Many payors, including Medicare, do not accept three-digit codes when higher levels of specificity exist. Never use 0 or 9 as "fillers" to add fourth or fifth digits to codes.

Volume 1

Correct:
412 Old myocardial infarction

Incorrect:
412.0 or 412.00

DISCUSSION QUESTIONS

1. Information appearing in parentheses can be contradictory and confusing. Look in your ICD-9-CM and give examples of this. Also, discuss how the information in the parentheses, called nonessential modifiers, can help in code selection.

_____

_____

_____

2. How can you verify that the code you selected is at the highest specificity available?

_____

_____

_____

3. What problems can arise from coding from Volume 2 instead of using Volume 2 as an index to Volume 1?

    _____

    _____

    _____

Clinical Applications of Coding Rules

Diagnostic coding has rules that must be applied to a broad variety of diseases and conditions. The medical record tells a written story of what has occurred with a patient. The numeric and alphanumeric codes assigned by the medical coder must tell the same story in code. Although diagnostic coding rules for inpatient and outpatient services are similar in some areas, they are very different in others. In some cases the rules directly contradict each other. The areas where inpatient and outpatient services differ are explained here and in a chart in *Code It Right*'s appendix. The most important factor in ICD-9-CM coding, whether outpatient or inpatient, is understanding the rules. Knowing how to correctly sequence and report diagnostic codes must be the goal for all coders. For official guidelines consult the *Federal Register, Coding Clinic,* or the *AHIMA Journal.*

PHYSICIAN CODING

The first code sequenced in order of importance in outpatient coding is the primary diagnosis. Other codes follow according to specified outpatient coding rules. The definition of the primary diagnosis and the coding rules are as follows:

Primary Diagnosis

The primary diagnosis is the code reflecting the current, most significant reason for the current services or procedures provided.

Secondary Coexisting Diseases and Conditions

Diseases and conditions that coexist during an encounter and affect the management of the patient's care should be sequenced after the primary diagnosis. When coding pre-existing conditions, make certain the diagnostic code assigned identifies the current reason for medical management.

Rule-Out Statements

Rule-out statements such as "probable," "possible," "questionable," "rule-out," and "suspected" are not coded in an outpatient setting. ICD-9-CM has no codes for rule-out statements, so do not code diagnoses documented as such. This has taken on new importance with the current HCFA-1500 form that has no space for written descriptions.

With today's advances in computerized recordkeeping, coding a suspected carcinoma or possible HIV-positive status as if they exist can raise a red flag in a patient's insurance record that is very difficult to remove. A patient's insurance denial could be traced back to a "rule-out" diagnosis wrongly coded, and your practice could be held legally responsible for the patient's ensuing insurance woes. The current HCFA-1500 form and an understanding of proper coding methodology require the coder to report complaints or symptoms rather than coding a rule-out statement.

OBJECTIVES

Determine and code primary, or principal, and secondary diagnoses

Select codes when no definitive diagnosis has been made

Correctly sequence diagnoses in cases of multiple injuries, complications, or multiple complaints

KEY POINT

Diseases and conditions that coexist during an encounter affecting the management of the patient's care should be sequenced after the primary diagnosis.

Coding Symptoms

When the health record provides a diagnosis qualified as "probable" or "rule-out," the presenting complaint symptom or sign should be reported instead. Volume 1, Chapter 16 contains codes for signs, symptoms, and ill-defined conditions. Use codes 780–799 for generalized complaints, signs, and symptoms until a definitive diagnosis is made.

Encounters for Circumstances Other Than Disease or Injury

Codes for reporting encounters for circumstances other than disease or injury, such as general medical exams, are included in ICD•9•CM. These codes frequently referred to as V-codes are found in the Supplementary Classification of Factors Influencing Health Status and Contact with Health Services (V01.0–V82.9)

HOSPITAL FACILITY CODING

The principal diagnosis in inpatient diagnostic coding is the first code sequenced. Other codes then follow according to inpatient coding rules. The principal diagnosis definition, coding rules, and further explanations are as follows:

Principal Diagnosis

The principal diagnosis is designated and defined as the condition established after study to be chiefly responsible for occasioning the admission of the patient to the hospital for care.

Secondary, Coexisting Diseases and Conditions

Other diagnoses are designated and defined as all conditions that coexist at the time of admission, that develop subsequently, or that affect the treatment received and/or the length of stay. Diagnoses that relate to an earlier episode which have no bearing on the current hospital stay are to be excluded.

Rule-Out Statements

"Rule-out," "possible," "probable," "suspected," and "questionable" statements are coded as if they exist and until they are ruled out. Remember this applies only to inpatient coding and there are exceptions to this rule, specifically related to HIV status coding. In addition, most acute care facilities have strict policies and procedures related to recording unsubstantiated diagnoses. This helps minimize overcoding in the absence of a definitive diagnosis.

Coding Symptoms

Signs and symptoms are coded when there is no other definitive diagnosis or cause listed for the condition.

Contrasting Diagnoses

Diagnoses that are contrasting should be coded as if the conditions were confirmed. The diagnoses should be sequenced according to the circumstances of the admission.

When a symptom is followed by contrasting diagnoses, the symptom is sequenced first. Contrasting diagnoses are considered to be suspected conditions and are sequenced as secondary diagnoses.

For example, if the record states chest pain due to coronary artery disease versus gastroesophageal reflux, the chest pain would be sequenced first. The coronary artery disease and the gastroesophageal reflux would be coded as secondary diagnoses.

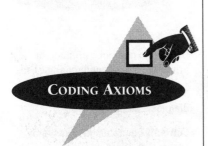

CODING AXIOMS

In **outpatient** coding, always code symptoms, not suspicions, when no definitive diagnosis has been confirmed.

In **inpatient** coding, an admitting diagnosis is always coded. It may or may not agree with the principal diagnosis because the principal diagnosis is the main reason the patient was admitted to the hospital, after study.

In outpatient and inpatient coding, the complication is not listed as the primary or principal diagnosis unless it meets the definition of a primary or principal diagnosis. To be listed first, the complication must be the reason for the hospital admission or physician encounter.

The physician does not always write the diagnoses in the medical record in the correct sequence. The primary or principal diagnosis may not be the first one listed by the physician.

Codes of Equal Importance

If two or more diagnoses of equal importance are listed, the principal diagnosis becomes the one for which definitive treatment was provided, either surgical or nonsurgical. If a definitive procedure was not performed, use the diagnosis that was the most resource intensive as the principal diagnosis.

OUTPATIENT AND INPATIENT COMMON CODING GUIDELINES

The medical coder must determine the primary outpatient or principal inpatient diagnosis and sequence them in the correct order using the appropriate coding rules and principles. The order that the physician writes the diagnoses in the medical record may not determine the primary or principal diagnosis. The medical coder should determine the correct order before listing the codes. Some outpatient and inpatient coding rules and guidelines are the same. If the primary or principal diagnosis based on documentation in the record cannot be determined, query the physician.

Unspecified Codes

Unspecified codes and general terms may not clarify the medical necessity issue; therefore, be as specific as possible in describing the patient's condition, illness, or disease.

Usually, categories will have two nonspecific selections. One will define a code as "unspecified." Use these codes when the diagnosis has not been finalized. The other code identifies "other specified," indicating that although a diagnosis has been made, there is no code identifying it more specifically.

In some cases, the index directs the reader from a very specific diagnosis to a less specific code. In these cases, the diagnosis is generally a contemporary diagnosis that has not yet received its own code, or a rare condition that may never be specified with its own code. For instance, the index directs:

DEFINITIONS

Unspecified codes: reported when the diagnosis has not been finalized.

Other specified: reported when a diagnosis has been made and there is no code identifying it more specifically.

Volume 2
Syndrome
Alice in Wonderland 293.89

The actual description of this code is less specific.

Volume 1
293.8   **Other specified transient organic mental disorders**
    293.89   **Other**

When a specific diagnosis is not yet determined clinically, "unspecified" codes are available. An unspecified diagnosis may be the only information available at the patient's first outpatient visit. When specific clinical information is determined, however, and the diagnosis is documented in the patient's chart, assign more definitive codes. Inpatient coders should not assign an unspecified code unless absolutely necessary. Whenever possible, both outpatient and inpatient coders should request more information from the physician about an unspecified code to determine and assign a more definitive diagnosis. A patient's diagnosis may change several times through the course of outpatient treatment as additional and more specific information becomes available.

Coexisting Conditions

Some patients present with coexisting conditions that affect the management of care. These conditions should be reported as supplemental information in order of importance. The order of importance may be partially based on the resources and the time it takes to complete the care. The HCFA-1500 form used to report physician outpatient services allows you to list up to three supporting diagnostic codes to establish clear medical necessity. When more information is available describing the necessity of outpatient treatment, include this documentation (operative reports, clinical reports and records, etc.) with your reimbursement claim. The inpatient UB-92 form allows you to report six diagnosis codes. The principal diagnosis is always listed first with secondary codes listed subsequently in the order they were sequenced.

Multiple Injuries

To report multiple injuries, list the conditions treated by the physician in order of importance, with the major problem listed first. As a rule of thumb, when medical and surgical problems are being managed, list the surgical problem first. Logically, the rule is secondary to the severity of the injuries being treated. In outpatient and inpatient coding the most severe injury is the primary or principal diagnosis.

Multiple Diseases

For multiple diseases, code only the disease and conditions that have an impact on the management of the patient. List the major management problem first based on the criteria of a primary outpatient or principal inpatient diagnosis.

DISCUSSION QUESTIONS

1. What are the reasons that "rule-out" diagnoses should not be coded as actual diagnoses for outpatient and physician services? What should the coder do instead?

   _____

   _____

   _____

2. When a patient has a secondary disease like diabetic retinopathy, what is the minimum number of codes that should appear on the claim? How should the codes be sequenced?

   _____

   _____

   _____

3. Discuss how multiple complaints or multiple injuries should be reported.

   _____

   _____

   _____

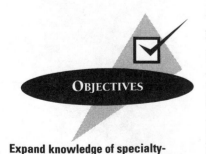

OBJECTIVES

Expand knowledge of specialty-specific coding issues

Special Coding Situations

The preceding information in this chapter was designed as a general introduction for new coders or a basic review for experienced ones. However, there are many special coding situations that you may encounter. The remainder of this chapter provides special instructions for some of these situations and some specialty-specific scenarios.

ACUTE AND CHRONIC DISEASES

Some diseases have both acute (subacute) and chronic manifestations. These acute and chronic phases may exist alone or together. When the diagnosis states that the patient has both the acute and chronic conditions and no single code exists for the combined acute and chronic disease, the acute condition is listed as the primary diagnosis and the chronic condition listed as a secondary or coexisting condition. For example, a diagnosis of acute and chronic cystitis requires two codes. Code 595.0 for acute cystitis would be listed as the primary or principal diagnosis, and code 595.2 for other chronic cystitis would be listed as a secondary or coexisting condition.

Chronic diseases often require long-term care and they may be coded as often as the patient is treated for the chronic condition. However, in the case of outpatient coding, do not code the chronic condition when it does not affect the current management of the patient.

HUMAN IMMUNODEFICIENCY VIRUS (HIV)

HIV infection is an exception to the inpatient coding rule which states that "probable," "suspected," "questionable," and "still to be ruled out" diagnoses are coded as if they existed. HIV infection is only reported when confirmed by either a positive serology report or the physician's diagnostic statement that the patient is HIV positive or has an HIV related illness.

The HIV code should be selected as follows:

Code 042 — Human Immunodeficiency Virus [HIV] Disease. Assign code 042 for patients with a current HIV related illness or any prior diagnosis of HIV related illness. Once the patient has developed an HIV related illness, the patient should be assigned code 042 on every subsequent admission.

Code V08 — Asymptomatic Human Immunodeficiency Virus [HIV] Infection. Patients with physician documented asymptomatic HIV infections who have never had an HIV related illness should be assigned code V08.

795.71 — Nonspecific Serologic Evidence of Human Immunodeficiency Virus [HIV]. Patients with nonspecific serologic evidence of HIV infection but with inconclusive HIV test resulsts should be assigned code 795.71.

Sequencing of HIV codes follows the guidelines for selection of principal diagnosis. Patients who are admitted for treatment of an HIV related illness are assigned two codes. Code 042 is assigned as the principal diagnosis followed by additional diagnoses for all reported HIV related conditions. Patients with HIV who are admitted for an unrelated condition such as a traumatic injury should have the code for the injury assigned as the principal diagnosis. Code 042 would be reported as an additional diagnosis.

HIV infection in pregnancy, childbirth, and the puerperium is reported with a principal diagnosis of 647.6_, with 042 listed second.

Testing for HIV in an asymptomatic patient who is concerned about his/her HIV status is reported with code V73.89, screening for other specified viral disease.

CIRCULATORY DISORDERS

Diseases of the circulatory system are covered in categories 390-459. This section contains two areas which cause confusion. The first, hypertensive disease, was covered earlier in the chapter. The second area frequently causing confusion relates to the coding of myocardial infarctions (MIs).

MIs are classified as acute, category 410, when the documented duration is eight weeks or less. After that period the condition is classified as chronic and code 414.8, *Other specified forms of chronic ischemic heart disease,* should be assigned. "Old" healed MIs are assigned code 412. This eight-week rule combined with the fifth digits for episode of care can cause difficulty to both the coder and the insurance payor. According to ICD-9-CM, the acute diagnosis is used throughout the entire eight-week phase of treatment. If the patient is dismissed from the hospital and then readmitted during the eight-week time with another new MI, the fifth digit 1 is assigned, indicating an initial episode of care. However, if the second admission is related to the previous admission and not for a new MI, it is a subsequent episode of care and would be assigned the fifth-digit 2.

MENTAL DISORDERS

Coding mental disorders is complicated by the availability of another set of widely used codes, the *Diagnostic and Statistical Manual, Fourth Edition* (DSM-IV). Coders are advised to use DSM-IV as a reference aid to arrive at a diagnosis, but ICD-9-CM should be used for the actual coding. Chapter 5 of ICD-9-CM was developed with the assistance of the American Psychiatric Association in an effort to provide consistency and accuracy in the use these diagnostic codes. The codes are recognized by payors and help avoid confusion and claim denials.

Appendix B in Volume 1 is a glossary of mental disorders. It defines the terms used in categories 290–319 and was created to standardize the terminology in reporting these services. The coder does not use the glossary to select codes, but simply follows what the physician has reported in the clinical record. Obviously, the physician must be exact in documentation and specify the complete condition of the patient.

Also note that many of the codes in Chapter 5 require fifth digits.

BURNS

Coding burns is another situation where a single code cannot adequately describe the entire condition to a payor. Burns are coded by site, by severity or degree of burn, and by the percent of total body surface burned.

Categories 940–947 include the location (site) of the burn within the main term. Fourth digits identify the severity of the burn. Many burns require a fifth digit for further site specificity.

Category 948 is unique within the ICD-9-CM text since it measures the extent of body surface involved in a burn. Use 948 in combination with categories 940–947 when the site is specified. Fourth-digit classification for code 948 indicates the percent of body surface burned regardless of the degree of burn. For third-degree burns there is a fifth digit to be determined. Although the full range of fifth digits

CODING AXIOM

Burns are coded by site, by severity or degree of burn, and by the percent of total body surface burned.

Rule of Nines for Burns

Head and Neck (9%)

Front (18 %)

Arm (9%)

Back (18 %)

Arm (9%)

Perineum (1%)

Leg (18 %)

Leg (18 %)

is defined, not all apply to each fourth digit. Applicable fifth digits are listed in brackets below the fourth-digit classification. Fifth digits indicate what percentage of the body received third-degree burns. If no third-degree burn exists use a fifth digit 0, indicating 10 percent or less.

Confusion may arise in determining the correct percentage of total body surface involved. It is logical to assume that if the whole leg is burned, it involves 100 percent of the leg. But accurate coding requires that you determine the percent of total body surface, not just that of the leg. The leg actually represents only 18 percent of the total body surface. The "Rule of Nines" diagram on the previous page provides an easy method to calculate total body burn percentages for adults.

In summary, guidelines for coding burns are:

- Use code categories 940–947 to code the burn by body location
- Select the fourth digit from the codes listed according to the degree of burn
- Use additional fifth digits as designated with applicable codes to indicate the specific body site
- Use code category 948 to identify the percent of body burned
- Select the fourth digit from the codes listed according to the percentage of body surface area burned
- Use an additional fifth digit to specify the percent of body surface with third degree burns (Note that the fifth digit 0 identifies less than 10 percent or an unspecified third-degree burn)

PREGNANCY, CHILDBIRTH AND THE PUERPERIUM

Coding obstetrical care is difficult. It requires use of codes from both Chapter 11, Complications of Pregnancy, Childbirth, and the Puerperium (630-677) and from the Supplementary Classification of Factors Influencing Health Status and Contact with Health Services (V22.0-V24.2, V27.0-V27.9).

During the antenatal period, when there are no complicating factors, the diagnosis code selected should be a V code for supervision of a normal or high-risk pregnancy (V22.0-V23.9).

When the patient presents with complications during any stage of pregnancy — antepartum, labor and delivery, or postpartum — codes should be selected from categories 630-676. All but four codes in this section require fourth- or fifth-digit specificity. There are also special instructional notes scattered throughout the section so be sure to pay special attention to Volume 1.

For codes in categories 640-676, fifth-digits relate specifically to the episode of care, and appropriate digits are enclosed within brackets located directly below the subcategory code. Patients presenting with risks that would influence their care generally require some type of special service. These problems must be well documented in the patient's record. The patient who is at risk during the prenatal period may have an uncomplicated delivery. Conversely, the patient who has no problem during the prenatal period may have a complicated delivery. The stage where the risk or complication occurs is the factor influencing the final code selection. Fifth-digit subclassifications are as follows:

CODING AXIOM

During the antenatal period, when there are no complicating factors, the diagnosis code selected should be a V code for supervision of a normal or high-risk pregnancy (V22.0-V23.9).

When the patient presents with complications during any stage of pregnancy – antepartum, labor and delivery, or postpartum – codes should be selected from categories 630-676. The stage where the risk or complication occurs is the factor influencing the final code selection.

0   Unspecified as to episode of care or not applicable

1   Delivered with or without mention of antepartum condition

2   Delivered with mention of postpartum condition

3   Antepartum condition or complication (not delivered during current episode of care)

4   Postpartum condition or complication (not delivered during current episode of care)

The postpartum period begins immediately after delivery and continues for six weeks following delivery. Any postpartum complication occurring within the six week period should be reported with a code from Chapter 11 (630–676). Pregnancy related complications after the six week period may be assigned a code from Chapter 11 if the physician specifies that the condition is pregnancy related.

Be aware of a situation encountered with the following categories:

Volume 1
645 Prolonged pregnancy
657 Polyhydramnios
670 Major puerperal infection
672 Pyrexia of unknown origin during the puerperium

ICD-9-CM indicates that these codes require a fifth digit but provides no fourth digit; there is only a statement at the end of each of the code ranges specifying *Use 0 as fourth-digit for this category*. Therefore, as the statement specifies, place a zero in the fourth position, and select the appropriate fifth digit for these coding categories from those listed in the note for the individual subsections.

Another situation where special coding rules apply involves the pregnant patient requiring medical care for a problem unrelated to her pregnancy. For example, if a pregnant patient is seen for an upper respiratory infection (URI), code the URI, 465.9, as the primary reason for the encounter. List code V22.2 Pregnant State, Incidental, as the second code. Code V22.2 used secondary to a nonobstetric diagnosis code alerts the payor that the visit is not for normal antepartum care which the physician may also be supplying.

Codes V27.0-V27.9, Outcome of Delivery, can also cause confusion. These codes are never used as the primary diagnosis, providing only supplemental information regarding the status of the infant. They are used in conjunction with codes from categories 640-676 and are used to record the status of the infant on the mother's record. These codes indicate whether the birth was live or stillborn as well as whether it was a single, twin, or other multiple birth.

Because codes related to pregnancy, delivery, and postnatal services are usually reported as a single global service, it is not normally necessary to report postpartum services separately. However, when routine postpartum care requires separate reporting, it should be coded with V24.0-V24.2.

NEWBORN CODING AND PERINATAL CONDITIONS

The primary diagnosis for a newborn, born during the current episode of care, is always a code from categories V30-V39, liveborn infant. This is because the primary reason for the hospital admission and medical care is the birth. Fourth digits are available to indicate whether the birth was in the hospital, prior to admission to the hospital, or outside the hospital and not admitted. Fifth digits indicate whether the birth was by cesarean delivery or without mention of cesarean delivery. For healthy newborns, a code from the liveborn infant categories may be the only code recorded.

Codes from categories V30-V39 are used only for infants born during the current admission, and should be recorded only at the facility where the birth occurred. If the infant has perinatal conditions that require transfer to another facility during the same episode of care or if the infant is discharged and readmitted to the same hospital, the condition necessitating the transfer or the readmission should be listed as the primary diagnosis.

While a code from categories V30-V39 may be the only code required for healthy infants, any infant with perinatal conditions complicating care will require additional codes to describe these circumstances. These codes are found in categories 760-779 and describe conditions which originate in the perinatal period. The perinatal period is considered to extend through the fourth week (28 days) following delivery.

An introductory note in this section for newborn coding can cause some confusion. It states that these codes include "conditions which have their origin in the perinatal period even though death or morbidity occurs later." The issue here is: When did the problem begin? For example, encounters with a child who has convulsions originating during the perinatal period and continues to be seen for a year for this problem are coded as 779.0 *Convulsions in newborn*.

Be sure to read the *includes* and *excludes* notes throughout this section and, most importantly, remember that these codes describe the infant's condition, not the mother's.

NEOPLASM CODING

The Neoplasm Table has been described earlier in this chapter. Instructions on the use of this table and special considerations related to neoplasm coding are presented here.

In order to select a code from the correct category of neoplasm, the coder must identify whether the neoplasm is benign, malignant, unspecified, or of uncertain behavior. This information may be presented several ways as described in the following paragraphs.

The treating physician may provide a complete description of the neoplasm in the physician's notes. For example, the following description allows the correct code to be selected directly from the neoplasm table "primary malignant neoplasm upper outer quadrant left breast." However, the treating physician might also describe the same neoplasm as follows: "adenocarcinoma upper outer quadrant left breast." How does the coder determine that the term adenocarcinoma refers to a malignant neoplasm? In this case it is necessary to first locate the term adenocarcinoma in the alphabetic index. The term adenocarcinoma provides an instructional note to "see also neoplasm, malignant, by site." Since the term "breast" does not appear as a modifier, the "see also note" should be followed. We now know that the neoplasm is malignant, but is it primary, secondary, or a

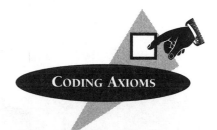

CODING AXIOMS

All but four codes in the obstetrical care section of ICD-9-CM require fourth- or fifth-digit specificity.

Perinatal codes describe the infant's condition, not the mother's.

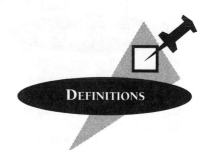

DEFINITIONS

Remember to read the *includes* and *excludes* notes when describing the infant's condition.

Includes appears immediately under a three-digit code title to provide further definition or to give an example of the category contents.

Excludes indicates terms that are not to be coded under the referenced term, as they are listed elsewhere.

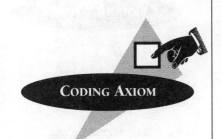

Whenever possible, use the pathology report for outpatient and inpatient coding to histologically verify the tumor type.

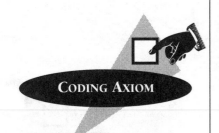

Family history of malignant neoplasm codes are used as a secondary diagnosis in outpatient and inpatient coding. The primary diagnosis is usually listed first, such as a screening Pap smear, with a family history of a malignant neoplasm of the cervix in an outpatient setting. Or, in an inpatient setting, the principal diagnosis may be listed as a malignant neoplasm of the cervix with a family history of malignant neoplasm of the cervix.

Ca in situ? The absence of the terms "metastatic to" or "Ca in situ" provide the answer. This is a primary malignant neoplasm and should be coded as 174.4.

If the treating physician fails to provide a complete description of the neoplasm, the pathology report frequently provides the missing information. Even when the treating physician provides a complete description, the pathology report should be reviewed to confirm the diagnosis. Some facilities will not allow coding of a malignancy unless the diagnosis has been confirmed by a pathology exam.

Sequencing of malignant neoplasm codes in the case of metastatic neoplasms is the next problem encountered by coders as it is necessary to record codes for both the primary and secondary sites.

Malignant indicates a tumor that has the potential to spread. When a neoplasm has metastasized (meaning the neoplasm has spread to a new location) the new growth is secondary to the primary (original) site. The rule in these cases is to determine the primary and secondary sites, then code first the site requiring patient care. If the initial or primary cancer is still active and represents the reason for the day's service, report the code for the primary site first. If a secondary growth is the primary reason for patient care, choose a code from the Secondary column of the table, list it first, then determine the code for the primary neoplastic site and list it second.

When a primary and secondary malignant neoplasm are present, the primary site must be reported, even if it was not the site treated. When information regarding the primary site is not available, ask the physician for clarification, or refer to previous medical records for information (e.g., staff notes, pathology report). Be specific about the tumor type and primary and/or secondary site(s). Use 199.1 *Malignant neoplasm without specification of site, other* only after determining that information is not available by questioning the physician or by checking previous records. Payors will often question a claim when the primary site is unknown. This could result in claims being delayed due to a request for clarification by the payor.

If the neoplasm has been removed or is in remission and the physician specifies the patient has a history of malignant neoplasm, use a V code (V10.00–V10.9 *Personal history of malignant neoplasm*). The V code is supplemental information and is listed after the code specifying the reason for the current visit.

V codes are also used as the primary diagnosis for patients who are receiving either radiotherapy, V58.0, or chemotherapy, V58.1, for treatment of a malignant neoplasm. The code for the malignant neoplasm should be listed as a secondary diagnosis. Therefore, the breast cancer patient described above who receives adjunctive chemotherapy to treat the malignancy would have the following codes assigned for encounters for chemotherapy:

V58.1   **Encounter for chemotherapy**
174.4   **Malignant neoplasm female breast upper-outer quadrant**

It is important not to confuse a diagnosis of a malignant neoplasm with the situation where the possibility of a malignant neoplasm is being evaluated. Patients often present with signs, symptoms, and complaints which require the physician to consider the possibility of a malignancy as one of several diagnoses. In these cases, the presenting problem should be coded. For example, on initial visit, the patient presents with a complaint of rectal bleeding.

Even though the physician begins a workup to determine the cause of the bleeding and indicates that the work-up is being done to "rule-out" a malignancy, the code for this visit should be 569.3 *Hemorrhage of rectum and anus*, not a malignant neoplasm code.

In addition, two other categories are available for coding workups for malignant neoplasms. The first, V71.1 *Observation for suspected malignant neoplasm*, should be used when persons presenting without signs or symptoms are suspected of having a malignant neoplasm, but after further diagnostic evaluation are not found to have a malignancy.

The second category is V76 *Special screening for malignant neoplasms*. Codes from this category can be used alone for routine screening for malignant neoplasms. For example, the diagnosis for a routine sigmoidoscopy in an asymptomatic patient would be V76.41 *Screening for malignant neoplasm of the rectum*. However, if the patient does have a related symptom or condition, such as change in bowel habits, this condition should be coded secondarily .

In the course of diagnosing and treating a malignant neoplasm, the codes selected will change. Treatment of neoplasms generally involves evaluation, biopsy or surgical excision, and postoperative services or other aftercare (chemotherapy, radiation therapy). Specific guidelines apply to each level of treatment and service.

During the evaluation phase, the patient usually presents with signs or symptoms which indicate that a neoplasm of some type must be ruled out. Initial evaluation codes should identify the nature of these signs, symptoms, or conditions. Examples of categories and codes which might be used to describe these signs, symptoms, or conditions include:

780–799	Symptoms, signs, and ill-defined conditions
V71.1	Observation for suspected malignant neoplasm
V76	Special screening for malignant neoplasms

At the time of biopsy or surgical excision, a more definitive diagnosis can be made. Once diagnosis of a neoplasm is made, preferably supported by a pathology report, the correct code should be selected from the neoplasm table.

The final phase of treatment involves postoperative or other aftercare. If the neoplasm is completely surgically excised, a V code should be sequenced first. Examples of applicable V codes include V58.3 *Attention to surgical dressings, and sutures*, V58.49 *Other specified aftercare following surgery*, and V67.0 *Follow-up examination following surgery*. Report the neoplasm code second. If the patient requires additional treatment with chemotherapy use V58.1 as the primary diagnosis. For radiation therapy use V58.0 as the primary diagnosis. Sequence the neoplasm code second.

The following is an example of coding for cancer treatment:

Clinical Scenario

On initial exam, a male patient presents with signs of rectal bleeding. The physician schedules an endoscopy for the following week. Multiple biopsies confirm cancer in several locations in the left colon and rectosigmoid junction. Immediate surgery follows. The physician performs a partial colectomy and proctectomy. While the physician follows the patient through the postoperative period, the patient begins a course of chemotherapy with an oncologist. One year after surgery, the physician finds no signs of recurrence of the tumor. The following ICD-9-CM codes identify the steps of the patient's treatment.

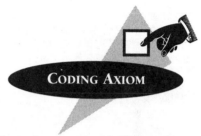

CODING AXIOM

Diagnostic codes selected will change in the course of diagnosing and treating a malignant neoplasm:

- Treatment generally involves evaluation, biopsy, or surgical excision.

- Initial evaluation codes should identify the nature of signs, symptoms, or conditions.

- Biopsy or surgical excision provides a more definitive diagnosis.

- The final treatment phase involves postoperative or other aftercare.

Outpatient

Initial visit

569.3   Hemorrhage of rectum and anus

Endoscopy visit

569.3   Hemorrhage of rectum and anus (preoperative diagnosis)

153.2   Malignant neoplasm of descending colon (not billed until confirmed by pathology report)

154.0   Malignant neoplasm of rectosigmoid junction (not billed until confirmed by pathology report)

Inpatient

Operative diagnosis

153.2   Malignant neoplasm of descending colon

154.0   Malignant neoplasm of rectosigmoid junction

Outpatient

Follow-up diagnosis

V58.3   Attention to surgical dressings and sutures

153.2   Malignant neoplasm of descending colon (secondary diagnosis)

154.0   Malignant neoplasm of rectosigmoid junction (secondary diagnosis)

If malignancy is no longer present

V58.3   Attention to surgical dressings and sutures

V10.05   Personal history of malignant neoplasm of large intestine

V10.06   Personal history of malignant neoplasm of the rectosigmoid junction

Outpatient - (Oncologist)

Chemotherapy visit

V58.1   Encounter for chemotherapy (primary diagnosis)

153.2   Malignant neoplasm of descending colon (secondary diagnosis)

154.0   Malignant neoplasm of rectosigmoid junction (secondary diagnosis)

Personal history of malignant noeplasm category V10, is not reported even if site has been eradicated or excised when adjunctive therapy is being provided.

Outpatient (Physician)

One-year follow-up

V71.1   Observation for suspected neoplasm

V10.05   Personal history of malignant neoplasm of large intestine

V10.06   Personal history of malignant neoplasm of the rectosigmoid junction

POISONING AND ADVERSE EFFECTS

Correctly coding poisonings and adverse effects requires a thorough understanding of the definitions. In addition, since both poisonings and adverse effects require more than one code to describe the condition, sequencing rules must also be memorized.

Poisoning

A poisoning is defined as occurring whenever an error is made in drug prescription or administration. A poisoning can be accidental, intentional (suicide attempt or assault), or undetermined. Terms normally associated with a poisoning include: poisoning, overdose, wrong substance given or taken, and intoxication.

At least three codes are required to correctly report a poisoning:

DEFINITIONS

Poisoning occurs whenever an error is made in drug prescription or administration.

Adverse effects occur when a drug is correctly prescribed and administered but the patient has an adverse reaction despite correct use.

1. Identify the drug which has caused the poisoning in the Table of Drugs and Chemicals. The first code sequenced will be from the poisoning column and identifies the drug or chemical.

2. The second code indicates the condition (e.g., coma or stupor) resulting from the poisoning.

3. The third code (an E code) identifies the cause of poisoning as accidental, suicide attempt, assault, or undetermined. The E code should be selected from the appropriate column of the Table of Drugs and Chemicals.

Poisoning Scenario

A patient received trimethobenzamide HCl capsules for nausea and vomiting. At home, she accidentally left the open pill bottle on the bathroom counter. Her two-year-old daughter saw the bottle, dumped out the capsules, and swallowed them. Within a few minutes, the patient noted that "it was awfully quiet in the house" and found the child unconscious on the bathroom floor. She rushed the child to the emergency department, where the child was treated and admitted to the hospital.

963.0	**Poisoning trimethobenzamide HCl**
780.01	**Coma**
E858.1	**Accidental poisoning by systemic agents**

Adverse Effect

An adverse effect occurs when a drug was correctly prescribed and administered but the patient has an adverse reaction to it despite correct use. Terms commonly associated with an adverse effect include: adverse reaction, side effect, sensitivity, and idiosyncratic reaction. Adverse effects occur due to individual differences among patients, including genetic factors, disease state, age, and sex.

To code an adverse effect first identify the effect as tachycardia, hallucinations, vomiting, respiratory failure, gastritis, etc. The effect is sequenced first. Next identify the drug or medicinal substance causing the adverse effect and select the E code in the Table of Drugs and Chemicals from the column titled Therapeutic Use. Sequence the E code second.

Adverse Effect Scenario

A 14-year-old female patient with strep throat is treated with erythromycin due to a stated allergy to penicillin. Two days later the patient is seen in the ER with severe generalized abdominal pain. Diagnosis is acute gastritis due to sensitivity to erythromycin.

535.00	**Acute gastritis w/o mention of hemorrhage**
E930.3	**Adverse effect due to erythromycin**

SURGICAL AND POSTOPERATIVE COMPLICATIONS

The majority of codes for surgical and postoperative complications are found in categories 996-999. Sequencing rules for coding surgical and postoperative complications do not differ from general coding rules. For outpatient coding the code reflecting the current, most significant reason for the current episode of care should be coded first. For inpatient coding, the condition leading to admission to the hospital is sequenced first.

Clinical Scenario 1

A patient with primary malignant neoplasm of the corpus uteri is seen in the physician's office for a preoperative history and physical for a planned vaginal hysterectomy. During the hysterectomy the urinary bladder is nicked requiring immediate repair by a urologist. Two

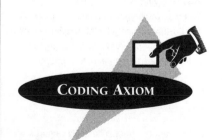

CODING AXIOM

Sequencing rules for coding surgical and postoperative complications do not differ from general coding rules. For outpatient coding, the most significant reason for the visit should be coded first. For inpatient coding, the condition leading to admission to the hospital is sequenced first.

days following the surgery on the same admission, the patient develops a postoperative wound infection. The diagnosis codes and sequencing are as follows:

182.0	Malignant neoplasm of corpus uteri
998.2	Accidental puncture or laceration during a procedure
998.59	Other postoperative infection

In this case the reason for the admission was treatment of the malignant neoplasm of the uterus. The accidental laceration and postoperative infection are coded secondarily because they are complications that arose during the hospital stay.

Clinical Scenario 2

A patient one-week status post hysterectomy for malignant neoplasm of the uterus is seen on an urgent basis by her gynecologist due to complaints of fever, nausea, and vomiting. Because of an inability to empty her bladder prior to discharge, the patient had been sent home with an indwelling urinary catheter. Upon examination the patient is found to have abdominal tenderness. A urine sample taken from the catheter is positive for red and white blood cells. A urine culture is taken and the patient is given a prescription for antibiotics. The physician diagnoses a bladder infection caused by the indwelling urinary catheter.

996.64	Infection due to indwelling urinary catheter

Only the infection is coded since it is the reason for the outpatient care.

INJURY

Codes for injuries are listed in the alphabetic index by type of injury. Notes can be found throughout the alphabetic index with alternative terms to be searched and definitions of the types of injuries included under the various terms. The tabular list also includes definitions and specific instructions for coding injuries.

In the case of the patient presenting with multiple injuries, a separate code should be assigned for each injury. To report multiple injuries, list the conditions treated by the physician in order of importance, with the major problem listed first. As a rule of thumb, when medical and surgical problems are being managed, list the surgical problem first. However, do not assume that the surgical problem is always the most severe. A patient presenting with an intracranial injury, managed medically, and a fractured phalanx, managed surgically, should have the intracranial injury listed as the primary or principal diagnosis.

While there are categories available for coding of multiple injuries, use these categories only when the information is not available to code each injury separately. Occasionally, multiple injury codes are assigned when it is more convenient to record a single code for data retrieval purposes.

Beginning coders assert that the most difficult part of assigning injury codes is knowing what terms to search for in the alphabetic index. Following is a list of common injury terms and the types of injuries included under each term:

Contusion. Includes bruise and hematoma without a fracture or open wound. If a fracture or open wound is identified at the same site, code only the fracture or open wound.

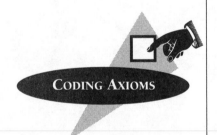

CODING AXIOMS

To look up injuries in Volume 2, choose the most appropriate category: *Foreign body, Wound, Injury, Blast injury, Blunt trauma, Bruising, Crushing, Hematoma, Laceration, Rupture, Tear, Puncture, Concussion, Traumatic rupture.* Next, find the subterm that describes the organ or site injured.

There is no time limit between the acute phase and the late effect.

To code a late effect accurately requires two codes — the residual effect and the cause of the late effect.

Crush. Includes only crushing injuries that are not complicated by concussion, fractures, injury to internal organs, intracranial injury.

Dislocation. Includes displacement and subluxation. Dislocations may be open or closed. Closed dislocations include those described as complete, partial, simple, uncomplicated. Open dislocations include those described as compound, infected, or with foreign body. A dislocation not indicated as closed or open is classified as closed.

Fracture. Fractures may be open or closed. Injuries described as fracture dislocations are coded as fractures. Open fractures include those described as compound, infected, missile, puncture or with foreign body. Closed fractures include those described as comminuted, depressed, elevated, fissured, greenstick, impacted, linear, march, simple, slipped epiphysis, and spiral. A fracture not indicated as open or closed is classified as closed.

Injury, blood vessel. Includes injuries to blood vessels described as arterial hematoma, avulsion, cut, laceration, rupture, traumatic aneurysm, and traumatic fistula.

Injury, internal. Includes all injuries to internal organs such as the heart, lung, liver, kidney, and pelvic organs. Types of injuries to internal organs include laceration, tear, traumatic rupture, penetrating wounds, blunt trauma, crushing, blast injuries, and open wounds to internal organs with or without a fracture in the same region.

Injury, intracranial. Includes concussion, cerebral laceration and contusion, and intracranial hemorrhage. The injuries may be open or closed. Intracranial injuries with skull fractures are found under fracture.

Injury, superficial. Includes injuries described as abrasion, insect bite (nonvenomous), blister, and scratch.

Sprain/Strain. Includes injuries to the joint capsule, ligament, muscle, and tendon described by the following terms: avulsion, hemarthrosis, laceration (closed), rupture, and tear. Open lacerations of these structures should be coded as open wounds.

Wound, open. Includes all open wounds not involving internal organs. Included are wounds to skin, muscle, tendon described as animal bite, avulsion, cut, laceration, puncture wound, and traumatic amputation. Open wounds may be uncomplicated or complicated. Complicated injuries must include mention of delayed healing, delayed treatment, foreign body, or major infection.

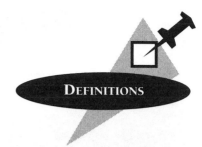

DEFINITIONS

Closed fractures are fractures in which the overlying skin is intact. They may be described in medical records as:

comminuted	depressed
elevated	fissured
greenstick	

Open fractures occur when an open wound extends through the skin down to the level of the fracture. They may be described in medical records as:

compound	puncture
infected	missile
with foreign body	

Clinical Scenario 1

An auto accident victim is admitted to the hospital with multiple injuries, including a cardiac contusion, nonpenetrating open wound to the abdominal wall, and fractures of the middle phalanx of both the fourth and fifth fingers. The patient is initially admitted to the ICU for observation for the cardiac contusion. The wound of the abdominal wall is repaired at the bedside. The nondisplaced phalanx fractures are splinted and may require surgical pinning at a later time.

861.01	**Contusion heart without mention of open wound into thorax**
879.2	**Open wound of abdominal wall, anterior, without mention of complication**
816.01	**Closed fracture middle phalanx/phalanges**
E812.9	**Motor vehicle accident, NOS**

LATE EFFECTS

A late effect is a residual condition occurring after the acute phase of an illness or injury. The original illness or injury is healed, but a chronic or long-term condition remains. In the following examples, each late effect appears in bold type while the underlying cause (etiology) is in italics.

> **Malunion** *fracture* of the left ankle
> Traumatic **arthritis** following *fracture* of the left wrist
> **Hemiplegia** following *cerebrovascular thrombosis* one year before
> **Scarring** of the left leg due to third degree *burns*
> **Contracture** of the left heel tendons due to *poliomyelitis*

There is no time limit between the acute phase and the late effect. The residual condition may be apparent in four to six months, or there may be a lapse of one year or more between the illness or injury and the current encounter. Late effects are listed in Volume 2 of ICD-9-CM.

> **Volume 2**
> **Late**
>   effect(s) (of)
>   burn (injury classifiable to 948-949) 906.9
>   eye (injury classifiable to 940) 906.5

A late effect requires two codes — the residual effect and the cause of the late effect. The residual condition is sequenced first when it is the primary or principal reason for the patient encounter or procedure. The late effect code is used to specify the etiology and is not a principal diagnosis. In inpatient coding a late effect code is not coded until one year or longer after the initial condition.

> **Incorrect**
> 905.4   **Late effect of fracture of lower extremities**
> 824.5   **Fracture of ankle, bimalleolar, open**

> **Correct**
> 733.81   **Malunion of fracture**
> 905.4   **Late effect of fracture of lower extremities**

A late effect code may be used as a principal diagnosis to specify the cause of the late effect when no residual effects are specified. However, the attending physician (or the documentation) should be consulted to obtain a more specific diagnosis. ICD-9-CM codes should not be assigned for diagnoses or conditions that are no longer detectable (e.g., fracture, cerebrovascular thrombosis, poliomyelitis).

DIABETES MELLITUS

The fifth digit subclassifications for diabetes mellitus (used with category 250) identify the type of diabetes as well as whether the condition is controlled or uncontrolled:

> 0   **Type II (non-insulin dependent type) (NIDDM type) (adult-onset type), or unspecified type, not stated as uncontrolled**
> 1   **Type 1 (insulin dependent type) (IDDM) (juvenile type), not stated as uncontrolled**
> 2   **Type II (non-insulin dependent type) (NIDDM type) (adult-onset type), or unspecified type, uncontrolled**
> 3   **Type I (insulin dependent type) (IDDM) (juvenile type), uncontrolled**

KEY POINT

Late effects categories

These codes are three-digit categories and may require additional digits.

137   Late effects of tuberculosis
138   Late effects of acute poliomyelitis
139   Late effects of other infectious and parasitic diseases
268   Rickets, late effect
326   Late effects of intracranial abscess or pyogenic infection
438   Late effects of cerebrovascular disease
677   Late effects of complication of pregnancy, childbirth, or the puerperium
905   Late effects of musculoskeletal and connective tissue injuries
906   Late effects of injuries to skin and subcutaneous tissues
907   Late effects of injuries to the nervous system
908   Late effects of other and unspecified injuries
909   Late effects of other and unspecified external causes

These classifications can cause confusion. For example, it's possible for individuals with Type II, adult-onset diabetes to require insulin for control of the condition. The rule in this case is to select the fifth-digit subclassification based on the onset of the disease not on the patient's insulin status. Therefore, the patient with Type II, adult-onset diabetes who is insulin dependent would be assigned the fifth-digit 0 or 2.

DISCUSSION QUESTIONS

1. When are myocardial infarctions classified as acute and when are they classified as chronic?

   _____

   _____

2. When should you use the *Diagnostic and Statistical Manual, Fourth Edition* (DSM-IV) in coding mental disorders?

   _____

   _____

   _____

3. List the criteria for coding burns.

   _____

   _____

   _____

4. When a pregnant patient comes to your office with a problem unrelated to her pregnancy how should the visit be coded?

   _____

   _____

   _____

5. Explain the special circumstances with rule-out statements in outpatient and inpatient coding for cancer treatment.

   _____

   _____

Specialty-Specific Scenarios

The following scenarios are designed by specialty to help you make the transition from documentation to correct code choices.

OB/GYN SCENARIO — INPATIENT

A 37-year-old had a normal spontaneous vaginal delivery (NSVD) with a third degree perineal laceration on Thursday at the hospital. Her attending OB/GYN physician delivered the baby boy, who weighed 10 lb. 3 oz., and repaired the patient's perineal laceration. In the medical record staff notes, the physician describes the delivery and repair of the perineal

OBJECTIVES

See the practical application of ICD-9-CM coding logic

Identify the special circumstances and rules of specialties

laceration; he also mentions that the baby is "large for dates." The pediatrician caring for the baby specifies in the record the baby is exceptionally large.

Common Coding Errors:

Mother's record

650	**Normal delivery**
664.21	**Third-degree perineal laceration**
V27.0	**Single liveborn**

Baby's record

V30.00	**Single liveborn, born in hospital, delivered, without mention of cesarean section**

Accurate Coding:

Mother's record

664.21	**Third-degree perineal laceration**
656.61	**Excessive fetal growth**
V27.0	**Single liveborn**

Baby's record

V30.00	**Single liveborn, born in hospital, delivered, without mention of cesarean section**
766.0	**Exceptionally large baby**

Although there was a normal spontaneous vaginal delivery, it was complicated by a third degree perineal laceration and the baby is exceptionally large. Category 650 specifies it cannot be used with any other code in the range 630–676 when describing conditions during the same operative session. The baby's record should include the significant finding by both the obstetrician and pediatrician (baby was large for dates). The diagnosis met the criteria of 766.0 which specifies an implied birth weight of 4500 grams or more. On the baby's record, code V30.00 should be used as the principal diagnosis and any coexisting conditions should be sequenced in order of importance.

DERMATOLOGY SCENARIO — OUTPATIENT

A 32-year-old female was seen by a dermatologist for acne she has been experiencing since the delivery of her baby six months ago. In obtaining the patient's medical history, the dermatologist notes in the medical record that the patient has a history of infertility, and had elevated blood pressure readings during her pregnancy. The dermatologist obtains a blood pressure of 118/76, makes a diagnosis of acne, and prescribes a medication for the acne. In listing diagnoses, the dermatologist writes in the medical record: Acne, previous history of infertility, and history of elevated blood pressure readings during last pregnancy.

Common Coding Errors

706.1	**Acne**
V13.2	**Personal history of other genital system and obstetric disorders**
796.2	**Elevated blood pressure reading without diagnosis of hypertension**

Accurate Coding

706.1	**Acne**

Acne is the only significant problem found in the examination. The patient's history of infertility and of elevated blood pressure readings do not affect the management of the patient's acne, and her blood pressure is currently normal.

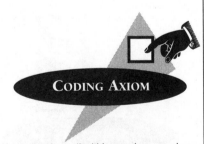

CODING AXIOM

If a patient's medical history plays no role in the management of a current condition, do not code that history.

ORTHOPEDIC SCENARIO — INPATIENT

A patient with severe, progressive, infantile scoliosis undergoes attempted spinal instrumentation. The procedure is terminated prematurely due to severe hypotension.

The patient is taken into the operating room where the anesthesiologist administers general anesthesia intravenously. The surgeon preps and drapes the patient before the anesthesiologist interrupts the procedure due to an apparent allergic response to the anesthesia manifested by severe hypotension. The patient is stabilized by the anesthesiologist. The surgeon elects to discontinue the procedure.

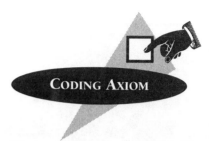

CODING AXIOM

The sequencing of codes is important. The coding rule for an adverse effect of a drug in therapeutic use requires the manifestation be listed first and then the E code.

Common Coding Errors

737.32	Progressive infantile idiopathic scoliosis
V64.3	Procedure not carried out for other reason
458.9	Hypotension, unspecified

Accurate Coding

737.32	Progressive infantile idiopathic scoliosis
458.9	Hypotension, unspecified
E938.3	Adverse effect, intravenous general anesthetics
V64.3	Procedure not carried out for other reason

The sequencing of codes is very important. After the principal diagnosis, the coding rule for an adverse effect of a drug in therapeutic use requires the manifestation be listed first and then the E code. The hypotension and the procedure not being carried out are "due to" the adverse effect of the anesthesia.

CARDIOLOGY SCENARIO — OUTPATIENT

A 65-year-old male with a history of angina asks to be worked into the office schedule of his cardiologist because of tightness in his chest and night sweats. The cardiologist reviews past and present medical history that is significant for a past history of a myocardial infarction (MI) four years ago. An extended examination of head, heart, lungs, and abdomen is obtained. As a part of the exam, the cardiologist provides a 12-lead ECG and an echocardiography with pulsed wave doppler and color flow mapping in the office. The patient is diagnosed as having acute unstable angina with an impending MI and a personal history of an MI. He is immediately admitted to the cardiac care unit of the local hospital.

Common Coding Errors

411.1	Intermediate coronary syndrome

Accurate Coding

411.1	Intermediate coronary syndrome
412	Old myocardial infarction

The old myocardial infarction is coded because it is significant and does affect the management of the patient.

GENERAL SURGERY SCENARIO — INPATIENT

A 43-year-old male is seen in the emergency department for abdominal pain and fever. The emergency room physician requests a general surgeon consultation. The patient history is significant for a transplanted kidney two years prior to the current ED visit. On examination, the patient is found to have right upper quadrant abdominal pain, nausea, and vomiting. Liver enzymes are elevated. The preoperative diagnosis is abdominal pain, R/O acute cholecystitis with cholelithiasis. The patient is taken to the operating room and surgery is performed by the physician. The postoperative diagnosis is choledocholithiasis with acute cholecystitis. The patient is placed on postoperative antibiotics. During the hospital stay the physician diagnoses him with hypokalemia, which is treated with IV potassium. The patient is discharged.

Common Coding Errors

Preoperative diagnosis

789.01	Abdominal pain, right upper quadrant
574.00	Acute cholelithiasis, without mention of obstruction

Postoperative diagnosis

574.30	Acute choledocholithiasis, with acute cholecystitis
V42.0	Kidney transplant status

Accurate Coding

Preoperative diagnosis

574.00	Acute cholelithiasis, without mention of obstruction

Postoperative diagnosis

574.30	Acute choledocholithiasis, with acute cholecystitis
V42.0	Kidney transplant status
276.8	Hypopotassemia

The preoperative diagnosis of abdominal pain should not be coded because it is due to and is a symptom of the cholelithiasis. The hypokalemia is coded because it is a condition that developed during the hospitalization, and the patient was treated for the condition.

OPHTHALMOLOGY SCENARIO — OUTPATIENT

A 35-year-old female makes an appointment with an ophthalmologist in relation to her diagnosis of adult onset insulin-dependent diabetes. On the day of the appointment the physician records the patient's complaints, obtains a history, and performs a complete ophthalmological examination noting the diagnoses in the medical record as diabetic cataract and early background diabetic retinopathy.

Common Coding Errors

250.00	Diabetes mellitus without mention of complication, type II
366.41	Diabetic cataract
362.01	Background diabetic retinopathy

Accurate Coding

250.50	Diabetes with ophthalmic manifestations, type II
366.41	Diabetic cataract
362.01	Background diabetic retinopathy

Both the diabetic cataract and background diabetic retinopathy specify that diabetes with ophthalmic manifestation be coded first. The diabetes code 250.5 notes, *Use an additional code to identify manifestation, as: cataract (366.41), retinopathy (362.01–362.02)*. All codes from category 250, *diabetes mellitus*, require a fifth digit to specify the diabetes as Type I or II and controlled or uncontrolled.

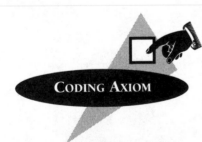

CODING AXIOM

When selecting the primary diagnosis associated with a complication of diabetes, remember the primary diagnosis should reflect that complication (e.g., diabetes with ophthalmic manifestations (250.5x) with diabetic retinopathy, or diabetes with renal manifestations (250.4x) with diabetic intercapillary glomerulosclerosis). A fifth digit specifies whether the patient is type I or II, and controlled or uncontrolled.

PATHOLOGY SCENARIO — INPATIENT

A frozen section taken from a patient is submitted to a hospital pathology department from the hospital surgical suite. The section is labeled "right upper outer quadrant breast tissue from a 45-year-old woman." A preliminary diagnosis is made by the pathologist of malignant neoplasm of right breast. A right radical mastectomy with excision of regional lymph nodes is performed by the surgeon. The right breast tissue along with the surgically removed lymph nodes are submitted for pathology. The pathologist's final diagnosis is infiltrating duct carcinoma of the right upper outer quadrant breast with metastasis to right axillary lymph nodes labeled 1–4.

Common Coding Errors

Preoperative diagnosis

174.4   **Malignant neoplasm of female breast, upper outer quadrant**

Postoperative diagnosis

196.3   **Secondary malignant neoplasm of lymph nodes of axilla and upper limb**

174.4   **Malignant neoplasm of female breast, upper outer quadrant**

Accurate Coding

Preoperative diagnosis

174.4   **Malignant neoplasm of female breast, upper outer quadrant**

Postoperative diagnosis

174.4   **Malignant neoplasm of female breast, upper outer quadrant**

196.3   **Secondary malignant neoplasm of lymph nodes of axilla and upper limb**

When both a primary and secondary site of a neoplasm are present, sequencing depends on the site being treated. Since the definitive procedure, radical mastectomy was done for the treatment of the malignant neoplasm of the breast, this code is sequenced first.

RADIOLOGY SCENARIO — OUTPATIENT

A 55-year-old woman is referred to your free-standing clinic for a mammogram. The gynecologist's request for the mammogram states the patient has a history of fibrocystic disease of the breast, with a 1 cm lump in the right upper-inner quadrant breast. The mammogram is performed to rule-out malignant neoplasm. The bilateral mammogram is inconclusive and the radiologist receives authorization to do an ultrasound on the right breast. The ultrasound allows the radiologist to better visualize the lump through very dense breast tissue and fibrocystic disease. The radiologist's final diagnosis is bilateral fibrocystic disease breast, mass upper-inner quadrant right breast. The radiologist requests a repeat examination in six months to evaluate any changes in the breast mass.

Common Coding Errors

174.2   **Malignant neoplasm female breast, upper-inner quadrant**

610.1   **Diffuse cystic mastopathy**

V72.3   **Gynecological examination**

Accurate Coding

611.72   **Lump or mass in breast**

610.1   **Diffuse cystic mastopathy**

Rule-out statements are not used for outpatient coding. The symptom of lump or mass in the breast should be used as the primary diagnosis because it is the reason the patient was

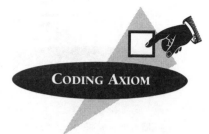

CODING AXIOM

When both a primary and secondary site of a neoplasm are present, sequencing depends on the site being treated.

seen. The diffuse cystic mastopathy should be coded since the mastopathy was significant and affected the management of the patient. The encounter being coded is the radiology service not the gynecological service, so do not use the gynecological exam code.

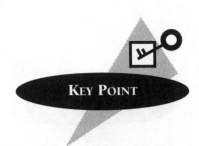

Advanced Coding Practice

CODING PRACTICE 1

A 16-year-old male, the unrestrained driver in a motor vehicle accident, sustained the following injuries:

- Depressed skull fracture of the parietal bone with subdural hemorrhage
- Ruptured spleen without penetrating wound
- Bladder laceration without penetrating wound
- Closed fracture of the pelvis multiple sites with disruption of pelvic circle

The patient car was struck from the side by a truck at a busy intersection. The patient was unconscious at the time of admission and did not regain consciousness until 3 days after the accident. All injuries required surgical intervention.

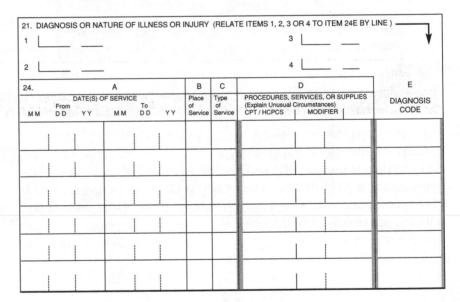

CODING PRACTICE 2

A newborn is delivered by cesarean section at a rural hospital. The newborn is 38 weeks gestation but is small for dates weighing only 4 lbs 2 oz. The newborn develops respiratory distress syndrome and is transferred to a tertiary care hospital. At the tertiary care facility the infant is also treated for transient hyperbilirubinemia.

Code the newborn diagnoses for each admission.

21. DIAGNOSIS OR NATURE OF ILLNESS OR INJURY (RELATE ITEMS 1, 2, 3 OR 4 TO ITEM 24E BY LINE)

1 |___ ___ | 3 |___ ___ |

2 |___ ___ | 4 |___ ___ |

24.	A				B	C	D		E
	DATE(S) OF SERVICE				Place	Type	PROCEDURES, SERVICES, OR SUPPLIES		DIAGNOSIS
	From		To		of	of	(Explain Unusual Circumstances)		CODE
MM	DD	YY	MM	DD	YY	Service	Service	CPT / HCPCS	MODIFIER	

Chapter Review

Diagnostic codes assist the reviewer in identifying the medical necessity of services provided to a patient by describing the circumstances of the patient's condition. Applying these principles to your diagnostic coding methodology will help ensure that the diagnostic codes selected properly demonstrate the written information in the medical record and that they accurately report the patient's course of treatment. Be aware of the many special coding situations that you may encounter.

2 CPT Introduction & Modifiers

CPT History

Physicians' Current Procedural Terminology (CPT) is a standardized system of five-digit codes and descriptive terms used to report the medical services and procedures performed by physicians. In addition, it is used to report the technical or facility component of most outpatient services including laboratory, radiology, and same day surgery. It was developed and is updated and published annually by the American Medical Association (AMA) and includes procedures that are consistent with contemporary medical practice by physicians in many locations. CPT codes communicate to providers, patients, and payors the procedures performed during a medical encounter. Accurate CPT coding is crucial for proper reimbursement from payors and for compliance with government regulations.

The first edition of *Current Procedural Terminology* was published by the AMA in 1966 as a companion piece to *Current Medical Terminology* (CMT), a manual of preferred medical nomenclature then in its third edition. The diminutive first edition of CPT (5 x 7 inches, 163 pages) contained a listing of four-digit codes and brief descriptions to report a full range of medical procedures and services. Each code was cross-referenced to then-available diagnostic codes: *Standard Nomenclature of Diseases and Operations* (SNDO) and the *International Classification of Diseases, Adapted* (ICDA). Editors of the first edition cited a variety of sources in developing the work, including the Social Security Administration, the *Blue Shield Manual of Statistical Requirements*, and *the Relative Value Studies of the California Medical Society*. The four-digit codes do not approximate those of today's CPT. That task was reserved for the editors of the second edition, published in 1970.

The 1970 edition of CPT marked the genesis of the coding manual so familiar to today's medical office workers. Many of the five-digit codes and expanded descriptions in this work remain unchanged to this day. The number of codes far exceeded those available to users of the first edition and guidelines to the various sections appeared for the first time. The second edition was developed with assistance from a handful of members of medical professional societies, a practice that would evolve into the 75-member CPT Advisory Committee listed in CPT.

The third edition of CPT was first published in 1973 and offered new features such as alphabetic modifiers and starred procedures marked with an asterisk. Deleted codes (but not new codes) could be found in an appendix. This edition also saw the medical codes moved to the front of the code listings, a benchmark that would stand for almost 20 years until the introduction of the evaluation and management codes in 1992.

The fourth edition of CPT, published in 1977, began the custom of significant yearly revisions, usually concentrated within a small number of sections. Since then, medical office coders across the country have made an annual ritual of analyzing the code changes and the related effects on

OBJECTIVES

Differentiate the origin and objectives of CMT and CPT

Understand the importance of CPT and how it is used

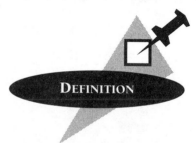

DEFINITION

CPT code: A five-digit identifying code number followed by a written narrative description of the procedure. CPT codes are developed and maintained by the American Medical Association.

Parallel procedural coding systems have been in place in medical reimbursement circles for decades. ICD-9-CM Volume 3 procedure codes are used by hospitals to report inpatient services. CPT covers outpatient services and inpatient services performed by physicians.

coding and billing for their practices. With printing runs approaching 400,000 copies, CPT is now among the largest-selling medical reference publications, long after its companion manual, CMT, has ceased publication.

WHO USES CPT?

CPT is the most widely accepted procedure coding system in the United States. In fact, Medicare and state Medicaid carriers are required by law to use these codes for the payment of health insurance claims, and most commercial insurance payors likewise use CPT. Common exceptions are state medical associations and workers' compensation plans that have developed their own procedure coding systems or use relative value studies for claims payment. These other systems vary, so request information as needed from the plans or associations in your area. Another procedural coding system in wide use today is ICD-9-CM Volume 3, used for hospital inpatient coding. See Chapter 9 in *Code It Right* for information on ICD-9-CM procedural coding.

Although they are required by most insurance companies, the mere existence of CPT procedure codes does not imply coverage under any given insurance plan. In other words, just because there is a CPT code for a current medical procedure does not mean that a payor is obligated to reimburse physicians for that service.

DISCUSSION QUESTIONS

1. How did today's CPT evolve and how are the codes created and maintained?

    _____

    _____

    _____

2. Who is required by law to use CPT codes?

    _____

    _____

    _____

CPT Conventions

CPT ALPHABETICAL REFERENCE INDEX

Effective CPT coding will be achieved when you are thoroughly familiar with CPT's contents and conventions.

As with ICD-9-CM, the CPT coding process begins with a careful examination of the medical record to determine primary and secondary procedures as well as any modifying or extenuating circumstances. The alphabetical CPT index is the starting point of all CPT coding, but do not select codes solely on the basis of information in the index — it is only a reference to the full listing of codes.

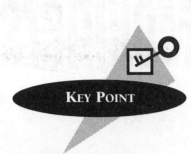

KEY POINT

For questions about CPT content, contact:

The Department of Coding & Nomenclature
American Medical Association
515 North State Street
Chicago, Illinois 60610
1-800-621-8335

OBJECTIVES

Understand the format and conventions of CPT, including indented codes and parenthetical phrases

Differentiate among new, revised, and deleted code symbols

Determine how to quickly locate codes through the index

THE INTRODUCTION

Understanding the complex CPT coding process begins with a careful study of the introduction. Understanding the CPT format and its support tools ensures accurate coding and streamlines claims processing. Essential information found in the introduction includes format and guidelines. The listing of a service or procedure and its code number in a specific section of CPT does not restrict its use to a specific specialty group. Any service or procedure code may be used to designate the services rendered by any qualified physician.

SECTIONS

CPT is arranged in six major sections as follows:

> Evaluation and Management (99201–99499)
> Anesthesiology (00100–01999)
> Surgery (10040–69990)
> Radiology (including nuclear medicine, radiation oncology, and diagnostic ultrasound) (70010–79999)
> Pathology and Laboratory (80049–89399)
> Medicine (90281–99199)

The six major sections of CPT are further arranged in subsections. Subsections pertaining to a section are listed within the section guidelines. For example, the radiology subsections are:

> Diagnostic Radiology
> Diagnostic Ultrasound
> Radiation Oncology
> Nuclear Medicine

Six appendices then follow the sections:

> Appendix A — Modifiers
> Appendix B — Summary of Additions, Deletions and Revisions
> Appendix C — Update to Short Descriptors
> Appendix D — Clinical Examples Supplement
> Appendix E — Summary of CPT Add-on Codes
> Appendix F — Summary of CPT codes exempt from Modifier -51

> Appendixes E and F are new features in CPT 1999.

FORMAT

Because many of the codes within a given section repeat some common portion of a procedure's description, CPT's printed format has been designed to save space. In the example below, 42104 and 42106 share the common description of *Excision, lesion of palate, uvula*. The difference between the codes is that 42104 is reported for excisions which do not require closure (suturing) of the surgically created wound, while 42106 is reported when simple primary closure is required. The key to interpreting these codes correctly is the semicolon (;) in 42104. The semicolon separates the common portion of the description from the portion unique to that code. Whenever a code is indented, you must always refer to the preceding unindented code for the common portion of the description. Thus, the indented 42106 code does not repeat the common portion (that part immediately before the semicolon), but instead supplies its own unique information.

42104   Excision, lesion of palate, uvula; without closure
42106   with simple primary closure

The complete description of 42106 is *Excision, lesion of palate, uvula; with simple primary closure.*

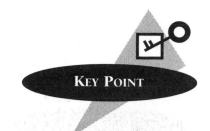

KEY POINT

Procedures are listed in the CPT index by:

- Procedure or service
- Organ or other anatomic site
- Condition
- Key synonyms
- Key eponyms (disease or procedure named after a person, e.g., Moh's technique)
- Abbreviations

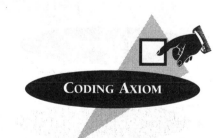

CODING AXIOM

An indented code always includes the common portion of the preceding unindented code description prior to the semicolon.

GUIDELINES

Guidelines appear at the beginning of each of the six major sections of CPT. The information contained in the guidelines provides definitions, explanations of terms, and factors relevant to the section. Each guideline must be reviewed to obtain a complete understanding of the proper use of the codes listed in the section; generally, information listed in the guidelines is not repeated within the section, subsection, or within the code range.

Guidelines also appear at the beginning of subsections located within the major sections of CPT. They provide information unique to a particular range of codes. Guidelines are also found within the code ranges in a subsection. Information specific to a given code may be included as a parenthetical phrase following the code. Revised text in guidelines, notes, and parenthetical phrases is enclosed by "▶◀" symbols.

> **67335**   Placement of adjustable suture(s) during strabismus surgery, including postoperative adjustment(s) of suture(s) (List separately in addition to code for specific strabismus surgery)
>
> (Use ▶67335 only◀ for codes for conventional muscle surgery, 67311–67334, to identify number of muscles involved)

Information specific to one code or a range of codes that has been deleted may be included as a parenthetical phrase in code number order. The parenthetical phrase may also contain directions on where to go to find the correct code.

> **22548**   Arthrodesis, anterior transoral or extraoral technique, clivus–C1-C2 (atlas-axis), with or without excision of odontoid process
>
> (22550, 22552, 22555, 22560, 22561, 22565 have been deleted. For intervertebral disk excision by laminotomy or laminectomy, see 63020–63042. For arthrodesis, see 22548–22632)

CODE CHANGES

To keep up with the dynamic nature of medicine, the AMA revises and publishes CPT on an annual basis. Appendix B consists of a summary of additions, deletions, and revisions to the current edition. Of these three types of changes, only partial descriptions of new codes appear in Appendix B making it necessary to refer to the main body of CPT for the full narrative description. Since code narrative changes state only that the terminology has been revised, you must compare the new edition to the previous one to identify how the code descriptions have been changed. The descriptions of codes in Appendix B listed with an asterisk have not been substantially altered. In most instances only placement of the semicolon has changed.

New codes are identified by a solid circle.

> ●**38792**   Injection procedure; for identification of sentinel node

Revised codes are identified by a solid triangle.

> ▲**23040**   Arthrotomy, glenohumeral joint, including exploration, drainage, or removal of foreign body

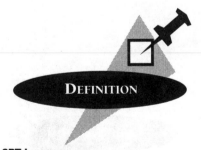

DEFINITION

CPT icons
- ● New codes
- ▲ Revised codes
- + Add-on codes
- ⊘ Modifier -51 exempt codes

Deleted codes are enclosed within parentheses.

> (68800 has been deleted. To report, use 68801)

Codes with minor grammatical changes are not identified in CPT with a symbol, but are identified in Appendix B with an asterisk (*).

Other CPT Icons

Two new icons were added to CPT 1999.

Add-on codes are identified by a **+** symbol.

> **+ 19001**   Puncture aspiration of cyst of breast; each additional cyst (List separately in addition to code for primary procedure)

Modifier -51 exempt codes are identified by a "⊘" symbol.

> **⊘ 20900**   Bone graft, any donor area; minor or small (eg, dowel or button)

Once you have updated the codes used in your office by referring to the newest edition of CPT, evaluate the fees assigned to all codes, not just the new codes.

DISCUSSION QUESTIONS

1. How does a coder read an indented code?

_____

_____

_____

2. Why shouldn't you assign a procedure code after reviewing the index alone?

_____

_____

_____

3. Where are guidelines located in CPT?

_____

_____

_____

Modifiers

Modifiers, introduced in the third edition of CPT, allow coders to indicate that a service was altered in some way from the stated CPT description without actually changing the basic definition of the service. This 1973 addition to CPT provided an easy-to-use variable to coding.

The 1999 edition of CPT reflects significant changes in modifiers. Applicable modifiers are no longer listed in the Guidelines of each CPT section. They can be found in Appendix A and those related to the multiple procedures can be found in the Surgery Guidelines. Appendix A is now divided into two sections. Modifiers for physician services are listed first and titled simply *Modifiers. Modifiers Approved for Ambulatory Surgery Center (ASC) Hospital Outpatient Use* are

OBJECTIVES

Review the effect CPT modifiers have on reimbursement

Know the proper use of modifiers and the definitions of frequently used modifiers

Understand when to report an unlisted procedure

CPT modifiers indicate that a service was altered in some way from the stated CPT description without actually changing the basic definition of the service.

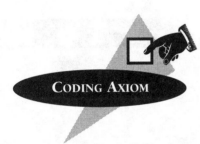

CODING AXIOM

Monitor reimbursements of all claims that include modifiers until you have determined a pattern of how their use affects payment. The effect of modifiers on reimbursement can be negotiated in contracts with payors.

Modifiers can indicate:
- A service or procedure represents only a professional component
- A service or procedure was performed by more than one physician
- Only part of a service was performed
- An adjunctive service was performed
- A bilateral procedure was performed
- A service or procedure was provided more than once
- Unusual events occurred
- A procedure or service was altered in some way

listed second and are divided into two subsections *CPT Level I Modifiers* and *Level II (HCPCS/National) Modifiers*.

Modifiers can be presented in one of two ways. They can be appended to a CPT code, as in 15000-22, or they can be listed separately, as in 15000 with 09922. To list separately, add 099 to the modifier number. For simplicity, *Code It Right* presents modifiers in the short form, as in -22.

MODIFIER IMPACT ON REIMBURSEMENT

Proper use of modifiers may have an impact on reimbursement. Modifiers can indicate the following:

- A service or procedure represents only a professional component
- A service or procedure was performed by more than one physician
- Only part of a service was performed
- An adjunctive service was performed
- A bilateral procedure was performed
- A service or procedure was provided more than once
- Unusual events occurred
- A procedure or service was altered in some way

It is important to remain current on the latest CPT guidelines regarding modifiers; and, it is equally important to become familiar with federal and commercial payors' guidelines. Monitor reimbursements of all claims that include modifiers until you have determined a pattern of how their use affects payment. The affect of modifiers upon reimbursement can be negotiated in contracts with payors.

Modifiers that usually affect reimbursement include the following:

-21	Prolonged Evaluation and Management Services
-22	Unusual Procedural Services
-26	Professional Component
-50	Bilateral Procedure
-51	Multiple Procedures
-52	Reduced Services
-53	Discontinued Procedure
-54	Surgical Care Only
-55	Postoperative Management Only
-62	Two Surgeons (formerly Cosurgery)
-66	Surgical Team
-80	Assistant Surgeon
-81	Minimum Assistant Surgeon
-82	Assistant Surgeon (when qualified resident surgeon not available)

May or May Not Affect Reimbursement — Modifiers that may or may not affect reimbursement, depending on the payor, include the following:

-23	Unusual Anesthesia
-47	Anesthesia by Surgeon
-56	Preoperative Management Only
-78	Return to the Operating Room for a Related Procedure During the Postoperative Period

Informational in Nature — The following modifiers are informational in nature and do not affect reimbursement. Since payors generally do not have specific guidelines for these modifiers, you must bill them consistently. It is a good idea to monitor the reimbursements received when using these modifiers.

-24	Unrelated Evaluation and Management Service by the Same Physician During a Postoperative Period
-25	Significant, Separately Identifiable Evaluation and Management Service by the Same Physician on the Day of a Procedure or Other Service
-32	Mandated Services
-57	Decision for Surgery
-58	Staged or Related Procedure or Service by the Same Physician During the Postoperative Period
-59	Distinct Procedural Service
-76	Repeat Procedure by Same Physician
-77	Repeat Procedure by Another Physician
-79	Unrelated Procedure or Service by the Same Physician During the Postoperative Period
-90	Reference (Outside) Laboratory
-99	Multiple Modifiers

MODIFIERS FOR PHYSICIAN SERVICES

-21 or 09921 Prolonged Evaluation and Management Services

Modifier -21 reports services that take more time or are greater than the highest level E/M code in a category.

- Modifier -21 may be reported only with CPT codes 99205, 99215, 99220, 99223, 99233, 99236, 99245, 99255, 99263, 99275, 99285, 99303, 99313, 99323, 99333, 99345, and 99350

- Modifier -21 is used to report physician face-to-face or floor/unit service(s); do not report with nonphysician service(s)

- Increased charge should be determined by the provider (Note: an additional value for this modifier has not been established)

Payors will determine a percentage increase based upon individual contracts, medical necessity, and documentation.

-22 or 09922 Unusual Services

Modifier -22 identifies unusual circumstances or medical complications requiring additional time, effort, or expense. This modifier supports increased reimbursement when justified by documentation establishing medical necessity. As a rule, payors allow 20 percent to 30 percent of the procedure allowance as additional reimbursement. The charge for the service should be determined by the physician.

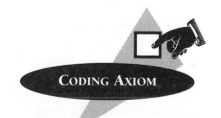

CODING AXIOM

Use modifier -22 when no other code can describe the complicated, unusual circumstances encountered, or when operative time is extended substantially.

Because modifier -22 is often used when complications are encountered during surgical procedures, medical necessity is substantiated by additional diagnostic codes that identify the complication. These diagnostic codes should reflect the operative condition and the complication(s) encountered during the surgery. The following example illustrates the use of modifier -22.

A 40-year-old morbidly obese male undergoes a cholecystectomy with cholangiography for a biliary calculus. Because of the patient's morbid obesity, the procedure is extremely difficult and requires unusual and prolonged dissection.

Modifier -22

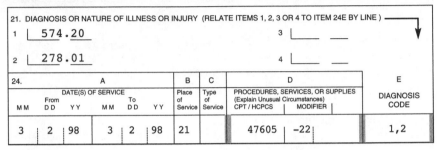

ICD-9-CM

574.20   Calculus of gallbladder without mention of cholecystitis or obstruction

278.01   Morbid obesity

CPT

47605-22   Cholecystectomy; with cholangiography — Unusual services

-23 or 09923 Unusual Anesthesia

Modifier -23 is neither appropriate with codes that state "without anesthesia" in the code description, nor with codes that report procedures or services usually performed under general anesthesia. Modifier -23 is appropriate with codes that report procedures or services usually performed without anesthesia or under local anesthesia.

-24 or 09924 Unrelated Evaluation and Management Service by the Same Physician During a Postoperative Period

Modifier -24 allows the physician to report a service performed during a postoperative period for reason(s) unrelated to the original procedure. Modifier -24 should be used only with E/M codes. Do not use this modifier with a CPT surgical code.

-25 or 09925 Significant, Separately Identifiable Evaluation and Management Service by the Same Physician on the Same Day of a Procedure or Other Service

Modifier -25 indicates that on a day a procedure or service identified by a CPT code was performed, the patient's condition required a significant, separately identifiable E/M service above and beyond the usual preoperative and postoperative care associated with the procedure that was performed. This modifier is not appropriate with an E/M code that has a minimum level of service. Assign the proper E/M code and amount as appropriate for the service rendered. Most payors will allow payment for significant E/M services on the day of a procedure. Documentation of unusual circumstances should be submitted with the claim.

-26 or 09926 Professional Component

Modifier -26 identifies the physician's component for procedures which have both a physician and a technical component. The physician component is reported separately when the physician provides only the supervision and interpretation portion of the procedure. The technical component includes reimbursement for the facility, equipment, film processing, and the technician. Typically, the reimbursement split for a two-component service is 60 percent technical and 40 percent professional; however, this split varies by payor and geographic location. See *Code It Right's* Radiology chapter for information regarding specific use of modifier -26 in radiology.

-32 or 09932 Mandated Services

Modifier -32 identifies services that are mandated by Medicare, a peer review organization, a private payor, or another local, state, or federal agency. Reimbursement may be made at 100 percent of the allowable amount for the service or procedure, such as confirmatory consultations and related diagnostic services. Deductibles or copayments may be waived by the payor. However, not all payors will reimburse for mandated services. They may determine the agency requesting the service is responsible for the payment.

-47 or 09947 Anesthesia by Surgeon

Modifier -47 identifies regional or general (not local) anesthesia administered by a surgeon. The charge for anesthesia is determined by the surgeon and is usually based on work increments instead of a percentage of the total charge for the surgical service. Reimbursement policies vary. Modifier -47 is used with surgical codes, never anesthesia codes. Generally, the procedure code is reported twice: first, without a modifier to report the surgical component; then second, with modifier -47 to report the anesthesia component. The following example illustrates the use of modifier -47.

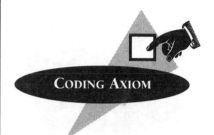

CODING AXIOM

Add modifier -47 to the base service when regional or general anesthesia is provided by the surgeon.

A 31-year-old carpenter sustains an injury to his left hand while working with a power saw at home. He severs a tendon to his index finger in "no man's land." The hand surgeon elects to do the surgery in his clinic's operating suite. The surgeon administers regional anesthesia then proceeds to debride all nonviable tissue. The surgeon repairs the tendon. A short-arm splint is applied.

ICD-9-CM Codes

883.2	Open wound of finger(s) with tendon involvement
E919.4	Accident caused by woodworking and forming machines
E849.0	Accident occurring at home

CPT Codes and Modifiers

26356	Repair or advancement, flexor tendon, in digital flexor tendon sheath (eg, no man's land); primary, each tendon
26356-47	Anesthesia administered by surgeon for flexor tendon repair

The CPT surgical package includes local and digital block anesthesia. Regional and general anesthesia provided by the surgeon may be separately reported by adding modifier -47 to the base service.

-50 or 09950 Bilateral Procedure

Modifier -50 identifies an identical procedure performed bilaterally during a single operative session, possibly through the same incision. To report bilateral procedures, list the appropriate code twice and append the modifier -50 to the second procedure code. Comparable HCPCS Level II (Medicare) modifiers are -LT and -RT.

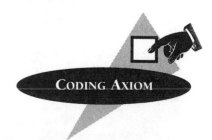

CODING AXIOM

Never use modifier -50 when a procedure code description specifically states that the procedure is bilateral, such as code 58700 *Salpingectomy, complete or partial, unilateral or bilateral (separate procedure).*

Medicare and some national payors are moving toward a single line entry to identify a bilateral procedure. Check with the payor to determine billing preference for this modifier.

Some payors allow 100 percent for each side if a separate incision is involved. Payors that do not allow 100 percent for the second side usually allow from 50 percent to 75 percent. Because of the varying allowances, monitor reimbursement to determine the percentage allowed for the second side. Bill all payors in full and let them apply reimbursement percentages. When billing Medicare, special rules apply. Establish policies for handling balances above third-party payor reimbursements and make patients aware of your policies. If you are contracted with a payor you usually can bill the patient the difference between the allowed charge and the amount paid by a payor, not the difference between the billed and the allowed.

The following case study illustrates how to bill using separate or single line entries for bilateral procedures.

A 55-year-old male undergoes a bilateral lumbar laminotomy with partial fasciotomy, foraminotomy, and excision of a herniated intervertebral disc for nerve root decompression due to displacement of an intervertebral disc.

KEY POINTS

The following guidelines make good billing and coding sense for modifier -51:

- List the procedure code with the highest value first when billing Medicare and commercial insurance payors.

- List additional procedures by descending value.

- Apply any modifiers as appropriate.

- Clearly differentiate in your operative reports procedures accomplished through separate incisions and procedures done through the same incision.

- Indicate if any portion of the procedure is planned for completion at a future operative session.

- Do not combine charges when coding multiple, unrelated procedures. List each procedure separately on the insurance claim form and indicate each charge.

- If a comprehensive procedure has a single CPT code, report that code rather than "unbundling" or listing the individual components or portions of the surgery.

Payor Requiring Separate Line Entries

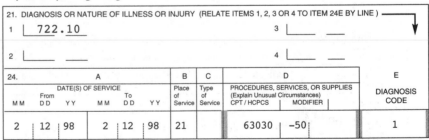

Payor Requiring Single Line Entries

ICD-9-CM

722.10 Lumbar intervertebral disc without myelopathy

CPT

63030-50 Laminectomy (hemilaminectomy), with decompression of nerve root(s), including partial facetectomy, foraminotomy and/or excision of herniated intervertebral disk; one interspace, lumbar — Bilateral procedure

-51 or 09951 Multiple Procedures

Modifier -51 designates multiple procedures that are rendered during the same operative session or on the same day. CPT states that modifier -51 should be used when a combination of surgical services, medical services, or surgical and medical services is provided. It is applicable when unrelated procedures are performed during the same operative session or when multiple related procedures are performed and there is no single inclusive code available. Do not append modifier -51 to those procedures designated as add-on (✚) or modifier -51 exempt (⊘). List the major procedure or service (most revenue intensive) first on the HCFA-1500 claim form, then attach modifier -51 to each applicable secondary procedure code. Most payors reimburse the primary procedure at 100 percent of the allowable and subsequent procedures at a reduced rate, usually 50 percent.

-52 or 09952 Reduced Services

Modifier -52 identifies when the physician elects to reduce or eliminate a portion of a service or procedure. Cover letters or operative reports are not necessary when modifier -52 is used since these claims are not usually sent to medical review. Cover letters and operative reports may impede claims processing. Physicians may find it helpful to provide the payor with an explanation of the reduced fee compared to the usual fee. The reduction in charge reflects the reduction or elimination of a portion of the usual service.

-53 or 09953 Discontinued Procedure

Modifier -53 indicates that the physician elected to terminate a surgical or diagnostic procedure. A surgical procedure may have been started, but because of extenuating or threatening circumstances discontinued. Modifier -53 is not used to report elective cancellation of a procedure prior to the anesthesia induction and/or surgical preparation in the operating suite.

The following example illustrates the use of modifier -53.

A patient with widely invasive anaplastic thyroid carcinoma undergoes an attempted surgical procedure. The surgical procedure is terminated due to an extensive, unresectable disseminated invasive tumor.

Discontinued Procedure

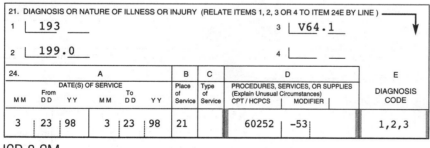

ICD-9-CM

193	Malignant neoplasm of thyroid gland
199.0	Disseminated malignant neoplasm
V64.1	Procedure not carried out because of contraindication

CPT

60252-53	Thyroidectomy, total or subtotal for malignancy; with limited neck dissection — Discontinued procedure

-54 or 09954 Surgical Care Only

Modifier -54 identifies when one physician performs a surgical procedure and another provides preoperative and/or postoperative management. The surgeon who performs the surgical procedure reports modifier -54. Both physicians need to determine percentages of the overall fee each will bill for their individual services (for example, 70 percent for the surgery and 30 percent for the postoperative care).

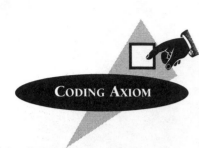

-55 or 09955 Postoperative Care Only

Modifier -55 identifies when one physician provides postoperative management after another physician has performed the surgical procedure. The physician providing postoperative management bills the surgical procedure code at the percentage agreed upon (see modifier -54) with modifier -55 attached.

-56 or 09956 Preoperative Management Only

Modifier -56 identifies a physician who is not performing the actual surgery though providing preoperative care during the preoperative time clause established by the payor. Use this modifier only with codes from the surgical and medicine sections.

-57 or 09957 Decision for Surgery

Modifier -57 identifies an evaluation and management service that results in the initial decision to perform surgery.

-58 or 09958 Staged or Related Procedure or Service by the Same Physician During the Postoperative Period

When reporting modifier -58, the physician may need to indicate that the procedure or service is: (a) planned prior to or at the time of the original procedure, or staged, (b) more extensive than the original planned procedure, or (c) for therapy following a diagnostic surgical procedure. Do not use this modifier to report the treatment of a problem that requires a return to the operating room (see modifier -78).

-59 or 09959 Distinct Procedural Service

Modifier -59 allows the physician to indicate that a procedure or service is distinct or independent from other services performed on the same day. Modifier -59 is appropriate for procedures or services that are not normally reported together, but are appropriate under the circumstances. CPT states that modifier -59 may represent a different session or patient encounter, different site or organ system, separate incision or excision, separate lesion, or separate injury (or area of injury in extensive injuries) not ordinarily encountered or performed on the same date by the same physician.

-62 or 09962 Two Surgeons

Modifier -62 indicates that the skills of two surgeons (sometimes with different skills) are required in the management of a single reportable surgical procedure. Each surgeon should report the cosurgery once using the same procedure code with modifier -62. Additional procedures performed during the same surgical session are reported based on the specific circumstances surrounding those procedures. If the two surgeons act as cosurgeons modifier -62 rules apply. If one or both surgeons perform additional separate services, each reports only those additional services provided. If one cosurgeon acts as an assistant for additional procedures, those services are reported with modifier -80 or -81.

The surgeons should agree on charges, procedure codes, and reimbursement percentage splits prior to submission. An additional percentage is usually allowed due to the more complex nature of procedures requiring two surgeons, and also since the surgeons usually provide assistant surgeon services in their capacity as cosurgeons. The additional percentage is usually 20 percent to 30 percent of that allowed. Because of the many variables, coordinate the physicians' billing, and submit complete and detailed documentation for each physician involved. Patient knowledge of the situation is essential; inform the patient of the cosurgery aspects and the billing issues.

Cosurgery usually includes one of the scenarios:

- Single-shared cosurgery
- Multiple-shared cosurgery
- Unrelated cosurgery

Modifier -62 is applied for the shared procedures, not the unrelated cosurgery. See the specialty coding scenarios at the end of the chapter for examples of single-shared cosurgery and unrelated cosurgery. The following is an example of single-shared cosurgery.

Single-Shared Cosurgery Scenario

A patient with an intraspinal lesion of the thoracic spine undergoes a complete vertebral corpectomy for excision of intradural malignancy of the spinal cord via a transthoracic approach. Two surgeons are required for this procedure. A thoracic surgeon performs the approach and closure while a neurosurgeon performs the corpectomy and excision of the intraspinal lesion.

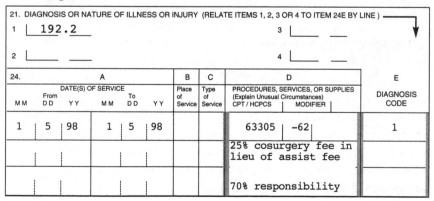

Thoracic surgeon

21. DIAGNOSIS OR NATURE OF ILLNESS OR INJURY (RELATE ITEMS 1, 2, 3 OR 4 TO ITEM 24E BY LINE)				
1	192.2		3	
2			4	

24.	A				B	C	D		E
	DATE(S) OF SERVICE				Place of Service	Type of Service	PROCEDURES, SERVICES, OR SUPPLIES (Explain Unusual Circumstances)		DIAGNOSIS CODE
MM	From DD	YY	To MM	DD YY			CPT / HCPCS	MODIFIER	
1	5	98	1	5 98			63305	-62	1
							25% cosurgery fee in lieu of assist fee		
							30% responsibility		

Neurosurgeon

21. DIAGNOSIS OR NATURE OF ILLNESS OR INJURY (RELATE ITEMS 1, 2, 3 OR 4 TO ITEM 24E BY LINE)				
1	192.2		3	
2			4	

24.	A				B	C	D		E
	DATE(S) OF SERVICE				Place of Service	Type of Service	PROCEDURES, SERVICES, OR SUPPLIES (Explain Unusual Circumstances)		DIAGNOSIS CODE
MM	From DD	YY	To MM	DD YY			CPT / HCPCS	MODIFIER	
1	5	98	1	5 98			63305	-62	1
							25% cosurgery fee in lieu of assist fee		
							70% responsibility		

ICD-9-CM

192.2 Malignant neoplasm spinal cord

CPT

63305-62 Vertebral corpectomy, (vertebral body resection), partial or complete, for excision of intraspinal lesion, single segment; intradural, thoracic by transthoracic approach — Two surgeons

Modifier -76 is easily misused, so note the following applications of other modifiers:

- A staged or related procedure or service by the same physician during the postoperative period is reported with modifier -58

- A return to the operating room for a related procedure during the postoperative period is reported with modifier -78

- An unrelated procedure or service by the same physician during the postoperative period is reported with modifier -79

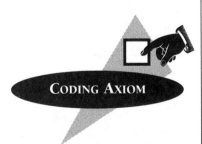

CODING AXIOM

Use modifier -77 to clarify that a procedure has been repeated by a different physician.

Use modifier -78 for related procedures performed in the operating room within the assigned postoperative period of a surgical procedure.

Use modifier -80 for assistant surgeon services.

-66 or 09966 Surgical Team

Modifier -66 identifies complex procedures that require the concomitant services of several physicians, often of different specialties, plus other highly skilled, specially trained personnel, and various types of complex equipment. Team surgery is usually confined to organ transplants and replantations. Identify these circumstances for team surgery by listing all procedures as though one physician performed all procedures and add modifier -66 to each procedure code used. The surgeons should agree on charges, procedure codes, and reimbursement splits prior to claims submission. Because of the many variables, coordinate the physicians' billings, and submit complete and detailed documentation. Also, include a cover letter explaining the reimbursement distribution for each member of the team. The total of charges for all procedures performed may be increased up to 50 percent for team surgery. The reimbursement is divided among the surgeons contingent upon actual fees, complexity of procedures, and medical review.

-76 or 09976 Repeat Procedure by Same Physician

Modifier -76 indicates that a basic procedure is repeated by the same physician subsequent to the original service. Use this modifier to identify the procedure as a repeat rather than a duplicate service or billing error. Payors may require additional documentation to establish medical necessity. The following is an example of a repeat procedure.

A lumbar puncture is attempted on a 3-year-old child with suspected meningitis. It fails. Later in the day, the child undergoes a repeat lumbar puncture that documents meningitis.

Repeat Procedure

21. DIAGNOSIS OR NATURE OF ILLNESS OR INJURY (RELATE ITEMS 1, 2, 3 OR 4 TO ITEM 24E BY LINE)			
1. 322.9		3.	
2.		4.	

24.	A						B	C	D		E
	DATE(S) OF SERVICE						Place of Service	Type of Service	PROCEDURES, SERVICES, OR SUPPLIES (Explain Unusual Circumstances)		DIAGNOSIS CODE
	From MM DD YY			To MM DD YY					CPT / HCPCS	MODIFIER	
	3	1	98	3	1	98	21		62270*	−53	1
	3	1	98	3	1	98	21		62270*	−76	1

ICD-9-CM

322.9 Meningitis, unspecified

CPT

62270*-53 Spinal puncture, lumbar, diagnostic — Discontinued procedure
62270*-76 Spinal puncture, lumbar, diagnostic — Repeat procedure by same physician

-77 or 09977 Repeat Procedure by Another Physician

Modifier -77 indicates that a basic procedure performed by one physician is repeated by a different physician. This modifier is usually used during the postoperative period of the basic procedure. The second physician adds the modifier to the procedure code used by the first physician. It is appropriate to use modifier -22 when the procedure is unusually complicated or modifier -52 when only a portion of the procedure is repeated. The ICD-9-CM diagnostic codes must substantiate the medical necessity of repeating the procedure. Because insurance payors often require additional documentation to establish medical necessity, it is advisable to submit the operative report with a cover letter.

-78 or 09978 Return to the Operating Room for a Related Procedure During the Postoperative Period

Modifier -78 reports related procedures performed in the operating room within the assigned postoperative period of a surgical procedure. CPT does not specify that the related procedure be performed by the initial physician.

-79 or 09979 Unrelated Procedure or Service by the Same Physician During the Postoperative Period

Modifier -79 notifies payors that the procedure was performed during the postoperative period of another procedure but is not related to that surgery. The diagnostic codes must document the medical necessity of the service, so the ICD-9-CM codes are usually different for the two procedures. Do not use modifier -79 to report staged or related procedures or services performed by the same physician during the assigned postoperative period of a procedure, see modifiers -58 and -78.

-80 or 09980 Assistant Surgeon

Modifier -80 identifies surgical assistant services when applied to the usual procedure code(s). Assisting physicians usually charge 16 percent to 30 percent of their full fee when providing assistant surgeon services. The assistant surgeon should use the same ICD-9-CM and CPT code(s) as the primary surgeon. The following case study illustrates billing for a primary surgeon and assistant.

A 53-year-old male underwent coronary artery bypass surgery of three coronary arteries using venous grafts for coronary atherosclerosis. The surgery required an assistant surgeon.

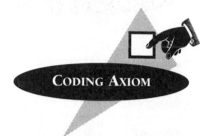

CODING AXIOM

The assistant surgeon should use the same ICD-9-CM and CPT code(s) as the primary surgeon.

Primary Surgeon

21. DIAGNOSIS OR NATURE OF ILLNESS OR INJURY (RELATE ITEMS 1, 2, 3 OR 4 TO ITEM 24E BY LINE)						
1. 414.01				3.		
2.				4.		

24.	A			B	C	D		E
	DATE(S) OF SERVICE			Place of Service	Type of Service	PROCEDURES, SERVICES, OR SUPPLIES (Explain Unusual Circumstances)		DIAGNOSIS CODE
	From MM DD YY	To MM DD YY				CPT / HCPCS	MODIFIER	
	4 19 98	4 19 98		21		33512		1

Assistant Surgeon

21. DIAGNOSIS OR NATURE OF ILLNESS OR INJURY (RELATE ITEMS 1, 2, 3 OR 4 TO ITEM 24E BY LINE)						
1. 414.01				3.		
2.				4.		

24.	A			B	C	D		E
	DATE(S) OF SERVICE			Place of Service	Type of Service	PROCEDURES, SERVICES, OR SUPPLIES (Explain Unusual Circumstances)		DIAGNOSIS CODE
	From MM DD YY	To MM DD YY				CPT / HCPCS	MODIFIER	
	4 19 98	4 19 98		21		33512	-80	1

ICD-9-CM

414.01 Atherosclerosis of native coronary artery

CPT

33512-80 Coronary artery bypass, vein only; three coronary venous grafts — Assistant surgeon

-81 or 09981 Minimum Assistant Surgeon

Modifier -81 identifies minimal surgical assistant services. Although CPT modifiers identify services performed by physicians, this modifier is sometimes used to report non-physician surgical assistants (e.g., PA, LPN, RN). Some payors will reimburse for the service, usually allowing half the amount allowed for physician assistant surgeons.

-82 or 09982 Assistant Surgeon (when qualified resident surgeon not available)

Modifier -82 identifies situations when a qualified resident is unavailable to assist in surgery and another physician must be brought in to assist.

-90 or 09990 Reference (Outside) Laboratory

Modifier -90 is used by the physician's office billing for the laboratory procedures performed by an outside laboratory. The modifier appended to laboratory codes tells the third-party payor that the outside laboratory will not be filing claims for these services. Rather, the reimbursement will be forwarded to the outside laboratory by the physician's office. Do not report this modifier on Medicare claims. The performing laboratory should bill Medicare directly.

-99 or 09999 Multiple Modifiers

Modifier -99 identifies circumstances when two or more modifiers are necessary to delineate a service. Attach -99 to the procedure code and list all appropriate modifiers as subsequent line items.

Only the two-digit modifier appended to the procedure code will be accepted by Medicare. When multiple modifiers apply, each applicable modifier is appended to the code in a single line entry. Approved Medicare modifiers include selected CPT and HCPCS Level II modifiers. Definitions and instructions specific to hospital reporting have been developed and these may differ from those related to reporting of physician services.

MODIFIERS APPROVED FOR AMBULATORY SURGERY CENTERS (ASC) HOSPITAL OUTPATIENT USE

An addition to Appendix A in 1999 CPT is the list of Modifiers Approved for Ambulatory Surgery Centers (ASC) Hospital Outpatient Use. Modifiers were required on Medicare Ambulatory Surgery Center (ASC)/Hospital Outpatient claims beginning July 1, 1998. HCFA requires this information in order to fully develop hospital outpatient prospective payment systems. Check with fiscal intermediaries for any additional local guidelines regarding modifier use.

CPT Level I Modifiers

-50 Bilateral Procedure. Modifier -50 should be used to report bilateral procedures performed during the same surgical session. Medicare requires that bilateral procedures be reported as a single line entry. Report the appropriate five digit CPT code and append modifier -50 to designate that the same procedure was performed bilaterally. Procedures which are identified as bilateral in the code description and those which are identified as either unilateral or bilateral should not be reported with modifier -50.

-52 Reduced Services. Use modifier -52 to report services or procedures that were partially reduced or eliminated at the physician's discretion. Report the five digit CPT code identifying the intended service or procedure and append modifier -52 to indicate that the service was reduced.

2 CPT Introduction & Modifiers

For procedures or services which are partially reduced or cancelled as a result of extenuating circumstances or circumstances which threaten the well-being of the patient prior to or after the administration of anesthesia, see modifiers -73 and -74.

-59 Distinct Procedural Service. Use modifier -59 to indicate that a service or procedure was distinct or separate from other services provided on the same day. It should be used to designate a separate session or patient encounter, a different surgery or procedure, a different site or organ system, a separate incision/excision, a separate lesion, a separate injury or a separate area of injury in extensive injuries. Modifier -59 should be used only if a more descriptive modifier is not available or when it best describes the special circumstances.

-73 Discontinued Outpatient Hospital/Ambulatory Surgery Center (ASC) Procedure Prior to Administration of Anesthesia. Due to extenuating circumstances or those which threaten the well-being of the patient, the physician may cancel a diagnostic or therapeutic service or procedure prior to the administration of anesthesia. When cancellation of the procedure occurs subsequent to the patient's surgical preparation (including sedation and transfer to the room where the procedure is to be performed) but prior to the administration of anesthesia (local, regional, or general) append modifier -73 to the CPT code which would have been reported had the procedure been performed as planned. Modifier -73 applies only to facility reporting and should not be used by the physician. Physician reporting of a discontinued procedure should be reported with modifier -53. The cancellation of a procedure prior to the patient's preparation for surgery and prior to occupation of the surgical/special procedure room should not be reported.

-74 Discontinued Out-Patient Hospital/Ambulatory Surgery Center (ASC) Procedure After Administration of Anesthesia. Due to extenuating circumstances or those which threaten the well-being of the patient, the physician may cancel a diagnostic or therapeutic service or procedure subsequent to the administration of anesthesia. When cancellation occurs after the administration of anesthesia (local, regional, general) or after the procedure was started (incision made, intubation started, scope inserted, etc), append modifier -74 to the CPT code which would have been reported had the procedure been performed as planned. Modifier -74 applies only to facility reporting and should not be used by the physician. Physician reporting of a discontinued procedure should be reported with modifier -53.

-76 Repeat Procedure by the Same Physician. When a service or procedure is repeated by the same physician report the procedure twice and append modifier -76 to the second line item. Do not use the units field to report procedures performed more than once on the same day. Report a separate line item each time the procedure is repeated.

-77 Repeat Procedure by Another Physician. When a service or procedure is repeated by another physician report the applicable CPT code and append modifier -77.

Level II HCPCS/National Modifiers

-LT	Left side (Used to identify procedures performed on the left side of the body. Do not report -LT with bilateral procedures, use modifier -50 instead.)
-RT	Right side (Used to identify procedures performed on the right side of the body. Do not report -RT with bilateral procedures, use modifier -50 instead.)
-E1	Upper left, eyelid
-E2	Lower left, eyelid
-E3	Upper right, eyelid
-E4	Lower right, eyelid

-FA	Left hand, thumb
-F1	Left hand, second digit
-F2	Left hand, third digit
-F3	Left hand, fourth digit
-F4	Left hand, fifth digit
-F5	Right hand, thumb
-F6	Right hand, second digit
-F7	Right hand, third digit
-F8	Right hand, fourth digit
-F9	Right hand, fifth digit
-LC	Left circumflex coronary artery (Hospitals use with codes 92980-92984, 92995-92996)
-LD	Left anterior descending coronary artery (Hospitals use with codes 92980-92984, 92995-92996)
-RC	Right coronary artery (Hospitals use with codes 92980-92984, 92995-92996)
-QM	Ambulance service provided under arrangement by a provider of services
-QR	Repeat laboratory test performed on the same day
-QN	Ambulance service furnished directly by a provider of services
-TA	Left foot, great toe
-T1	Left foot, second digit
-T2	Left foot, third digit
-T3	Left foot, fourth digit
-T4	Left foot, fifth digit
-T5	Right foot, great toe
-T6	Right foot, second digit
-T7	Right foot, third digit
-T8	Right foot, fourth digit
-T9	Right foot, fifth digit

Unlisted Procedures

Each section of CPT — evaluation and management, anesthesiology, surgery, radiology, pathology and laboratory, and medicine — contains unlisted procedure codes. Use these codes when the procedure or service is not adequately described by an existing CPT code. Select the unlisted procedure code from the appropriate section. For example, a procedure on the elbow that cannot be reported with an existing CPT code or combination of codes would be reported with 24999 *Unlisted procedure, humerus or elbow.* If an existing CPT description closely describes the procedure performed, report that code with modifier -22 *Unusual services* or -52 *Reduced services.*

Unlisted codes are billed by report and extensive documentation is required for proper reimbursement. Insurance claims with unlisted codes take longer to process since they are usually sent for medical review individual consideration. Include cover notes and comprehensive operative reports with the claims submission.

Add-On and Modifier -51 Exempt Codes

In the 1999 edition of CPT two major changes occurred related to codes previously referred to as "in-addition-to" or subsidiary codes. Icons were added to specifically identify two types of services for which special coding rules apply.

Add-on procedures are identified with a **+** prior to the five-digit procedure code. This + identifies services which are always performed with another service or procedure. In other words, add-on procedures are always secondary procedures and should never be reported alone. However, unlike other secondary procedures, add-on procedures are never appended with modifier -51. In addition to adding the icon, CPT has standardized the terminology related to add-on procedures. All add-on procedures include the parenthetical statement (list separately in addition to code for primary procedure) as part of the procedure description.

Modifier -51 exempt procedures are similar to add-on procedures and are designated with a $\oslash$. Modifier -51 exempt procedures may be reported alone, but are usually components of a larger service. Modifier -51 exempt procedures include secondary services that are not directly related to the primary procedure.

For example, codes 36488-36491 report placement of central venous catheters. These services may be performed alone or they may be part of a larger service. When performed as part of a larger service such as the repair of a gastroschisis in a newborn (49605), central venous catheter placement involves a secondary service that is not directly related to the primary procedure.

DISCUSSION QUESTIONS

1. What is the purpose of modifiers?

    _____

    _____

    _____

2. List modifiers identifying multiple procedures and explain the differences.

    _____

    _____

    _____

3. Why does HCFA require the use of Ambulatory Surgery Center (ASC) codes?

    _____

    _____

    _____

4. What should you include in documentation for unlisted procedure codes in CPT?

    _____

    _____

    _____

5. When is it appropriate to report an unlisted procedure?

    _____

    _____

    _____

6. Explain how add-on codes are reported.

_____

_____

_____

7. How do add-on and modifier -51 exempt codes differ?

_____

_____

_____

8. No matter the coding system, how do you begin the actual coding process?

_____

_____

_____

OBJECTIVES

See the practical application of modifiers

Identify the special circumstances and rules of specialties

Specialty-Specific Scenarios

The following scenarios will help you make the leap from documentation to correct coding.

SINGLE-SHARED COSURGERY

General Surgery and Orthopedic Specialty Scenario

A general surgeon exposes a thoracic vertebral segment in which a staphylococcus aureus infection has invaded the bone. The orthopedic surgeon debrides and irrigates the bone and the general surgeon closes the incision.

General Surgeon (provides exposure and closure)

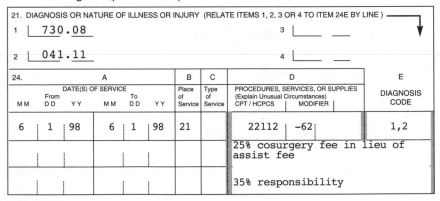

ICD-9-CM

730.08   Acute osteomyelitis, other specified sites
041.11   Staphylococcus aureus in conditions classified elsewhere and of unspecified site

CPT

22112-62   Partial excision of vertebral body, for intrinsic bony lesion, without decompression of spinal cord or nerve root(s), single vertebral segment; thoracic — Cosurgery

Orthopedist (provides debridement and irrigation)

21. DIAGNOSIS OR NATURE OF ILLNESS OR INJURY (RELATE ITEMS 1, 2, 3 OR 4 TO ITEM 24E BY LINE)
1 | 730.08   3 |___ ___
2 | 041.11   4 |___ ___

24.	A					B	C	D		E
	DATE(S) OF SERVICE					Place of Service	Type of Service	PROCEDURES, SERVICES, OR SUPPLIES (Explain Unusual Circumstances)		DIAGNOSIS CODE
	From			To				CPT / HCPCS	MODIFIER	
MM	DD	YY	MM	DD	YY					
6	1	98	6	1	98	21		22112	-62	1,2
								25% cosurgery fee in lieu of assist fee		
								65% responsibility		

ICD-9-CM

730.08   Acute osteomyelitis, other specified site

041.11   Staphylococcus aureus in conditions classified elsewhere and of unspecified site

CPT

22112-62   Partial excision of vertebral body, for intrinsic bony lesion, without decompression of spinal cord or nerve root(s), single vertebral segment; thoracic — Cosurgery

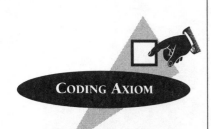

When performing unrelated cosurgeries on the same patient during the same operative session, each physician should report his or her service only without applying the cosurgery modifier.

OB/GYN SCENARIO—UNRELATED COSURGERY

While her gynecologist performed an abdominal hysterectomy and salpingo-oophorectomy for submucous leiomyoma of the uterus and severe polycystic disease of the ovaries, the patient also had an arthroplasty performed on her TMJ to remove bony ankylosis.

Gynecologist

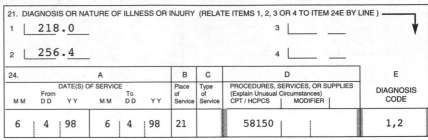

ICD-9-CM

218.0	Submucous leiomyoma of uterus
256.4	Polycystic ovaries

CPT

58150	Total abdominal hysterectomy (corpus and cervix), with or without removal of tube(s), with or without removal of ovary(s);

Otolaryngologist

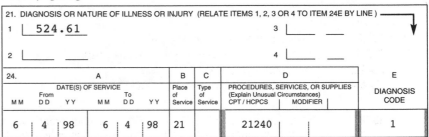

ICD-9-CM

524.61	Adhesions and ankylosis (bony or fibrous) of temporomandibular joint

CPT

21240	Arthroplasty, temporomandibular joint, with or without autograft (includes obtaining graft)

When unrelated cosurgeries are performed, each physician reports his or her service only and the cosurgery modifier is not applied.

PLASTIC SURGERY SCENARIO

A 35-year-old male was burned one year ago at work in a copper mine propane tank explosion. The man returns to surgery for severe fibrosis and scarring of the skin of the face. The preparation of the recipient site is very difficult and more time-consuming (one hour longer) than usual because of the location and severity of the scarring around the patient's mouth. A 10 cm excision of the scar tissue and a split thickness graft from the lower left abdomen are used to repair his face.

Plastic Surgery

21. DIAGNOSIS OR NATURE OF ILLNESS OR INJURY (RELATE ITEMS 1, 2, 3 OR 4 TO ITEM 24E BY LINE)		
1. 709.2	3. E923.2	
2. 906.5	4. E849.2	

24.	A DATE(S) OF SERVICE						B Place of Service	C Type of Service	D PROCEDURES, SERVICES, OR SUPPLIES (Explain Unusual Circumstances)		E DIAGNOSIS CODE
	From MM	DD	YY	To MM	DD	YY			CPT / HCPCS	MODIFIER	
	1	10	98	1	10	98	24		15120		1,2,3,4
	1	10	98	1	10	98	24		15000	-99	1,2,3,4
	1	10	98	1	10	98	24		09951		1,2,3,4
	1	10	98	1	10	98	24		09922		1,2,3,4

ICD-9-CM

709.2	Scar conditions and fibrosis of skin
906.5	Late effect of burn of eye, face, head, and neck
E923.2	Accident caused by explosive gases
E849.2	Place of occurrence, mine and quarry

CPT

15120	Split graft, face, scalp, eyelids, mouth, neck, ears, orbits, genitalia, hands, feet and/or multiple digits; first 100 sq cm or less, or one percent of body area of infants and children (except 15050)
15000-99	Surgical preparation or creation of recipient site by excision of open wounds, burn eschar, or scar (including subcutaneous tissues); first 100 sq cm or one percent of body area of infants and children — Multiple modifiers
09951	Multiple procedures
09922	Unusual procedural service

Multiple modifiers are required to describe this service and may be reported a number of ways. Modifier -51 should be assigned for multiple procedures. Modifier -22 is also appropriate because the surgeon specified that the surgery was difficult and took one hour longer than usual. One method of reporting would be to append the two-digit modifiers to the procedure, -99, -51, -22. However, since space is limited, the alternate method would be to append the two-digit modifier -99 to the procedure, and list the five digit modifiers 09951 and 09922 on separate lines.

CARDIOLOGY SCENARIO

This illustrates reporting of multiple procedures.

A 60-year-old heavy smoker with occlusive atherosclerosis of the abdominal aorta and the popliteal artery undergoes excision and direct repair of these areas.

Multiple Procedures

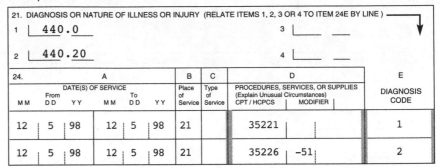

ICD-9-CM

440.0	Atherosclerosis of aorta
440.20	Atherosclerosis of native arteries of the extremities, unspecified

CPT

35221	Repair blood vessel, direct; intra-abdominal
35226-51	Repair blood vessel, direct; lower extremity — Multiple procedure

OPHTHALMOLOGY SCENARIO

The following case study illustrates coding for a surgeon and managing physician combination.

A 60-year-old female with type I diabetes and diabetic cataracts travels to a large city to have cataract surgery and returns to her rural community physician for follow-up treatment.

Cataract Surgeon

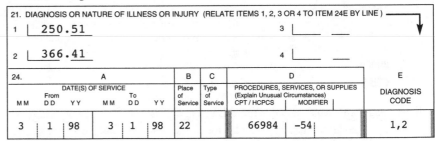

ICD-9-CM

250.51	Type I [insulin dependent type] [IDDM] [juvenile type] diabetes mellitus with ophthalmic manifestations, not stated as uncontrolled
366.41	Diabetic cataract

CPT

66984-54	Extracapsular cataract removal with insertion of intraocular lens prosthesis (one stage procedure), manual or mechanical technique (eg, irrigation and aspiration or phacoemulsification) — Surgical care only

General Ophthalmologist

21. DIAGNOSIS OR NATURE OF ILLNESS OR INJURY (RELATE ITEMS 1, 2, 3 OR 4 TO ITEM 24E BY LINE)		
1 | 250.51	3 |___ ___	
2 | 366.41	4 |___ ___	

24.	A					B	C	D		E
	DATE(S) OF SERVICE					Place of Service	Type of Service	PROCEDURES, SERVICES, OR SUPPLIES (Explain Unusual Circumstances)		DIAGNOSIS CODE
	From			To				CPT / HCPCS	MODIFIER	
MM	DD	YY	MM	DD	YY					
3	1	98	3	1	98	11		66984	-55	1,2
								Postoperative care rendered from 3/4/97 — 6/1/97		

ICD-9-CM

250.51 Type I [insulin dependent type] [IDDM] [juvenile type] diabetes mellitus with ophthalmic manifestations, not stated as uncontrolled

366.41 Diabetic cataract

CPT

66984-55 Extracapsular cataract removal with insertion of intraocular lens prosthesis (one stage procedure), manual or mechanical technique (eg, irrigation and aspiration or phacoemulsification) — Postoperative management only

PATHOLOGY SCENARIO

The police department uses a local hospital laboratory to perform a blood alcohol level on anyone who is suspected of drunk driving. A mandated blood alcohol test is performed by the laboratory.

Pathology

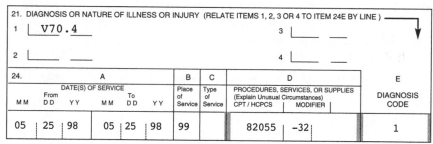

21. DIAGNOSIS OR NATURE OF ILLNESS OR INJURY (RELATE ITEMS 1, 2, 3 OR 4 TO ITEM 24E BY LINE)		
1 | V70.4	3 |___ ___	
2 |___ ___	4 |___ ___	

24.	A					B	C	D		E
	DATE(S) OF SERVICE					Place of Service	Type of Service	PROCEDURES, SERVICES, OR SUPPLIES (Explain Unusual Circumstances)		DIAGNOSIS CODE
	From			To				CPT / HCPCS	MODIFIER	
MM	DD	YY	MM	DD	YY					
05	25	98	05	25	98	99		82055	-32	1

ICD-9-CM

V70.4 Examination for medicolegal reasons

CPT

82055-32 Alcohol (ethanol); any specimen except breath — Mandated service

RADIOLOGY SCENARIO

A radiologist reads an outpatient two-view chest x-ray film on a patient who presents with diagnoses of cough and r/o pneumonia. No evidence of pneumonia is identified on the films.

Radiology

21. DIAGNOSIS OR NATURE OF ILLNESS OR INJURY (RELATE ITEMS 1, 2, 3 OR 4 TO ITEM 24E BY LINE)						
1	786.2		3			
2			4			

24.	A				B	C	D		E
	DATE(S) OF SERVICE				Place of Service	Type of Service	PROCEDURES, SERVICES, OR SUPPLIES (Explain Unusual Circumstances)		DIAGNOSIS CODE
	From		To				CPT / HCPCS	MODIFIER	
	M M	DD YY	M M	DD YY					
	09	12 98	09	12 98	22		71020	-26	

ICD-9-CM

786.2 Cough

CPT

71020-26 Radiologic examination, chest, two views, frontal and lateral; — Professional component

Advanced Coding Practice

CODING PRACTICE 1

A 70-year-old female Medicare patient trips on stairs at her apartment complex, falls forward, and fractures both wrists (distal radius). Closed reduction with manipulation is performed on both wrists. Three-view preoperative and postoperative x-rays are obtained of both wrists. The procedure is performed on an outpatient basis in same-day surgery. Code the procedure with modifiers approved for hospital outpatient services.

21. DIAGNOSIS OR NATURE OF ILLNESS OR INJURY (RELATE ITEMS 1, 2, 3 OR 4 TO ITEM 24E BY LINE)						
1			3			
2			4			

24.	A				B	C	D		E
	DATE(S) OF SERVICE				Place of Service	Type of Service	PROCEDURES, SERVICES, OR SUPPLIES (Explain Unusual Circumstances)		DIAGNOSIS CODE
	From		To				CPT / HCPCS	MODIFIER	
	M M	DD YY	M M	DD YY					

CODING PRACTICE 2

A 51-year-old presents with several skin lesions requiring treatment. Six skin tags are removed by scissor. In addition, two lesions suspected to be basal cell carcinoma, one on the left temple and the other on the left ear, are biopsied. Code the procedures with appropriate modifiers.

21. DIAGNOSIS OR NATURE OF ILLNESS OR INJURY (RELATE ITEMS 1, 2, 3 OR 4 TO ITEM 24E BY LINE)					
1	_____ ___		3	_____ ___	
2	_____ ___		4	_____ ___	

24.	A				B	C	D		E
	DATE(S) OF SERVICE				Place of Service	Type of Service	PROCEDURES, SERVICES, OR SUPPLIES (Explain Unusual Circumstances)		DIAGNOSIS CODE
	From		To				CPT / HCPCS	MODIFIER	
	MM DD YY		MM DD YY						

Chapter Review

A CPT code is a descriptor of a procedure with a five-digit identifying code number. CPT codes are developed and maintained by the AMA. Keep up with the dynamic nature of medicine by reviewing the AMA's CPT on an annual basis. Compare the new edition to the previous one to identify how the code descriptions have been revised. As with ICD-9, the CPT coding process begins with a careful examination of the medical record to determine primary and secondary procedures as well as any modifying or extenuating circumstances. The alphabetical CPT index is the starting point of all CPT coding, but do not select codes solely on the basis of information in the index — it is only a reference to the full listing of codes. CPT modifiers allow you to indicate that a service was altered in some way from the stated CPT description without actually changing the basic definition of the service. The list of modifiers was expanded in the 1999 edition and now includes Modifiers Approved for ASC Hospital Outpatient Use. Use unlisted procedure codes when the overall procedure and outcome of the surgery is not adequately described by an existing CPT code. New features in 1999 CPT include icons which identify add-on procedures and modifier -51 exempt procedures.

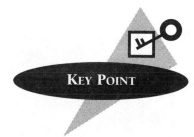

KEY POINT

Keep up with the dynamic nature of medicine by reviewing the updated CPT on an annual basis. CPT coding requires a careful examination of the medical record to determine primary and secondary procedures as well as any modifying or extenuating circumstances.

3 Evaluation & Management

EVALUATION AND MANAGEMENT CODE PLACEMENT

Evaluation and management (E/M) codes encompass services that are part of the 99000 series of CPT codes. Because the codes represent services (e.g., office, emergency department, inpatient visits) that are the most frequently performed by physicians, the codes have been placed, for convenience, at the beginning of the book.

Understanding how to report E/M services correctly is very important. Although E/M codes are not the most revenue intensive code set, they account for significant revenues to a practice because of their frequency.

E/M Service Guidelines

Guidelines for E/M services are presented in the same arrangement as in other sections of CPT. They are found at the beginning of the section and continue through some of the categories and subcategories. The guidelines are directions on how the codes within the section should be used and interpreted.

Evaluation and Management Category and Subcategory of Service

Evaluation and management services are arranged first in categories and then in subcategories, as follows:

Office or Other Outpatient Services
    New Patient
    Established Patient
Hospital Observation Services
    Observation Care Discharge Services
    Initial Observation Care
Hospital Inpatient Services
    Initial Hospital Care
    Subsequent Hospital Care
Hospital Observation or Inpatient Care Services (including admission and discharge services)
    Hospital Discharge Services
Consultations
    Office or Other Outpatient Consultations
    Initial Inpatient Consultations
    Follow-up Inpatient Consultations
    Confirmatory Consultations
Emergency Department Services
Critical Care Services
Neonatal Intensive Care

OBJECTIVES

Recognize the difference between a new and an established patient

Understand the key terms related to evaluation and management codes

Understand the three key components of E/M Service

Know the role contributing components play in E/M Service

Note that the E/M code section is divided into subsections by type and place of service

Determine a method of documentation for your office

KEY POINT

Guidelines provide information:

- Unique to the section
- Unique to a category
- Unique to a subcategory
- Unique to a specific code and/or codes

DEFINITIONS

A **new patient** is one who has not received any professional services from the physician, or another physician of the same specialty who belongs to the same group practice, within the past three years.

An **established patient** is one who has received professional services from the physician, or another physician of the same specialty who belongs to the same group practice, within the past three years.

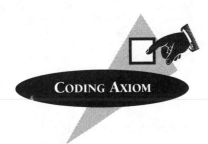

CODING AXIOM

E/M MODIFIERS

-21 Prolonged Evaluation and Management Services

-24 Unrelated Evaluation and Management Service by the Same Physician During a Postoperative Period

-25 Significant Separately Identifiable E/M Services by the Same Physician on the Same Day of a Procedure or Other Service

-32 Mandated Services

-52 Reduced Services

-57 Decision for Surgery

Nursing Facility Services
  Comprehensive Nursing Facility Assessments
  Subsequent Nursing Facility Care
  Nursing Facility Discharge Services
Domiciliary, Rest Home or Custodial Care Services
  New Patient
  Established Patient
Home Services
  New Patient
  Established Patient
Prolonged Services
  With Direct Patient Contact
  Without Direct Patient Contact
  Standby Services
Case Management Services
  Team Conferences
  Telephone Calls
Care Plan Oversight Services
Preventive Medicine Services
  New Patient
  Established Patient
  Individual Counseling
  Group Counseling
  Other
Newborn Care
Special E/M Services
Other E/M Services

Evaluation and Management Service Levels
E/M services within subcategories are arranged in levels, each with the same basic format:

- A unique code
- Place and/or type of service
- What is included in the service (content)
- The signs and symptoms (nature) of the presenting problem
- Time

NEW AND ESTABLISHED PATIENT SERVICE

Several code subcategories in the E/M section are based on the patient's status as being either new or established. CPT guidelines clarify this distinction by providing the following time references:

A new patient is one who has not received any professional services from the physician, or another physician of the same specialty who belongs to the same group practice, within the past three years.

An established patient is one who has received professional services from the physician, or another physician of the same specialty who belongs to the same group practice, within the past three years.

The new versus established patient guidelines also clarify situations that occur when one physician is on call or covering for another physician. In this instance, you are instructed to classify the patient encounter the same as if it were for the physician who is unavailable.

E/M SERVICE COMPONENTS

The components of history, examination, and medical decision making are keys to selecting the correct E/M codes. In most cases, all three components must be addressed in the documentation. However, in established, subsequent, and follow-up categories, only two of the three must be met or exceeded for a given code. Additional components — counseling, coordination of care, presenting problem, and time — will also be addressed in this chapter.

History — First Key Component

The history has four distinct elements consisting of the chief complaint; history of present illness; past, family, and/or social history; and a review of systems. Each of the elements are defined as follows:

- **Chief complaint (CC).** The patient's description of the problem, symptom, condition, diagnosis, or other factor that prompted the encounter.

- **History of present illness (HPI).** A chronological description of the patient's present illness from the first sign or symptom to the present or from the previous encounter to the present. It includes: location, quality, severity, duration, timing, context, modifying factors, associated signs/symptoms.

- **Review of systems (ROS).** An inventory of body systems obtained through a series of questions aimed at identifying additional signs/symptoms the patient may be experiencing. It includes: constitutional symptoms (fever, weight, loss, etc.); eyes/ears/nose/mouth, throat; cardiovascular; respiratory; gastrointestinal; genitourinary; musculoskeletal, integumentary (skin, breast); neurological; psychiatric; endocrine; hematologic/lymphatic; allergic/immunologic.

- **Past, family, and/or social history (PFSH).** Past history includes: prior major illnesses/injuries, prior operations, prior hospitalizations, current medications, allergies, immunization status, feeding/dietary status. Family history consists of a review of medical events in the family, including diseases which may be hereditary or place the patient at risk. Social history includes: marital status/living arrangements, current employment, occupational history, use of drugs/alcohol/tobacco, education, sexual history.

The history component in E/M is categorized by four levels:

Problem Focused — chief complaint; brief history of present illness or problem

Expanded Problem Focused — chief complaint; brief history of present illness; problem-pertinent system review

Detailed — chief complaint; extended history of present illness; problem-pertinent system review (with limited additional systems); pertinent past, family, and/or social history directly related to the patient's problems

Comprehensive — chief complaint; extended history of present illness; review of systems related to present illness/problems (with review of all additional body systems); complete past, family, and social history

DEFINITION

The **key components** in determining the correct level of E/M codes are: history, examination, and medical decision making.

A **presenting problem** is a disease, condition, illness, injury, symptom, sign, finding, complaint, or other reason for the patient encounter.

Chief Complaint (CC) is the patient's description of the problem, symptom condition, diagnosis, or other factor that prompted the encounter.

History of Present Illness (HPI) is a chronological description of the patient's present illness from the first sign or symptom to the present, or from the previous encounter to the present. It includes the following elements:

- location
- quality
- severity
- duration
- timing
- context
- modifying factors
- associated signs/symptoms

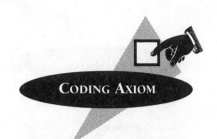

CODING AXIOM

Three subcomponents must be evaluated to determine the overall complexity level of the medical decision for E/M code selection. They are:

- Number of possible diagnoses and or management options.

- Amount and/or complexity of medical records, diagnostic tests, and/or other information that must be obtained, reviewed, and analyzed.

- Risk of significant complications, morbidity and/or mortality, and comorbidities, associated with the patient's presenting problem(s), diagnostic procedure(s) and/or possible management options.

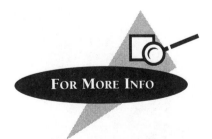

FOR MORE INFO

Documentation guidelines for Evaluation and Management (E/M) services are available from the AMA (by mail or the AMA website).

Physical Exam — Second Key Component

The physical examination is the process of investigating or inspecting any symptomatic or involved body areas and/or organ systems using a variety of methods and techniques for the purpose of diagnosing the complaint, sign, symptom, condition.

The physical exam component is similarly divided into four levels of complexity:

Problem Focused — a limited exam of the affected body area or organ system

Expanded Problem Focused — a limited examination of the affected body area or organ system and of other symptomatic or related organ systems

Detailed — an extended examination of the affected body area(s) and other symptomatic or related organ system(s)

Comprehensive — a complete single organ system specialty examination or a general multi-system examination

To correctly identify the number of body areas or organ systems for the second key component (physical examination), it is necessary to understand how the areas and systems have been defined in CPT.

Body areas:
- Head, including the face
- Neck
- Chest, including breasts and axilla
- Each extremity
- Genitalia, groin, buttocks
- Back
- Abdomen

Organ systems:
- Eyes
- Ears, nose, mouth and throat
- Cardiovascular
- Respiratory
- Gastrointestinal
- Hematologic/lymphatic/immunologic
- Genitourinary
- Musculoskeletal
- Skin
- Neurologic
- Psychiatric

Medical Decision Making — Third Key Component

Medical decision making is the third key component and refers to the complexity of establishing a diagnosis and/or selecting a management option. This component is more complicated to determine than are the history and exam components.

CPT lists four types of medical decision making: straightforward, low complexity, moderate complexity, and high complexity. Any level of medical decision making requires that two of three elements are met or exceeded. *Straightforward* decision making entails minimal risk of complications, and/or morbidity, or mortality; minimal complexity or no data; and a minimal number of diagnoses or management options. *Low complexity* entails low risk, limited complexity of the reviewed data, and a limited number of diagnoses. *Moderate complexity* entails moderate risk, moderate complexity of the reviewed data, and multiple diagnoses. *High complexity* entails high risk, extensive complexity of the reviewed data, and an extensive number of diagnoses.

Later in this chapter is a guide to selecting E/M codes. The key components are discussed there, particularly as they relate to the graphs that were developed to facilitate code selection.

Contributory Components

Counseling, coordination of care, and the nature of the presenting problem are not major considerations in most encounters, so they generally provide contributory information to the code selection process. The exception arises when counseling or coordination of care dominates the encounter (more than 50 percent of the time spent). In these cases, time determines the proper code. Documentation of the exact amount of time spent will substantiate your selected code. For office encounters, count only the time spent face-to-face with the patient and/or family; for hospital or other inpatient encounters, count the time spent in the patient's unit or on the patient's floor, but be sure the time spent and counted is directed at caring only for one patient. The time assigned by CPT to each code is an average and varies by physician.

Along with the time, the medical record should indicate what was discussed during the encounter. If a physician coordinates care with an interdisciplinary team of physicians or health professionals/agencies without a patient encounter, report it as a case management service.

CPT defines five types of presenting problems: minimal, self-limited or minor, low severity, moderate severity, and high severity. You should review the definitions of a presenting problem, but remember this information merely contributes to code selection — the presenting problem is not a key factor.

GUIDELINES

The AMA and HCFA developed documentation guidelines for E/M services. These guidelines supplement the information already found in CPT and are summarized here. The Guidelines developed by the AMA and HCFA have undergone substantial revision since their initial publication and are in the process of being revised again. Physicians may use either the 1995 or the 1997 Guidelines for Medicare purposes.

History Component Guidelines

- The chief complaint, review of systems, and the past, family, and/or social history may be included as separate elements of the history. Or, this information may be included in the description of the history of the present illness.

- A review of systems and/or a past, family, and/or social history obtained during an earlier encounter does not need to be re-recorded if there is evidence that the physician reviewed and updated the previous information. This may occur when a physician updates his or her own record, or in an institutional setting or group practice where many physicians use a common record. The review and update may be documented by describing any new review of systems and/or past, family, and/or social history information or noting there has been no change in the information and indicating the date and location of the earlier review of systems and/or past, family, and/or social history.

DEFINITIONS

Counseling is defined in CPT as a discussion with a patient and/or family concerning one or more of the following areas:

- Diagnostic results, impressions, and/or recommended diagnostic studies

- Prognosis

- Risks and benefits of management (treatment) options

- Instructions for management (treatment) and/or follow-up

- Importance of compliance with chosen management (treatment) options

- Risk factor reduction

- Patient and family education

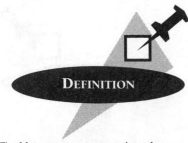

The **history** component consists of:

- Chief complaint (CC)
- History of present illness (HPI)
- Review of systems (ROS)
- Past, family, and social history (PFSH)

An extended history of present illness has been expanded to include information about chronic or inactive conditions.

- The review of systems and/or past, family, and/or social history may be recorded by ancillary staff or on a form completed by the patient. To document that the physician reviewed the information, there must be a notation supplementing or confirming the information recorded by others.
- If the physician cannot obtain a history from the patient or other source, the record should describe the patient's condition or other circumstance that precludes obtaining this information.
- The medical record should clearly reflect the chief complaint.
- To qualify for brief history of present illness, the medical record should describe one to three elements of the present illness.
- To qualify for extended history of present illness, the medical record should describe four or more elements of the present illness or associated comorbidities.
- To qualify for problem pertinent review of systems, the patient's positive responses and pertinent negatives for the system related to the problem should be documented.
- To qualify for extended review of systems, the patient's positive responses and pertinent negatives for two to nine systems should be documented.
- To qualify for complete review of systems, at least 10 organ systems must be reviewed. Those systems with positive or pertinent negative responses must be individually documented. For the remaining systems, a notation indicating all other systems are negative is permissible. In the absence of such a notation, at least 10 systems must be individually documented.
- At least one specific item from any of the three history areas must be documented for a pertinent past, family, and/or social history.
- At least one specific item from two of the three history areas must be documented for a complete past, family, and/or social history for the following categories of E/M services: office or other outpatient services, established patient; emergency department; subsequent nursing facility care; domiciliary care, established patient; and home care, established patient.
- At least one specific item from each of the three history areas must be documented for a complete past, family, and/or social history for the following categories of E/M services: office or other outpatient services, new patient; hospital observation services; hospital inpatient services, initial care; consultations; comprehensive nursing facility assessments; domiciliary care, new patient; and home care, new patient.

Examination Component Guidelines

- Specific abnormal findings and relevant negative findings of the examination of the affected or symptomatic body area(s) or organ system(s) should be documented. A notation of "abnormal" without elaboration is insufficient.
- Abnormal or unexpected findings of the examination of the unaffected or asymptomatic body area(s) or organ system(s) should be described.
- A brief statement or notation indicated "negative" or "normal" is sufficient to document normal findings related to unaffected area(s) or asymptomatic organ system(s).
- Examinations are divided into two different types, general multi-system examinations or single organ system examinations. Either type of examination can be performed by

any physician in any specialty. The type is based upon clinical judgment, the patient's history, and the nature of presenting problems.

- Specific elements have been identified for each type of examination and for each specialty. The elements for each are not included in this book as the tables are too lengthy to be reproduced here. Obtain a copy of the complete Documentation Guidelines for specific details about each type of examination.

Medical Decision Making Component Guidelines

Make sure the following components are documented:

Number of diagnoses or management options
- An assessment, clinical impression, or diagnosis for each encounter. This information may be explicitly stated or implied in documented decisions regarding management plans and/or further evaluation.

- The initiation of, or changes in, treatment. Treatment includes a wide range of management options including patient instructions, nursing instructions, therapies, and medications.

Amount/complexity of data reviewed
- In cases of referrals or consultations, who requests the advice, and to which provider the referral or consultation is made.

- If a diagnostic service is ordered, planned, scheduled, or performed at the time of the E/M encounter, the type of service (e.g., lab or x-ray).

- The review of lab, radiology, and/or other diagnostic tests. An entry in a progress note such as "WBC elevated" or "chest x-ray unremarkable" is acceptable.

- A decision to obtain old records or a decision to obtain additional history from the family, caretaker, or other source to supplement that obtained from the patient.

- Relevant findings from the review of old records, and/or the receipt of additional history from the family, caretaker, or other source. If there is no relevant information beyond that already obtained, that fact should be documented. A notation of "old records reviewed" or "additional history obtained from family" without elaboration is insufficient.

- The results of discussion of laboratory, radiology, or other diagnostic test with the physician who performed or interpreted the study.

- The direct visualization and independent interpretation of an image, tracing, or specimen previously or subsequently interpreted by another physician.

Risks of Complications, Morbidity, Mortality
- Comorbidities, underlying diseases, or other factors that increase the complexity of medical decision making by increasing the risk of complications, morbidity, and/or mortality.

- If a surgical or invasive diagnostic procedure is ordered, planned, or scheduled at the time of the E/M encounter, the type of procedure (e.g., laparoscopy).

- If a surgical or invasive diagnostic procedure is performed at the time of the E/M encounter, the specific procedure.

- The referral for, or decision to perform, a surgical or invasive diagnostic procedure on an urgent basis.

DEFINITION

Past, Family, and/or Social History (PFSH) consists of a review of these three areas:

- Past history (prior major illnesses/injuries, prior operations, prior hospitalizations, current medications, allergies, immunization status, feeding/dietary status)

- Family history (review of medical events in the family, including diseases which may be hereditary or place the patient at risk)

- Social history (marital status/living arrangements, current employment, occupational history, use of drugs/alcohol/tobacco, education, sexual history)

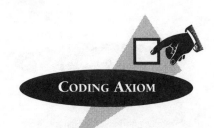

Place of Service Distinctions

Non-hospital based emergency or urgent care centers report outpatient evaluation and management service codes. Special services adjunctive codes 99052, 99054, and 99058 can be reported separately if applicable. To report non-hospital based emergency or urgent care visits involving more time, use modifier -21 or prolonged service codes (99354, 99355, 99358, 99359).

Contributing Factors

If the physician elects to report the level of service based on counseling and/or coordination of care, the total length of time of the encounter (face-to-face or floor time, as appropriate). The record should describe the counseling and/or activities to coordinate care.

Guidelines Summary

Don't let this overview of the 1997 guidelines be your only resource as these guidelines are currently being revised. The jointly developed E/M framework is available from the AMA (by mail or the AMA website). A summary of changes that are likely to be part of the formal guidelines are as follows:

- Clarify that a code may be selected and documented based on counseling/coordination of care, without reference needed to any other dimension of code selection (i.e., history, exam, and medical decision making).

- Emphasize that for established patients, only two of the three key components need be performed (i.e., history, examination, complexity of medical decision making).

- Simplify history selection by allowing documentation of two of the three history areas (HPI, ROS, and PFSH) instead of requiring all three to be documented.

- Add a note that, when a history can not be obtained due to the patient's condition (e.g., inability to communicate, urgent, emergent situation), the history is deemed "comprehensive" for coding and documentation purposes.

- Simplify examination criteria by eliminating confusing instructions (e.g., "perform all elements", shaded and unshaded boxes), while enhancing clinical flexibility by eliminating rigid distinctions between general multi-system versus single system examinations.

- Simplify the medical decision making component by eliminating one level of complexity (straightforward) - the proposed levels are: low, moderate, and high complexity.

- Simplify the medical decision making component by allowing the highest complexity element (i.e., the number of diagnoses/risk of complications, diagnostic procedures/tests and or data to be reviewed, or management options) to drive the level of medical decision making selection. This change eliminates the need to make a separate selection from the table of risk and then entering that decision into another matrix.

In addition to the noted changes in the glossary, clarifications in the proposed guidelines also include the following:

- These documentation guidelines are not applicable to the Preventive Medicine Services, Critical Care, or Neonatal Intensive Care codes

- Any record format for documenting history (including preprinted history forms completed by the patient and reviewed by the physician) is acceptable

- The chief complaint and reason for the encounter requirements are not applicable to inpatient hospital services

- Definitions of chief complaint, reason for encounter, and brief/extended history of present illness have been added

PLACE OF SERVICE DISTINCTIONS

The E/M code section is divided into subsections by type and place of service. Keep the following in mind when coding each service setting:

- A patient is considered an outpatient at a healthcare facility until formal inpatient admission occurs.

- Physicians, regardless of specialty, may use 99281–99285 for reporting emergency department services within hospital-based facilities.

- Consultation codes are linked to location.

- Initial hospital inpatient and hospital observation codes as well as initial nursing facility visit codes include evaluation and management services provided elsewhere (office visit codes or emergency department) by the admitting physician on the same day.

DOCUMENTATION

Physicians and staff members have developed numerous methods to document professional services, and there is no single "right" way as long as all pertinent components of the codes are documented. Some physicians check off a CPT code on an encounter form, while others make clinical notations in the patient's chart for the coding personnel to translate into codes. With the current E/M codes, however, translating the three key components into a CPT code can be more complicated and time-consuming than many physicians will want to deal with at the time of the encounter. By the same token, standard chart notes may not provide enough information for a coder to determine the medical decision making component.

The question then is what device will best communicate the necessary information from the examination room to the coding personnel. The following methods may help you bridge this communication barrier. Figure 3.1 presents a layout that can be turned into an ink stamp for inclusion in chart notes. Figure 3.2 shows one way to incorporate the information into an encounter form. Figure 3.3 is an example of one type of guide that can be used to determine the correct level of E/M service for new patient office visits. Some offices may

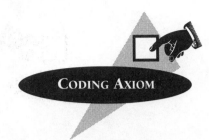

A complete clinical picture must be recorded in the patient's medical record before consulting any coding reference.

prefer to develop a separate E/M routing form that can be clipped to the patient's chart. Because the information in these examples is abridged for space considerations, physicians and coders alike should understand the E/M definitions before using such devices.

Date _____	☐ Kept	☐ Late	☐ Missed

History		**Exam**	
☐	Problem Focused	☐	
☐	Exp Prob Focused	☐	☐ New Patient
☐	Detailed	☐	☐ Est Patient
☐	Comprehensive	☐	

Medical Decision	**Number Dx/Tx Options**	**Amount of Data**	**Risk M&M**
☐ Straightforward	Min	Min	Min
☐ Low Complexity	Low	Low	Low
☐ Moderate Complexity	Mult	Mod	Mod
☐ High Complexity	Ext	Ext	High

☐ **Counseling**	☐ **Consult**	☐ **Observation**
Time_____min	Referring Dr._____	

Figure 3.1

CPT		Description				ICD•9	
Code	Mod	Hx	Ex	MDM	Time	Rank	Charge
New Office or Outpatient Services (assess 3 of 3)							
99201		PF	PF	S	10		
99202		EPF	EPF	S	20		
99203		D	D	LC	30		
99204		C	C	MC	45		
99205		C	C	HC	60		
Established Office or Outpatient Services (assess 2 of 3)							
99211		"NURSE VISIT"			5		
99212		PF	PF	S	10		
99213		EPF	EPF	LC	15		
99214		D	D	MC	25		
99215		C	C	HC	40		

Figure 3.2

Use of forms 3.1 and 3.2 do not themselves document the required elements of the three key components.

3 of 3 (key)	Level/Definition	99201	99202	99203	99204	99205
HISTORY	**Comprehensive** CC; extended HPI; complete ROS, complete PFSHx				▓	▓
	Detailed CC; extended HPI; extended ROS; pertinent PHx, FHx and/or SHx			▓		
	Expanded Problem Focused CC; brief HPI; problem pertinent ROS		▓			
	Problem Focused CC; brief HPI	▓				
EXAMINATION	**Comprehensive** Complete single system specialty Ex or complete multi-system Ex				▓	▓
	Detailed Extended Ex of affected area(s) and other symptomatic or related systems			▓		
	Expanded Problem Focused Limited Ex of affected area(s) and other symptomatic or related organ systems		▓			
	Problem Focused Ex limited to affected body area or organ system	▓				
MEDICAL DECISION MAKING (two subcomponents must be met or exceeded)	**High Complexity** Extensive Dx or Tx options; extensive amount/complx. of data; high risk					▓
	Mod. Complexity Multiple Dx or Tx options; moderate amount/complx. of data; moderate risk				▓	
	Low Complexity Limited Dx or Tx options; limited amount/complx. of data; low risk			▓		
	Straightforward Minimal Dx or Tx options; min or no amount/complx. of data; minimal risk	▓	▓			
TIME (min)	**Face to Face** Estimates only; use when counseling/coordination of care dominate 50% of encounter	10	20	30	45	60
PRESENTING PROBLEM (See key on pg. 3) Severity		sl/m	ls ms	ms	ms hs	ms hs

Figure 3.3

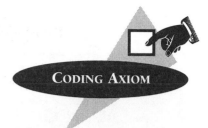

E/M documentation guidelines for Medicare claims combine revised and new definitions that clarify coding objectives both for present use and for future revisions.

DISCUSSION QUESTIONS

1. What distinguishes a new patient from an established patient?

_____

_____

_____

2. List the three key components of E/M service.

_____

_____

_____

3. What role does the presenting problem play in code selection?

    _____

    _____

    _____

4. Name the four levels of complexity in a physical exam.

    _____

    _____

    _____

5. Explain the impact of place of service settings on classifying services.

    _____

    _____

    _____

6. What is the biggest obstacle in documenting an encounter?

    _____

    _____

    _____

OBJECTIVES

Match clinical documentation to the proper codes

Recognize and apply differences among the E/M subcategories

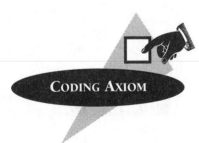

CODING AXIOM

The notes for initial hospital observation care include the following instructions:

• Use these codes to report the encounter(s) by the supervising physician when the patient is designated as "observation status"

• These codes include initiation of observation status, supervision of the health care plan for observation, and performance of periodic reassessments

• See office and other outpatient consultation codes to report observation encounters by other physicians

E/M Subcategories

The E/M section is broken down into subcategories by type and place of service. This section of *Code It Right* provides an overview of these subcategories. E/M codes are intended to standardize the way physicians, coders, and claims processors code patient visits. The varied choices presented by E/M codes result in more consistent billing patterns.

OFFICE OR OTHER OUTPATIENT SERVICES

Use the office or other outpatient services codes (99201–99215) to report the services for most patient encounters. CPT does not provide instructions for reporting multiple office or outpatient visits provided by the same physician on the same calendar date. The most common practice is to report a single visit code per day, evaluating all services provided during that day to arrive at the correct level of service. Prolonged service codes may be used to report services beyond the usual.

HOSPITAL OBSERVATION SERVICES

Codes 99217–99220 report E/M services provided to patients designated or admitted as "observation status" in a hospital. It is not necessary that the patient be located in an observation area designated by the hospital to use these codes; however, whenever a patient is placed in a separately designated observation area of the hospital or emergency department, these codes should be used.

Initial Observation Care

When a patient is admitted to observation status in the course of an encounter in another site of service (e.g., hospital emergency department, physician's office, nursing facility), all related E/M services provided by that physician on the same day are included in the admission for hospital observation. Only one physician can report initial observation services. Do not use these observation codes for post-recovery of a procedure that is considered a global surgical service.

Observation Care Discharge Services

Use 99217 only if discharge from observation status occurs on a date other than the initial date of observation status. The code includes final examination of the patient, discussion of the hospital stay, instructions for continuing care, and preparation of discharge records. If a patient is admitted to and subsequently discharged from observation status on the same date, report the service observation/inpatient hospital care codes 99234–99236. These codes were added in 1998 for patients who are admitted and discharged on the same date.

HOSPITAL INPATIENT SERVICES

The codes for hospital inpatient services report admission to a hospital setting, follow-up care provided in a hospital setting, observation or inpatient care for same day admission and discharge and hospital discharge day management. For inpatient care, the time component includes not only face-to-face time with the patient, but also any unit/floor time related to the patient's care. This time may include family counseling or discussing the patient's condition with the family, establishing and reviewing the patient's record, documenting within the chart, and communicating with other healthcare professionals, such as other physicians, nursing staff, respiratory therapists, and so on.

Initial hospital care codes (99221–99223) should be used by the admitting physician to report the first hospital inpatient encounter. All evaluation and management services provided by the admitting physician in conjunction with the admission regardless of the site of the encounter are included in the initial hospital care service. Services provided in the emergency room, observation room, physician's office or nursing facility specifically related to the admission cannot be reported separately. Physicians, other than the admitting physician, should not use initial hospital care codes, but should report their services with the appropriate consultation or subsequent hospital care codes.

Codes 99238 and 99239 report hospital discharge day management, but exclude discharge of a patient from observation status. Discharge services for newborns or neonates may be reported with 99238 or 99239 for lengths of stay of more than one day. When concurrent care is provided on discharge day by a physician other than the attending physician, report these services using subsequent hospital care codes.

In 1998, a new subcategory was added to Hospital Inpatient Services for reporting either observation or inpatient care services for patients admitted and discharged on the same date of service. This category titled Observation or Inpatient Care Services (including Admission and Discharge Services) is reported with codes 99234–99236. These codes are reported once and include all care provided by the admitting physician whether initiated at another site, within the observation unit, or on an inpatient basis.

CONSULTATIONS

Consultations are provided at the request of another physician or other appropriate source for the purpose of rendering an opinion or advice regarding the evaluation and management of a specific problem.

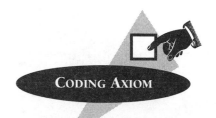

CODING AXIOM

Observation services are included in the inpatient admission service when provided on the same date. Use initial hospital care codes for services provided to a patient who, after receiving observation services, is admitted to the hospital on the same date—the observation service is not reported separately. If not admitted on an inpatient status, observation services for more than one day are reported as 99499 for each day the patient is in observation status except the discharge day which should be reported with 99217. Codes 99218–99220 should not be reported to describe these services.

If the patient is admitted to a facility on the same day as any related outpatient encounter, report the total care as one service with the appropriate initial hospital care code.

An **emergency department** is an organized hospital-based facility for the provision of unscheduled episodic services to patients who present for immediate medical attention. The facility must be available 24 hours a day.

Critical care is the care of unstable, critically ill patients in a variety of medical emergencies that requires the constant attendance of the physician (e.g., cardiac arrest, shock, bleeding, respiratory failure, postoperative complications, critically ill neonate). The physician need not be constantly at bedside, but is engaged in physician work directly related to the individual patient care.

A **consultation** is a type of service provided by a physician whose opinion or advice regarding evaluation and/or management of a specific problem is requested by another physician or other appropriate source.

CODING AXIOM

Care provided in the ED setting for convenience should not be coded as an ED service. Also note that more than one ED service can be reported per calendar day if medically necessary.

Consultations in CPT fall under four subcategories: office or other outpatient consultations, initial inpatient consultations, follow-up inpatient consultations, and confirmatory consultations. Again, if counseling dominates the encounter, time determines the correct code in three of the four subcategories. Confirmatory consultations have no times established.

The general rules and requirements of a consultation are:

- Requests for consultation must come from an attending physician or other appropriate source, and the necessity for this service must be documented in the patient's record.

- The consultant may initiate diagnostic and/or therapeutic services, such as writing orders or prescriptions and initiating treatment plans.

- The opinion rendered and services ordered or performed and the physician ID number must be documented in the patient's medical record and a report of this information communicated to the requesting provider.

- Report separately any identifiable procedure or service performed on, or subsequent to, the date of the initial consultation.

- When the consultant assumes responsibility for the management of any or all of the patient's care subsequent to the consultation encounter, consult codes are no longer appropriate. Depending on the location, identify the correct subsequent or established patient codes.

- Confirmatory consultations may be requested by the patient and/or family or may result from the second (or third) opinion required by the patient's insurance company.

EMERGENCY DEPARTMENT SERVICES

Emergency department (ED) service codes do not differentiate between new and established patients and are used by hospital-based and nonhospital-based physicians.

Time is not a descriptive component for the emergency department levels of E/M services since services are on a variable basis and usually involve multiple encounters with several patients over extended periods of time.

Use 99218–99220 to report evaluation and management services provided in the observation area of a hospital. Use 99291 and 99292 to report critical care provided in the emergency department.

An E/M service can be billed by a physician in addition to a surgical procedure when a separately identifiable E/M service is rendered. For example, if a physician sutures a scalp wound and performs a full neurological exam for a patient with head trauma, it would be proper to bill the surgery and the E/M service. This circumstance would be reported by adding modifier -25 to the appropriate E/M code. It would not be correct, however, if the evaluation only required identifying the need for sutures and confirming immunization status.

Associated with ED services is 99288 *Physician direction of emergency medical systems (EMS) emergency care, advanced life support*. The physician must be located in the ED or critical care department; be in two-way voice communication with the ambulance or rescue personnel outside the hospital; and direct the performance of necessary medical procedures.

CRITICAL CARE SERVICES

Critical care is not specific to a location such as an ICU or CCU. Rather it is determined by the patient's critical condition requiring this type of physician care. Therefore, routine visits to a stabilized patient in an ICU are not necessarily critical care.

Any services performed that are not listed in the margin as a coding axiom can be reported in addition to critical care E/M. Services such as endotracheal intubation (31500) and the insertion and placement of a flow directed catheter (e.g., Swan-Ganz, 93503) may be reported separately. Append modifier -25 to the critical care code to indicate a separate service was performed if the procedure performed is not a starred procedure and has a global follow-up period associated with it.

Critical Care Services Guidelines

* Critical care codes include evaluation and management of the critically ill or injured patient, requiring constant attendance of the physician.

* Care provided to a patient who is not critically ill but happens to be in a critical care unit should be identified using subsequent hospital care codes or inpatient consultation codes as appropriate.

* Critical care of less than 30 minutes should be reported using an appropriate E/M code.

* Critical care codes identify the duration of time spent by a physician on a given date, even if the time is not continuous. Code 99291 reports the first hour and is used only once per date. Code 99292 reports each additional 30 minutes of critical care per date.

* Critical care of less than 15 minutes beyond the first hour or less than 15 minutes beyond the final 30 minutes should not be reported.

* Refer to CPT for examples of correct reporting of critical care services.

NEONATAL INTENSIVE CARE

Codes 99295–99298 report services provided by a physician directing care of a critically ill neonate or infant usually in a neonatal intensive care unit (NICU). Code 99298 was added in 1999 to report subsequent evaluation and management services provided to infants recovering from very low birth weights (less than 1500 grams).

Initial NICU care does not include physician standby services (99360), attendance at delivery and initial stabilization (99436), or newborn resuscitation (99440) when the physician's presence for the delivery and resuscitation is required prior to transfer of the infant to the NICU. In addition, codes for prolonged physician services (99356 and 99357) may be used if prolonged, face-to-face services are required, prior to admission to NICU.

Neonatal intensive care includes initiation and management of mechanical ventilation or CPAP; umbilical, central, or peripheral vessel catheterization; oral or NG tube placement; endotracheal intubation; lumbar puncture; suprapubic bladder aspiration; bladder catheterization; surfactant administration; intravascular fluid administration; transfusion of blood components; vascular punctures; monitoring of vital signs; bedside pulmonary function tests; monitoring and interpretation of blood gases or oxygen saturation. Parent counseling and personal direct supervision of the healthcare team in the performance of cognitive and procedural activities are also included. Also included are additional services referred to in the introductory matter to neonatal intensive care codes or in a parenthetical

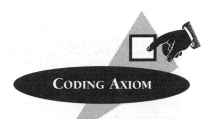

CODING AXIOM

The following services are included in critical care and should not be reported separately when performed during the critical period by the physician providing critical care.

The interpretation of:

* Cardiac output measurements (93561 and 93562)

* Chest x-rays (71010 and 71020)

* Blood gases

* Information stored in computers (e.g., ECGs, blood pressures, hematologic data) (99090)

* Gastric intubation (91105)

* Temporary transcutaneous pacing (92953)

* Ventilator management, (94656, 94657, 94660, 94662)

* Vascular access procedures (36000, 36410, 36415, 36600)

Neonatal intensive care codes represent care starting the date of admission to the NICU, and only one code may be reported per patient per date. Once the neonate is no longer considered to be critically ill, report services with subsequent hospital care codes.

note following the code itself. Report separately any services provided that are not specifically mentioned with each code or in the instructional notes.

NURSING FACILITY SERVICES

Nursing facility E/M services can be provided in skilled (SNFs), intermediate (ICFs), or longterm (LTCFs) facilities. They have been grouped into three subcategories: comprehensive nursing facility assessments (99301–99303), subsequent nursing facility care (99311–99313) and nursing facility discharge services (99315–99316). Included in these codes are E/M services provided to patients in psychiatric residential treatment centers. These facilities must provide a "24-hour therapeutically planned and professionally staffed group living and learning environment." Report other services, such as medical psychotherapy, separately when provided in addition to E/M services.

DOMICILIARY, REST HOME, OR CUSTODIAL CARE SERVICES

These codes (99321–99333) report care given to patients residing in a long-term care facility that provides room and board, as well as other personal assistance services. The facility's services do not include a medical component and typical times have not been established.

HOME SERVICES

Services and care provided at the patient's home or other private residence are reported from this subcategory. Typical times have been established for this code group for 1998.

Some physicians do not know that home visits are a reportable service. While not all payers will reimburse for physician home services, it is important to document home visits and submit a claim. Payers, if educated about the specific circumstances, may be willing to consider claims for home visits.

PROLONGED SERVICES

This section of E/M codes includes three service categories.

Prolonged Physician Service with Direct Patient Contact

These codes report services involving direct patient contact beyond the usual service, with separate codes for office or outpatient encounters (99354 and 99355) and for inpatient encounters (99356 and 99357). Prolonged physician services are add-on services and should be listed separately in addition to the E/M service. The codes report the total duration of face-to-face time spent by the physician on a given date, even if the time is not continuous.

Code 99354 or 99356 reports the first hour of prolonged service on a given date, depending on the place of service, with 99355 or 99357 used to report each additional 30 minutes for that date. Services lasting less than 30 minutes are not reportable in this category, and the services must extend 15 minutes or more into the next time period to be reportable. For example, services lasting one hour and 12 minutes are reported by code 99354 or 99356 alone. Services lasting one hour and 17 minutes are reported by the code for the first hour plus the code for an additional 30 minutes. CPT provides a table illustrating correct coding by time spent.

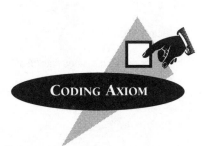

CODING AXIOM

Document home visits and submit a claim although not all payers reimburse for physician home services. Payers may consider claims for home visits depending on the documentation of specific circumstances.

Prolonged Physician Service without Direct Patient Contact

These prolonged physician services without direct patient contact are used before and/or after face-to-face patient care and may include review of extensive records and tests, and communication (other than telephone calls, 99371–99373) with other professionals and/or the patient and family. These are beyond the usual services and include both inpatient and outpatient settings. Report these services in addition to other services provided, including any level of E/M service.

Use 99358 to report the first hour and 99359 for each additional 30 minutes. All aspects of time reporting are the same as explained above for direct patient contact services.

Physician Standby Service

Code 99360 reports when a physician is requested by another physician to be on standby, and the standby physician has no direct patient contact. The standby physician may not provide services to other patients or be proctoring another physician for the time to be reportable. Also, if the standby physician ultimately provides services subject to a surgical package, the standby is not separately reportable.

This code reports cumulative standby time by date of service. Less than 30 minutes is not reportable and a full 30 minutes must be spent for each unit of service reported. For example, 25 minutes is not reportable and 50 minutes is reported as one unit (99360 x 1).

CASE MANAGEMENT SERVICES

Physician case management is a process of involving direct patient care as well as coordinating and controlling access to the patient or initiating and/or supervising other necessary healthcare services. Case management services include team conferences (99361–99362) and telephone calls (99371–99373).

CARE PLAN OVERSIGHT SERVICES

Codes 99374–99380 report the services of a physician providing ongoing review and revision of a patient's care plan involving complex or multidisciplinary care modalities. Care plan oversight services are reported separately from any necessary office/outpatient, hospital, home, nursing facility, or domiciliary services. Only one physician may report these codes per patient per 30-day period. Also, low intensity and infrequent supervision services are not reported separately.

PREVENTIVE MEDICINE SERVICES

Preventive medicine evaluation and management codes (99381–99397) are the most frequently used codes in this subsection. They are used to report periodic preventive medicine evaluation and management of infants, children, adolescents, and adults. Examples of services reported with these codes include: well-child exams, annual gynecologic exams, other annual or periodic exams specifically focused on promoting health and preventing illness.

Preventive medicine evaluation and management services can be reported with problem-oriented evaluation and management services (99201–99215) if the abnormality encountered or the pre-existing condition addressed during the preventive medicine exam requires significant additional work. Report with modifier -25 to indicate that a separately identifiable evaluation and management service was provided.

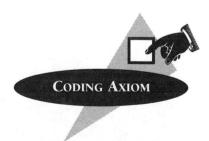

CODING AXIOM

Do not use care plan oversight services codes for supervision of patients in nursing facilities or under the care of hospice and home health agencies unless the patient requires recurrent supervision of therapy.

Codes 99381–99397 include counseling, anticipatory guidance, and risk factor reduction provided at the time of the preventive medicine service. Use codes 99401–99429 only when reporting counseling and risk factor reduction provided at a separate encounter. Report all ancillary lab, x-ray, and other procedures additionally.

NEWBORN CARE

Codes 99431–99440 describe care provided to normal or high-risk newborns in several different settings. The codes identify specific locations, such as the hospital or birthing room, or other than hospital or birthing room.

Discharge services provided to newborns admitted and discharged on the same date should be reported with 99435. Discharge services to newborns discharged on a date subsequent to the admission date should be reported with codes 99238–99239.

SPECIAL EVALUATION AND MANAGEMENT SERVICES

This series of codes (99450–99456) reports physician evaluations performed in order to establish baseline information for insurance certification and/or work related or other medical disability. These E/M codes are used only when no active management of the patient's problem is undertaken during the encounter.

OTHER EVALUATION AND MANAGEMENT SERVICES

Code 99499 is an unlisted code to report other E/M services not specifically defined in CPT.

DISCUSSION QUESTIONS

1. Where do most requests for a consultation originate?

   _____

   _____

   _____

2. When are observation services included in the inpatient admission service?

   _____

   _____

   _____

3. What is meant by the phrase "direct patient contact?"

   _____

   _____

   _____

4. Prolonged service codes are add-on services. When should they be reported?

   _____

   _____

   _____

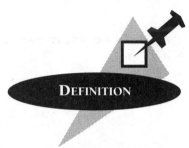

DEFINITION

Special E/M services codes are used to establish baseline information prior to the issue of life or disability certificates.

5.   Define Preventive Medicine Services.

_____

_____

_____

Assigning E/M Codes

With adequate documentation and a general idea of the E/M subcategories, your next step is to match the patient encounter information to the codes. The following sections examine the E/M codes by subcategory. Most subcategories include a graph to the key components of those E/M codes and a medical scenario that illustrates how the components combine to indicate the proper code for that scenario.

The key components of history, physical examination, and medical decision making govern the selection of most E/M codes. The box at the lower right-hand corner of each graph shows the number of key components that must be met or exceeded for that subcategory. Two contributing factors — time and the nature of the presenting problem — are also presented in these charts.

To determine the level of history, examination, and medical decision making, the coder must have documentation that supports these levels. Refer to the following charts to match services to the appropriate level. The four options in assessing both the history and examination components are labeled "Problem Focused," "Expanded Problem Focused," "Detailed," and "Comprehensive." Note, however, that the definitions vary as a result of the different nature of the components. In short, a problem focused history is not the same as a problem focused examination.

Not surprisingly, the medical decision making component involves assessing several elements before determining the complexity of the entire component. Of the three decision-making components, two criteria must be met or exceeded to select a given level.

OBJECTIVES

Match patient encounter information to E/M codes

Examine E/M codes by subcategory

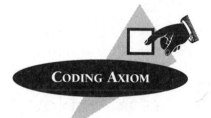

CODING AXIOM

Always treat each key component independently as you assess the extent of the service rendered.

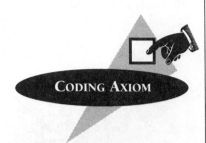

CODING AXIOM

Pay attention to the criteria required for assigning E/M codes. Some E/M categories require only two of the three key components for a given level of service while other E/M categories are charted according to time.

History

Comprehensive	Chief complaint; extended Hx of illness; complete system review; complete past, family and social history
Detailed	Chief complaint; ext. Hx of illness and ext. system review; pertinent past, family, and/or social history
Expanded Problem Focused	Chief complaint; brief Hx of present illness; problem pertinent system review
Problem Focused	Chief complaint; brief Hx of present illness or problem

Examination

Comprehensive	Complete single system specialty exam or complete multisystem exam
Detailed	Extended exam of affected area(s) and other symptomatic or related system(s)
Expanded Problem Focused	Exam extended to other symptomatic or related organ systems
Problem Focused	Exam limited to affected body area or organ system

Subcomponents Level

ext mult lim min	ext mod lim min	high mod low min	
			high complexity
			moderate complexity
			low complexity
			straight forward
Number of Diagnoses or Management Options	Amount and/or Complexity of Data Reviewed	Risk of Complications and/or Morbidity, Mortality	

Medical Decision Making
(Two subcomponents must be met or exceeded)

Abbreviation Key

Levels	Presenting Problem
CC — chief complaint	min. — minimal
Ex — examination	sl/m — self-limiting or minor
HPI — history of present illness	
	ls — low severity
PHx — past medical history	ms — moderate severity
	hs — high severity
FHx — family history	
SHx — social history	**Medical Decision Making**
PFSHx — past medical, family and social history	Dx — diagnoses
	Tx — treatment
ROS — review of systems	

Once you've measured the extensiveness or complexity of each component as supported in the medical record, compare your results with the requirements of each code in the appropriate graph. Remember, these are minimal qualifications. Instructions note that the key components must meet or exceed the indicated level. Therefore, your assessments need not (and probably won't) match exactly the requirements as illustrated in the graphs.

Note that some E/M categories are charted somewhat differently — according to time, for example — or are simply listed with abbreviated definitions. These categories do not lend themselves to the same organization of the other graphs.

The following medical scenarios are presented by specialty to help you make the leap from documentation to correct code choices. Examine the documentation provided, then apply that information to the requirements on the graph. We've highlighted the components as supported in the documentation and indicated the correct code. This hands-on approach should help you better understand the process of E/M code selection. Diagnosis coding has not been included on these pages, though individuals reading these sections are invited to practice these skills. Diagnosis coding answers are found in the appendix.

INTERNAL MEDICINE SCENARIO

Date of Service: March 26, 1997   Chief Complaint: Calf pain

Last Visit: August 17, 1990

History

HPI: Patient is a 60-year-old male with an 18-month history of gradually worsening bilateral calf claudication. Currently he can walk only one block before the claudication begins. The pain resolves after resting for three to five minutes. He denies rest pain, gluteal or thigh claudication, or impotence. He states he has a 100-pack-year smoking history and currently smokes one pack per day.

PMHx: Major medical — CAD, COPD
Surgical — 4 vessel CABG 1985
— Right inguinal hernia 1973
— Appendectomy 1949
Medications — none
Allergies — PCN rash

Family Hx — Father died of MI age 35, Mother died of colon cancer age 68
Social Hx — smokes 1 pack per day
ETOH: six-pack a day of beer; divorced retired engineer

Exam

VS: T — 37.0, BP — Right arm 147/90, Left arm 130/87;
HR: 78; RR: 18 regular
General: Thin man appearing much older than stated age
HEENT: Unremarkable
Neck: w/o masses or enlargements, soft carotid bruit on left
Chest: barrel chested, breath sounds w/ occasional rhonchi
CV: RRR, S_1 and S_2 nl

Pulses:	R	L	
	2+	1+	Carotid
	1+	1+	Radial
	1+	1+	Femoral
	0	0	Popliteal

	0	0	Dorsalis pedis
	0	0	Posterior tibial

Abd: scaphoid, bowel sounds active, soft, no hepato-splenomegaly
GU: nl ext male
Rectal: prostate firm, slightly enlarged, without masses; guaiac negative
Ext: LEs without deformity; mild trophic changes below knee; no ulceration; both feet cool and mottled
Neuro: alert & oriented; CN II through XII intact; decreased sensation below knee bilaterally

Segmental pressures:
R	L	
145	128	Arm
60	64	Ankle

Assessment/Plan

Peripheral vascular disease with claudication — Pt w/o rest pain or disabling symptoms. Patient will begin conservative treatment with walking program, medication and stop smoking. If problem worsens may need surgical intervention. Follow-up in one month.

ICD•9 Diagnosis Code

Office or Other Outpatient Services — New Patient

CPT defines a new patient as one who has not received any professional services from the physician, or another physician of the same specialty who belongs to the same group practice, in the past three years. These services are reported with 99201–99205.

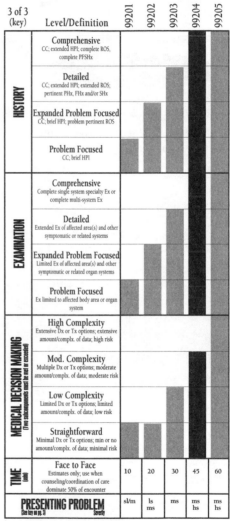

Correct code: 99204

Office or Other Outpatient Services — Established Patient

Office or other outpatient services for an established patient are reported with 99211–99215. Code 99211 is unique (even in the subcategory) because it does not require the key components. The service must be supervised by the physician, who does not have to be in the room but must be available on the premises.

DEFINITION

SOAP is a common documentation format consisting of the following elements:

S — symptoms

O — observation

A — assessment

P — plan

DERMATOLOGY SCENARIO

Date of Service: April 14, 1997   Place of Service: Dermatology Clinic

S   Recurrence of forearm rash

O   3 x 5 cm rash over volar mid-forearm with scaly, erythematous, raised papules

A   Recurrent eczematous dermatitis

P   Topical 1 percent cortisone cream — recheck in one week

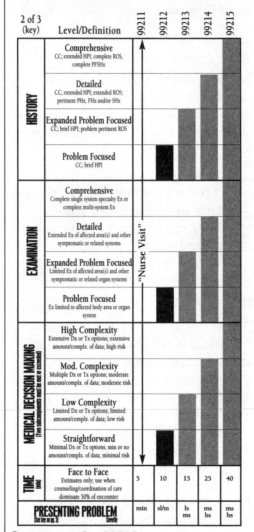

Correct code: 99212

ICD•9 Diagnosis Code

GYNECOLOGY SCENARIO
Date of Service: March 11, 1997   Place of Service: Emergency Department

History
HPI: Patient is a 16-year-old female with right-lower-quadrant abdominal pain. She was in her usual state of good health until approximately 9 a.m. today when she had sudden onset of pain. The pain is steady, does not radiate, and has not significantly changed since it began. She denies having any nausea, vomiting, or change in bowel habits. Her last menstrual period was two weeks prior and was described as normal.

PMHx: Major medical — Ø
Surgical — T&A age 7
Medications — Ø
Family/Social Hx — Both parents living without significant medical history.

ROS: — Unremarkable
Patient denies tobacco, ethanol, or nonprescription drug use. She states she is not sexually active.

Exam
General: slender girl in obvious discomfort
HEENT: normal exam
Neck: supple, w/o masses
Chest: breath sounds clear and equal, respiration unlabored
CV: RRR, S_1 and S_2 nl,
Abd: scaphoid, bowel sounds slightly hyperactive, no hepato-splenomegaly, no palpable masses, guarding over RLQ, no rebound, very tender to deep palpation inferior to McBurney's point
Pelvic: cervix nontender, no adnexal masses, tender in right adnexa
Rectal: no masses, no tenderness
Neuro: normal exam
Musculoskeletal: normal exam

Labs
UA: normal
HCG: pending
SMA-7: normal
CBC: Hct 45%, WBC mildly elevated with slight left shift, no bands

Radiology
Pelvic ultrasound: no masses, some free fluid in deep pelvis

Assessment
RLQ pain — onset and history not typical for appendicitis. Physical exam also not consistent for appendicitis. Other options include ruptured ovarian cyst, early PID, mittelschmerz, ruptured ectopic pregnancy, or ovarian torsion.

Plan
Will hold for observation with frequent abdominal examinations throughout the day. Check results of HCG to rule out pregnancy. If pain progresses, may need laparoscopy. Will repeat CBC in 4 hours.

ICD•9 Diagnosis Code

Initial Observation Care
These codes (99218–99220) report E/M services provided to patients admitted to observation status in a hospital. However, it is not necessary that the patient be located in a designated observation area.

Any other related E/M services provided on the same date as the observation are included in the observation code and cannot be billed separately. These codes should not be used for postoperative recovery of a global surgical procedure, and they can be billed by the admitting physician only.

Use initial hospital care codes rather than these codes to report services provided to patients who first receive observation services then are admitted as inpatients.

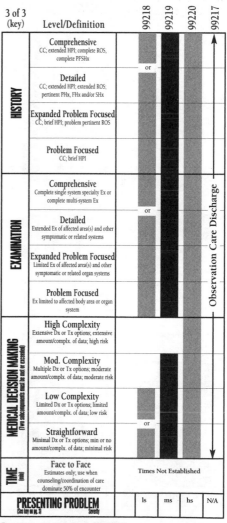

Correct code: 99219

Initial Hospital

These codes (99221–99223) identify services provided on the day of admission by the admitting physician. Only one initial hospital service can be billed for a patient for each hospital stay.

Code 99221 includes either a detailed or comprehensive history and examination. Codes 99222 and 99223 both require a comprehensive history and examination. Therefore, code determination is often based solely on the complexity of medical decision making for initial inpatient services.

Initial hospital care includes all related evaluation and management services provided in a calendar day by the physician, not a 24-hour period.

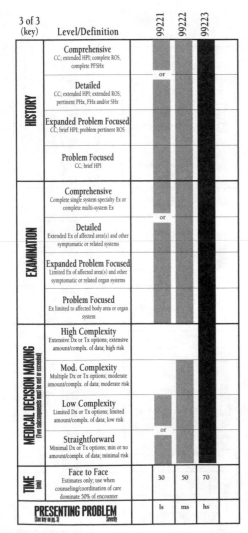

Correct Code: 99223

GENERAL SURGERY SCENARIO

Date of Service: March 3, 1997   Chief Complaint: Abdominal and back pain

History

HPI: Patient is a 50-year-old man with a long history of ETOH abuse. He developed steadily worsening abdominal pain early this a.m. This evening he developed severe nausea and vomiting. He presented to the ED at 10 p.m. where he was found to have a markedly increased serum amylase. He had one episode of pancreatitis one year ago that responded well to TPN.

PMHx: Major Medical
— Pancreatitis 2/95
— Pneumonia 4/88
— Glomerulonephritis 3/80
Surgical — ∅

Medications — ∅
Allergies — NKDA
Social Hx — widowed bookkeeper;
    ETOH: fifth/day; tobacco: 1.5 packs per
    day

ROS: All systems review unremarkable except for present illness.

Exam

VS: T — 37.8; BP — 100/70; HR — 96; RR — 26; Wt — 60 kg
General: Cachectic-looking man in abdominal distress
HEENT: unremarkable
Neck: Supple without THM or masses
Chest: BS clear and equal; without R,R or W
CV: RRR, S1 and S2 nl; pulses all +1

Abd: distended; bowel sounds absent; mild hepatomegally; tender to palpation in epigastrium; no palpable masses or splenomegally
GU: nl ext. male
Rectal: without masses, guaiac negative
Musculoskeletal: without deformity or C, C or E
Neuro: mildly disoriented; CN II through XII intact

Labs

CBC: Hct 50, WBC — 20,000
Calcium: elevated
SGOT: elevated
Serum albumin: decreased
UA: sp gr elevated
ABGs on room air: decreased pO_2 and saturation

X-ray: KUB — calcifications in epigastrium, air-fluid levels in bowel
US: nl gallbladder and ducts without stones; pancreas thickened, no evidence of pseudocyst

Assessment/Plan

1. Acute pancreatitis — in view of exam and labs, patient is severely dehydrated. Will rehydrate. Keep NPO and may need NG suction.

2. Hypoxemia — begin O_2 at 2 liters N.C. and recheck ABGs. If respiratory condition worsens may need intubation and mechanical ventilation. Begin IV analgesics.

3. Will check CT in 2–3 days to R/O pseudocyst.

ICD•9 Diagnosis Code

CARDIOLOGY SCENARIO

Date of Service: March 12, 1997   Hospital Day: #3

S   No complaints

O   Lungs: breath sounds clear and equal
CVS: RRR, S1 and S2 nl
Abd: soft, flat

A/P   Idiopathic cardiomyopathy—had a 40-minute discussion of biopsy and lab results with patient and family. Discussed natural progression of disease as well as treatment options with benefits and disadvantages of each.

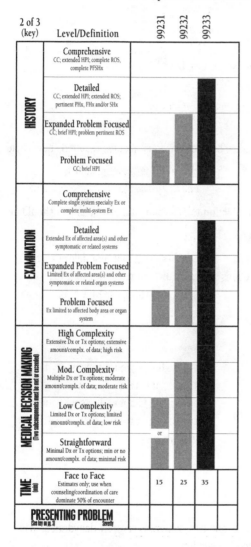

Correct Code: 99233[1]

[1]The major service was counseling, so the code is based on time.

ICD•9 Diagnosis Code

Subsequent Hospital Care

Codes 99231–99233 report the total services provided on each day in the hospital, including reviewing the medical record and analyzing diagnostic studies and test results. The physician must provide some patient care.

Same Day Admission and Discharge Services

These codes should be used to report observation or inpatient services when the patient is admitted and discharged on the same day. The unit of service is a calendar day, not a 24-hour period.

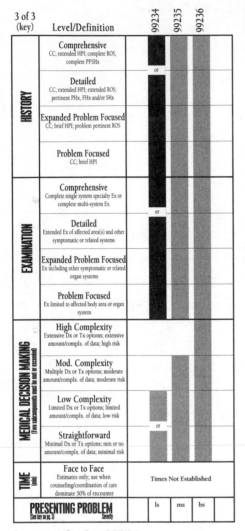

Correct Code: 99234

UROLOGY SCENARIO

History

HPI: The patient presented with severe right flank pain of several hours duration. Past history is significant for previous kidney stone requiring endoscopic retrieval.

Medications — Ø

ROS: Unremarkable

Family Hx: Brother has history of kidney stones.

Exam:

General: Slender male in obvious distress.

HEENT: Normal

Chest: Lung sounds clear.

Cardiovascular: Normal sinus rhythm.

Abdomen: Tender upper right quadrant. No masses. Bowel sounds normal.

Neuro: Normal.

Musculoskeletal: Normal.

Assessment

Symptoms consistent with ureteral calculus. Because previous calculus required endoscopic retrieval will admit and observe. Urine will be strained.

Re-evaluation

Stone passed. Will send for laboratory evaluation to determine if dietary changes should be made.

Discharge

Patient discharged to home with instructions regarding diet. To return for follow-up office visit in one week.

ICD•9 Diagnosis Code

ONCOLOGY

S   Continues to complain shortness of breath, especially on exertion.

O   Continuous pulse oximetry shows 90–95 percent saturation on 4 liters of oxygen per nasal cannula.

A   Interstitial pneumonitis due to adverse effect of methotrexate. Low-grade, non-Hodgkin's lymphoma.

P   After consulting with Pulmonary Medicine physician it is agreed the patient may be discharged to home on continuous oxygen, 4 liters per nasal cannula. Will arrange home oxygen services. Patient to follow-up in 3 days with oncologist for re-evaluation and chest x-ray. To continue oral prednisone, 60 mg. Patient given instructions on diet and exercise.

Time required for final evaluation of the patient, discharge instructions, coordination of home oxygen services, and coordination of care with pulmonary medicine 45 minutes. Correct code is 99239.

ICD•9 Diagnosis Code

Hospital Discharge Services

Report the discharge services of a multiple-day stay with 99238 and 99239. When admission and discharge occur on the same day, report with codes 99234–99236. The discharge service includes final hospital care, final examination, discussion of the hospital stay, instructions for continuing care, and preparation of discharge records. Report 99239 for more than 30 minutes.

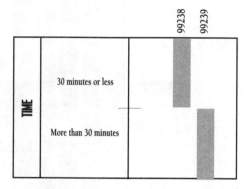

Correct Code: 99239

Office or Other Outpatient Consultations

This subcategory (99241–99245) makes no distinction between new and established patients. If the attending physician requests an additional opinion or advice for the same or for a new problem, these codes are appropriate for that service.

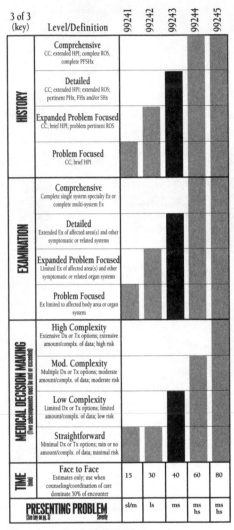

Correct Code: 99243

RHEUMATOLOGY SCENARIO

Date of Service: August 22, 1997   Place of Service: Rheumatology Clinic

Request for Consult

A rheumatologist was asked to evaluate a 48-year-old female with unrelenting shoulder arthralgia and decreasing ROM.

History

The patient had onset of arthralgia after a family vacation that required frequent lifting of heavy suitcases. The patient has been followed for six weeks by her primary care physician using Motrin and hot packs without improvement. Now the other shoulder is becoming stiff. The patient has a history of rheumatoid arthritis and increased difficulty with activities of daily living (ADLs) secondary to additional joint stiffness noted in her fingers and wrist.

Social History: She is unable to type at work without soaking her hands in warm water for 20 minutes each morning. She does not drink alcohol or smoke cigarettes.

Exam

In general, patient appeared to be in good health. Musculoskeletal examination of shoulders and all extremities performed. Range of motion of shoulders was very limited. AP and lateral x-ray views of shoulders obtained and reviewed.

Assessment/Plan

Patient has arthralgia of shoulders. Discussed several treatment options with the patient which include initiating physical therapy and changing her anti-inflammatory. Will consider injecting her shoulder(s) with cortisone and having a physiatrist workup if the symptoms do not improve after two weeks of physical therapy. Instructed patient to follow-up with her primary care physician in one week and to call with any additional questions or if her condition worsens.

The rheumatologist sent a letter to the primary care physician outlining the findings and suggested treatment plan.

ICD•9 Diagnosis Code

RADIOLOGY SCENARIO

Other sections of CPT besides the E/M section include codes for reporting special types of consultations. When a radiologist is asked to perform a consultation on an x-ray examination that was made elsewhere, the correct code to use is:

76140   Consultation on x-ray examination made elsewhere, written report

For radiology guidelines and codes, see Chapter 6 of *Code it Right*.

PATHOLOGY SCENARIO

The Clinical Pathology subsection of CPT is another place where consultation codes are located other than the E/M section. Consultations for Clinical Pathology are reported with codes:

80500   Clinical pathology consultation; limited, without review of patient's history and medical records

80502   comprehensive, for a complex diagnostic problem, with review of patient's history and medical records

However, if the consultation involves an actual examination and evaluation of the patient, codes 99241–99275 should be used to report the service.

For pathology guidelines and codes, see Chapter 7 of *Code it Right*.

X-ray Consultation (76140)

Clinical Pathology Consultations (80500–80502)

Initial Inpatient Consultations

These codes (99251–99255) apply to either new or established patients in a hospital or nursing facility. Report only one initial consultation per admission. If the attending physician requests additional opinions from the consultant on the same patient, report these services as follow-up inpatient consultations.

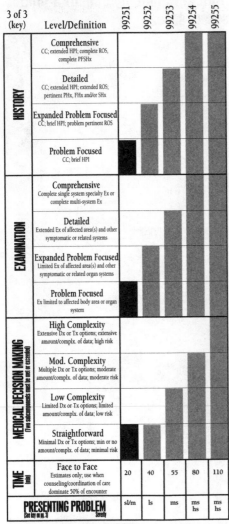

Correct Code: 99251

GENERAL SURGERY SCENARIO

Date of Service: June 2, 1997   Place of Service: Medical ICU, 11:20 p.m.

Request for Consult
I was asked by the attending physician to see this 42-year-old woman admitted to the MICU with rectal bleeding.

History
The patient was in her usual state of good health until this a.m. when she had a sudden urge to move her bowels at which time she passed a large quantity of blood. She was taken immediately to the ED by her husband. Her hematocrit in the ED was 29 percent and she was admitted to the MICU and transfused with three units PRBC. Following transfusion in the MICU her hematocrit one hour later was 33 percent. She was colonoscopied by GI and a moderate amount of blood was seen in the sigmoid colon but no site of bleeding was identified. No blood was seen proximal to the splenic flexure.

Her pertinent past medical history is unremarkable.

Exam
On exam her abdomen is flat and nontender, bowel sounds are hyperactive; no masses or organomegally noted. Rectal exam shows no masses. Labs show initial Hct 29 percent increased to 33 percent with 3 U PRBC. PT and PTT normal.

Assessment/Plan
Recommendations include:

- Transfuse 2 U PRBC now and stay 4 U ahead
- Selective SMA and IMA angiogram ASAP
- Red-cell scan if angiogram is negative
- If patient continues to bleed may need exploration with left colectomy

Discussed with MICU attending.

ICD•9 Diagnosis Code

CARDIOLOGY SCENARIO

Date of Service: April 16, 1997   Place of Service: SICU

Request for Consult

Asked to reevaluate this 55-year-old man who was admitted to the ENT service with uncontrolled epistaxis.

History

During his initial workup he was found to have frequent PVCs, and as per my initial consult he was started on lidocaine. His initial response to the therapy was good with only occasional PVCs. However, during the past 24 hours he has had increasing frequency of PVCs despite increasing doses of lidocaine. Of note: his epistaxis has been stable for the past 24 hours.

Exam

Lungs: bibasilar rales with rhonchi; breath sounds equal

CV: frequent premature beats; S_1 and S_2 nl; S_3 and systolic ejection murmur present

Extremities: pretibial edema to mid-leg

I/Os: Intake = 4000 cc IV; Output = 1000 cc uop

Wt: 73kg (up 2 kgs)

Labs

Hct 44 (down from 49 yesterday), Electrolytes — normal except K 3.1

Assessment/Plan

Initially controlled PVCs on low dose lidocaine, now with increasing PVCs. Patient has evidence of fluid overload with rales, rhonchi, S3 and decreased Hct despite no rebleeding. Would recommend diuresis today of at least 1000 cc. Note that K is low and this needs to be aggressively replaced today. If PVCs continue despite diuresis and K replacement, would consider changing drug therapy but not before other factors corrected.

ICD•9 Diagnosis Code

Follow-up Inpatient Consultations

Codes 99261–99263 apply exclusively to established patients and report services that either complete the initial consultation or were subsequent consultative services requested by the attending physician. These services include monitoring progress, recommending modifications in management, and giving advice on a new care plan in response to changes in a patient's status.

More than one follow-up inpatient consult may be billed per calendar day if medically necessary.

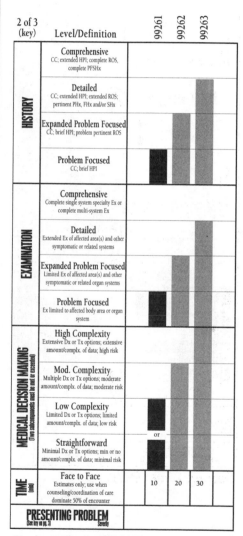

Correct Code: 99261

Confirmatory Consultations

Use codes 99271–99275 if the consultation is for a second or third opinion on the necessity or appropriateness of a previously recommended medical treatment or surgical procedure. In these cases, the requesting party is usually not a physician; it is usually the patient or insurance payer.

Confirmatory consultations are not linked to a location. Report any services subsequent to the visit with established patient or subsequent care codes. When this consultation is required by an insurer, list the proper code with modifier -32.

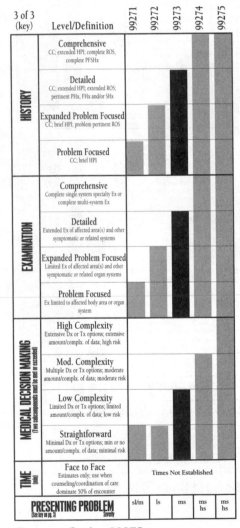

Correct Code: 99273

NEUROSURGERY SCENARIO

Date of Service: May 19, 1997   Place of Service: Neurosurgery Clinic

Request for Referral

Asked to see this 29-year-old to verify the need for surgery.

History

The patient has been evaluated by Dr. Osler who recommended cervical fusion for his chronic cervical disc degeneration and bilateral radiculopathy. The patient states he was without problems until he was involved in a serious auto accident six years ago. He sustained a cervical sprain, which was treated with a cervical collar and physical therapy. Four years ago he began developing paresthesias in the C_5 and C_6 distribution, first on the right, then bilaterally. He had cervical x-rays that showed 50 percent decrease in the C_4–C_5 and C_5–C_6 disc spaces. The symptoms progressed despite aggressive physical therapy until currently he has what he describes as unbearable burning pain at the base of his neck and along the radial side of both arms into his thumbs. He states he is unable to work due to the pain. He currently takes 20 aspirins daily. Dr. Osler has performed nerve conduction studies showing marked slowing in the musculocutaneous and median nerves bilaterally, consistent with C_5 and C_6 neuropathies.

PMHx: Major Medical — Rheumatic fever at age 6

Surgeries — T and A, age 8; ORIF ankle 1986

Meds — ASA, 20/day

Allergies — Sulfa-caused rash

Family Hx — Rheumatoid arthritis — mother

Social Hx — Single, carpenter, no ETOH or tobacco use

ROS:

ENT — frequent ear infections

RESP — ∅

CV — ∅

MS — ankle pain

Neuro — see HPI

Heme — ∅

Endo — ∅

GU — ∅

Exam

General: WN/WD man in NAD

HEENT: NC/AT, PERRLA, EOMI, Fundi benign

Neck: flexion 20 degrees, extension 10 degrees, rotation 10 degrees left and right; tender to palpation C_4–C_7

Chest: BS equal, clear; equal expansion

CV: RRR; pulses all 2+

Abd: soft, flat; bowel sounds active; no HSM

Rectal: normal tone; prostate firm, without masses

MS: 2+ weakness of muscles supplied by musculocutaneous, median, and radial nerves

Assessment/Plan

The patient clearly has C_5 and C_6 neuropathies most likely secondary to the post-traumatic degeneration of C_4–C_5 and C_5–C_6 discs. The nerve conduction studies are consistent with nerve root compression. I would recommend preoperative MRI to verify the actual mechanical compression and any spinal canal encroachment. After this, the patient is a good candidate for cervical fusion. I would not recommend a partial procedure such as foraminotomy alone due to the marked loss of height of both disc spaces.

ICD•9 Diagnosis Code

MEDICAL SPECIALTIES SCENARIO
Date of Service: August 17, 1997; 10:45 a.m.

Place of Service: ED

S Patient is a 14-year-old girl with a history of asthma who was without respiratory problems until early this a.m. when she was playing outside with friends. She began having difficulty breathing and is currently having extreme respiratory difficulty. Mother states she hasn't been taking her asthma medicines at home.

PMHx:

Major Medical — asthma

Allergies — NKDA

Medicine — albuterol inhaler, not using currently

O **Initial exam:**

Chest — retractions bilaterally; extreme respiratory effort apparent; decreased breath sounds with faint wheeze; no rales or rhonchi

CV: RRR; S_1 and S_2 nl, without RCGM

Pulse oximeter: 80 percent saturation on room air

A/P Acute asthma exacerbation. Will give racemic epinephrine and alupent inhalation treatment now. Recheck in 15 minutes.

Follow-up exam post-treatment
Breath sounds clear without wheezes. O_2 saturation 95 percent on room air. Patient discharged in good condition with inhaler and instructions to follow-up with family physician in a.m.

ICD•9 Diagnosis Code

Emergency Room Physician — Emergency Department Services (99281–99285)
CPT defines an emergency department as an organized hospital-based facility for the provision of unscheduled episodic services to patients who present for immediate medical attention. The facility must be available 24 hours a day.

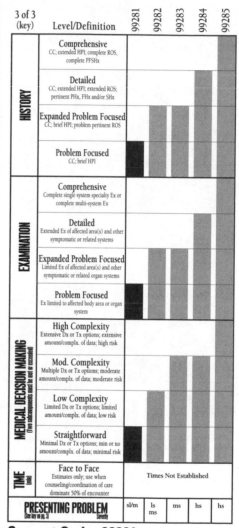

Correct Code: 99281

Critical Care Services

Critical care reporting is currently accomplished with two codes: 99291 reports the first hour of care provided on each date, and 99292 reports all additional time per 24-hour period, in 30 minute increments. Obviously, the physician must document this time carefully. Report separately any procedures not directly attendant to the critical care management, such as suturing lacerations and setting fractures.

CARDIOLOGY SCENARIO

A 60-year-old man is admitted to the CCU with chest pain. On the second hospital day, his physician examines him on morning rounds finding nothing remarkable. Two hours later the patient goes into cardiac arrest requiring resuscitation and stabilization totaling 90 minutes. Code the services for the physician after the initial morning visit.

99291 Critical care, evaluation and management of the unstable critically ill or unstable critically injured patient, requiring the constant attendance of the physician; first hour

99292 each additional 30 minutes (List separately in addition to code for primary service)

92950 Cardiopulmonary resuscitation (eg, in cardiac arrest)

Use the appropriate subsequent hospital care code to report services provided to a patient who is stable and no longer critically ill or injured.

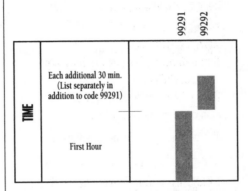

Critical care, evaluation and management of the unstable critically ill or unstable critically injured patient, requiring the constant attention of the physician.

Critical care is a global procedure and includes the performance of a variety of procedures attendant to the emergency care of the critical patient.

When providing critical care of less than 30 minutes total duration on a given date, report the services with the appropriate subsequent hospital care code (99231–99233).

Critical care is coded by time only, so there is no component graph.

ICD•9 Diagnosis Code

NEONATOLOGY SCENARIO

Admit Note

The patient is a full-term baby girl who was spontaneously delivered vaginally. APGAR scores were 6 and 8. This is the mother's first child and she has no history of problems during pregnancy. The baby was well until her second day of life when she began having episodes of respiratory distress described by her mother as appearing to be "gasping for breath." She was brought to the ED where evaluation showed her to be cyanotic with labored breathing with retractions. An arterial blood gas showed a PO_2 of 40. Neonatology was called to evaluate and treat the baby.

Exam

VS: T — 39.5 R ; BP — 60/40; HR — 120; RR — 30; Wt — 14.5 kg

HEENT:

Head — fontanelles open, soft and flat; mild caput

Eyes — anicteric

Ears — TMS flat

Mouth — without lesions

Neck: without masses

Chest: BS decreased both bases with coarse rhonchi. Intercostal retractions

COR: II/V, SEM, RRR

Abd: soft, without masses

Genitalia: nl ext. female

Rectal: patent anus

Extremities: without deformities, hips located bilaterally

Neuro: listless, poor suck reflex, decreased startle response

Labs

CBC: Hct elevated, WBC elevated with marked left shift

SMA 7: elevated Na and K, decreased HCO_2

ABGs on room air: PO_2 40, PCO_2 15

CXR: dense infiltrates bases bilateral with air bronchograms

Assessment

Pneumonia — aspiration vs. infectious

Plan

Admit to NICU. Begin O_2 40 percent mask, repeat ABGs, may need intubation if no improvement. Begin arterial line. Begin scalp vein IV fluids. Broad spectrum antibiotics. May need feeding tube if no improvement in 24 hours.

Code 99295 is correct because it reports the initial neonatal intensive care described in the scenario. All described procedures are included in initial neonatal intensive care and should not be coded separately.

The following procedures are also included as part of the global descriptors in neonatal intensive care services: umbilical, central, or peripheral vessel catheterization; endotracheal intubation; and lumbar puncture, and suprapubic bladder aspiration and others as listed in the CPT guidelines for neonatal intensive care. In addition, specific services are included in the parenthetical note following each NICU code. Any services performed which are not listed above or are not listed with each neonatal intensive care code should be reported separately.

ICD•9 Diagnosis Code

Neonatal Intensive Care Services

The codes to report neonatal intensive care services are not broken into components. Instead, 99295 reports the initial care, 99296 reports subsequent care provided to a critically ill unstable neonate, and 99297 reports the subsequent care provided to a critically ill stable neonate. A new code was added in 1999 to report E/M services for very low birthweight infants (less than 1500 grams). These infants require intensive care but do not require the same level of care as critically ill neonates. Report these codes only once per day per patient. Once the neonate is no longer considered to be critically ill and attains birthweight which exceeds 1500 grams, use Subsequent Hospital Care codes. When provided prior to admittance to a NICU, the following services may also be reported: prolonged physician services (99354–99359), physician standby (99360), and newborn resuscitation (99440).

Codes 99295, 99296, 99297, and 99298 include the following as necessary:

Initiation and management of mechanical ventilation or CPAP; umbilical, central, or peripheral vessel catheterization; oral or NG tube placement; endotracheal intubation; lumbar puncture; suprapubic bladder aspiration; bladder catheterization; surfactant administration; intravascular fluid administration, transfusion of blood components; vascular punctures; monitoring of vital signs; bedside pulmonary function tests; monitoring and interpretation of blood gases or O_2 saturation.

99295: Initial NICU care, per day, for evaluation and management of critically ill neonate or infant. Provided on date of admission to neonate requiring cardiopulmonary monitoring and support. Includes preoperative evaluation and stabilization of neonates with life threatening surgical or cardiac conditions.

99296: Subsequent NICU care, per day, for evaluation and management of critically ill and unstable neonate or infant. Provided on dates subsequent to the admission date. Most require frequent ventilator changes, intravenous fluid alterations and/or early initiation of parenteral nutrition. Includes neonates in the immediate postoperative period or those who become critically ill and unstable during the hospital stay.

99297: Subsequent NICU care, per day, for evaluation and management of critically ill though stable neonate or infant. Provided on dates subsequent to the admission date. Require less frequent changes in respiratory, cardiovascular, and/or fluid and electrolyte therapy.

99298: Subsequent NICU care, per day, for evaluation and management of the recovering very low birth weight infant (less than 1500 grams) provided on dates subsequent to the admission date. Very low birthweight infants who require less frequent changes in respiratory, cardiovascular, and/or electrolyte therapy than those induced under 99296 or 99297.

Correct Code: 99295

Comprehensive Nursing Facility Assessments

Comprehensive assessments may be performed in various locations such as hospital, office, nursing facility, domiciliary/non-nursing facility, or the patient's home. Nursing facility codes (99301–99303) apply to new and established patients, and more than one comprehensive assessment may be needed during the course of patient confinement.

All evaluation and management services provided on the same day as the comprehensive assessment are included in that care, such as care provided in the ED or physician's office. The only exception is when a patient is being discharged from the hospital and admitted to a nursing facility on the same day. In this situation, the discharge services may be reported separately.

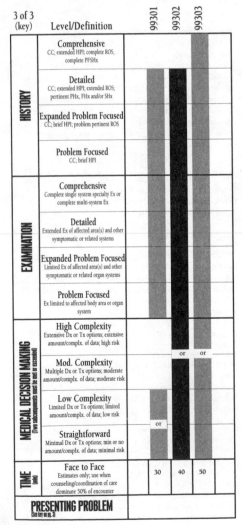

Correct Code: 99302

FAMILY PRACTICE SCENARIO

Date of Service: September 17, 1997

History

Patient is an 18-year-old boy injured in a motorcycle accident, sustaining a severe head injury with depressed skull fracture and intracerebral hemorrhage. He had elevation of his fracture and drainage of the subdural hematoma on June 30, 1996. He underwent a tracheostomy placement on July 10, 1996. He has been fed internally via a feeding tube since July 11, 1996. He spent the next several weeks in rehabilitation, but his injury was severe and he currently has an extremely low level of function with residual brain damage. He is being admitted to the nursing facility for long-term skilled nursing care. PFSH: No changes from original admission.

Exam

HEENT: Head — healed temporal surgical wound

Eyes — PERRLA; tracks poorly

Ears — TMs flat, pearly

Nose — feeding tube present in right nostril

Mouth — without lesions

Neck: midline tracheostomy in place

Chest: breath sounds clear, equal; without R,R or W

CV: RRR; S1 and S2 nl, without RCGM, pulses all full and equal

Abd: soft, flat; BS active; no HSM

GU: nl ext male; condom catheter in place

Rectal: tone decreased

Ext: without C, C or E; slight flexion contractures LEs

Neuro: responds to pain or loud stimuli only; CN II through XII intact; DTRs all brisk, equal; Babinski downgoing bilaterally

Labs

CBC — Hct 49 percent

SMA 20 — all normal

UA — normal

CXR — without infiltrates

KUB — tip of feeding tube in 2nd portion of duodenum

Assessment/Plan

Severe head injury with residual brain damage and extremely low level functioning. He will need:

- Ongoing physical therapy for ROM all joints
- Decubitus precautions
- Routine tracheostomy care
- Tube feedings
- Urinary catheter care with prophylactic antibiotics
- Oral care with nystatin
- Routine labs as per protocol

ICD•9 Diagnosis Code

INTERNAL MEDICINE SCENARIO

Date of Service: July 20, 1997

S   Patient has done well since last week. Her multiple sclerosis has not progressed significantly in past several weeks. No new problems.

O   **Lungs** — clear

   CV — RRR

   Abd — soft; BS active

   Ext — without ulceration or skin breakdown

   Neuro — MS unchanged; motor function without change

A/P   Stable and currently without any deterioration for past 4–6 weeks. Will continue all current care without change. Recheck in one week. She needs labs checked next visit.

ICD•9 Diagnosis Code

Subsequent Nursing Facility Care

Subsequent nursing facility care codes (99311–99313) describe the services provided to patients who do not require a comprehensive assessment — patients who have had no major or permanent change in status. All subsequent care services include reviewing the medical record, noting any changes since the last visit, and reviewing and signing orders.

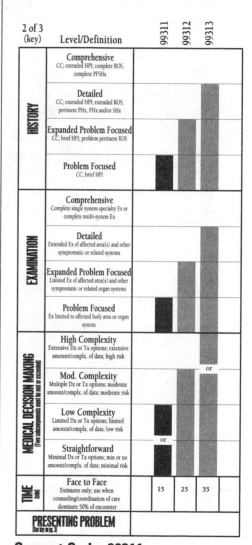

Correct Code: 99311

Nursing Facility Discharge Services

Nursing facility discharge day management services are assigned based on total physician time required to discharge the patient. Physician work related to discharge management includes: final exam of the patient, review of nursing facility stay, instructions for and arrangment of continuing care, preparation of discharge records, prescriptions, and referral forms.

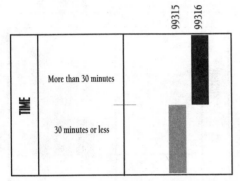

Correct Code: 99316

NURSING FACILITY DISCHARGE SERVICES

Internal Medicine/Orthopedics Scenario

This 78-year-old female status post hip fracture was admitted to a skilled nursing facility two weeks ago for continued rehabilitation and management of her CHF, anorexia, and malnutrition. She is now able to walk with the aid of a walker, her CHF is under good control with medications, and she has gained two pounds. She is being discharged and will be cared for by her daughter. Arrangements were made for home health services which will include continued physical therapy and nutrition management. The home health service met with daughter to discuss medication and nutrition needs as well as daily physical therapy.

Total discharge service time 40 minutes.

ICD•9 Diagnosis Code

GERONTOLOGY SCENARIO
Date of Service: July 7, 1997

Referral
Asked to see this 65-year-old, hemiplegic rest-home resident for evaluation and care of a left trochanteric skin breakdown.

History
The patient has been hemiplegic since a CVA five years prior to admission. He has had no prior skin breakdown problems.

Exam
Shows an erythematous, 2 x 3 cm area of skin immediately overlying the left greater trochanter.

Of note: There are no other areas of irritation over the sacrum or left ankle. The area of erythema shows no breakdown at this time and no underlying fluctuation or drainage.

Assessment
Early pressure sore of left trochanteric area without breakdown or ulceration at this point. Treatment includes avoidance of pressure to this area and duoderm wafer to skin. I will recheck in 48–72 hours.

ICD•9 Diagnosis Code

Domiciliary, Rest Home, or Custodial Care Services — New Patient

Codes 99321–99333 identify E/M services in a facility that provides room, board, and other personal assistance services, generally on a long-term basis. The facility's services do not include a medical component. These new patient codes are used when a patient has not received any professional services from the physician or another physician of the same specialty who belongs to the same group practice, within the past three years.

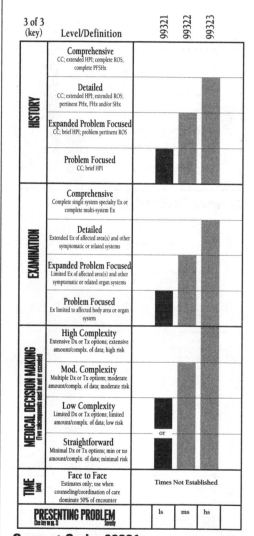

Correct Code: 99321

Domiciliary, Rest Home, or Custodial Care Services — Established Patient

Codes 99321–99333 identify E/M services in a facility that provides room, board, and other personal assistance services, generally on a long-term basis. The facility's services do not include a medical component. These established patient codes are used when a patient has received any professional services from the physician or another physician of the same specialty who belongs to the same group practice within the past three years.

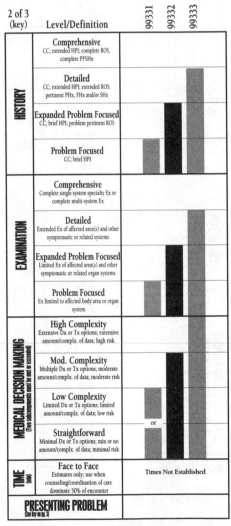

Correct Code: 99332

INTERNAL MEDICINE SCENARIO
Date of Service: April 21, 1997

History
Patient has developed increasing insulin requirements since last visit, currently requiring nearly twice the daily insulin as two weeks prior. Also, COPD has become more severe with increased respiratory rate and cough.

Exam
VS: T — 37.8; HR — 90; BP — 138/84; RR — 24

HEENT: Ears — TMs flat, pearly

    Sinuses — non-tender

    Mouth — without lesion or erythema

Chest: Asymptomatic BS decreased left lower base

CV: RRR

Abd: soft, flat; BS active

Skin: without breakdown

Assessment
Increasing insulin requirements over past week is worrisome. The left lower lung field exam is consistent with a localized pneumonia and this could be the source of the insulin resistance. Will check a CXR, draw a CBC, electrolytes, and blood, urine, and sputum cultures. Will then begin a broad spectrum oral antibiotic. I will recheck tomorrow or later today if patient worsens.

ICD•9 Diagnosis Code

FAMILY PRACTICE SCENARIO
New Patient
Home visit to a blind patient who has developed a cough and left earache. The physician conducts an examination of the respiratory system and checks the patient's ears. Assessment is URI with left otitis media. The patient is placed on an oral antibiotic.

MEDICAL SPECIALTIES/PEDIATRICS
Established Patient
The physician is called to the home of a family of established patient to discuss the post-concussion syndrome of their 13-year-old son. The child is examined due to a recent urinary tract infection and medication is reviewed.

Home Services — New and Established Patients (99341–99350)
The home services codes identify E/M services provided by a physician in a private residence. Procedures may be identified separately.

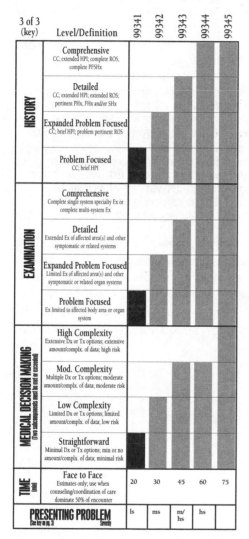

Correct Code: 99341

ICD•9 Diagnosis Code

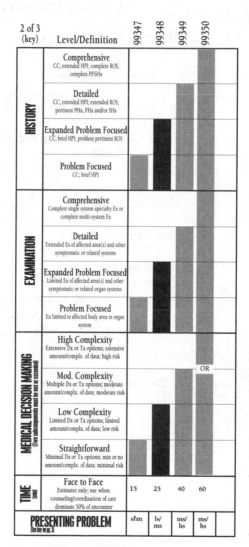

Correct Code: 99348

ICD•9 Diagnosis Code

Prolonged Services With Direct (Face-To-Face) Patient Contact

Codes 99354–99357 identify prolonged physician services requiring direct patient contact (face-to-face time) by the physician. These codes may be reported in addition to procedures performed in the care of the patient when the additional time spent monitoring the patient consists of a minimum of one hour of time over and above the usual service provided. The physician is dedicated to the management of the patient and should not be performing unrelated services.

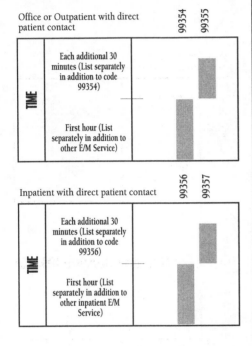

UROLOGY SCENARIO

A patient presents at the emergency department with multiple trauma. The ED physician examines the patient and calls in a urologist to evaluate the patient for suspected ruptured bladder. The patient is catheterized by the ED staff.

The urologist performs an abdominal tap (which shows frank blood), a comprehensive workup of the patient for admission, and monitors the patient for one hour while the operating room is prepared. The patient undergoes a simple partial cystectomy for ruptured bladder in the operating room and is subsequently admitted to the hospital.

The urologist's services:

51550	Cystectomy, partial; simple
49080*	Peritoneocentesis, abdominal paracentesis, or peritoneal lavage (diagnostic or therapeutic); initial
99223-25	Initial hospital care, per day, level 3; significant, separately identifiable evaluation and management service by the same physician on the same day of the procedure or other service
99356	Prolonged physician service in the inpatient setting requiring direct (face-to-face) patient contact beyond the usual service (e.g., maternal fetal monitoring for high risk delivery or other physiological monitoring, prolonged care of an acutely ill inpatient); first hour (List separately in addition to code for inpatient Evaluation and Management service)

Patient is being held in the ED pending surgery and admission. Therefore, even though the patient is receiving care in the ED, the patient is considered an inpatient.

Starred procedures are explained in the surgery chapter.

ICD•9 Diagnosis Code

INTERNAL MEDICINE SCENARIO

A 53-year-old female was admitted to the hospital for severe pleuritic chest pain over the past three days. The admission history and physical were performed by the medical service resident. The patient has multiple medical problems consisting of insulin dependent diabetes with nephropathy, neuropathy, retinopathy and autonomic insufficiency, and vascular insufficiency-status post left BK amputation. The patient was found to have acute uremic pericarditis and the internal medicine staff physician was contacted to direct the patient's care.

The internal medicine physician spent 30 minutes prior to seeing the patient reviewing extensive medical records from past hospitalizations, previous tests including labs, EKG, chest x-ray films, and cardiac echo. The physician found the patient uncooperative, refusing hemodialysis, and she would not answer direct questions. Following the 10 minutes spent with the patient the physician held a 30-minute conference with the patient's family (patient not present) regarding the patient's refusal of care and hemodialysis. The physician discussed the patient's condition and necessity of hemodialysis and renal replacement since the patient was not a good candidate for long-term hemodialysis.

Code 99358 alone reports the described service because 60 minutes was spent without the patient present. At least 75 minutes of service is necessary to also report 99359.

The 10 minutes spent with the patient face-to-face would not be coded. At least 30 minutes must be spent with the patient before code 99354 is reported.

ICD•9 Diagnosis Code

MULTIPLE SPECIALTIES SCENARIO

Code 99360 reports physician standby services involving prolonged attendance without direct patient contact. This service should be requested by another physician and is reported in 30-minute increments. A full 30 minutes must be provided for each unit of service reported. The standby physician may not provide care or services to other patients during the standby period.

Procedure code 99360 can be used by any physician on standby (e.g., for newborn resuscitation) per CPT (e.g., operative standby, standby for frozen section, for C-section/high risk delivery, for newborn care, EEG monitoring).

ICD•9 Diagnosis Code

Prolonged Services Without Direct (Face-To-Face) Patient Contact

Codes 99358 and 99359 identify prolonged physician services that do not require direct patient contact (face-to-face time) by the physician. These services may involve the review of extensive records and tests or communication with other professionals, the patient, or family. The codes may be reported in addition to other physician services, such as any level of E/M service. A service of less than 30 minutes total duration on a given date is not reported separately.

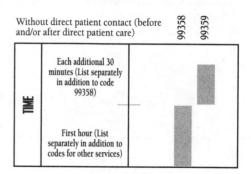

Physician Standby Service (99360)

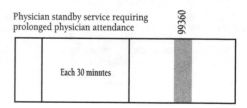

Case Management Services

Physician case management is the process of physician-directed care. This includes coordinating and controlling access to the patient or initiating and/or supervising other necessary healthcare services.

The case management codes for team conferences and telephone calls in CPT are currently reported with the numbers 99361–99373.

Medicare considers these services "bundled" into other medical services such as an office or hospital visit and, therefore, never pays for them separately. Private payers vary in their policies regarding these codes. Medicode recommends that you submit these codes to establish a billing pattern and draw attention to the need for these services.

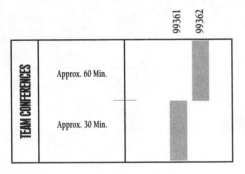

Telephone Calls by a physician to a patient or for consultation or medical management or for coordinating medical management with other healthcare professionals (eg, nurses, therapists, nutritionists, pharmacists, etc.):

99371:   simple or brief

99372:   intermediate

99373:   complex or lengthy

MULTIPLE SPECIALTIES SCENARIO

A patient on anticoagulant therapy has a protime test performed at a laboratory. The results are phoned to the physician. After careful review of the lab results and patient's chart, he phones the patient to adjust the medication.

Telephone Calls by a physician to patient or for consultation or medical management or for coordinating medical management with other healthcare professionals (e.g., nurses, therapists, nutritionists, pharmacists):

99371	simple or brief
99372	intermediate
99373	complex or lengthy

Correct Code: 99371

ICD•9 Diagnosis Code

REHABILITATION MEDICINE OR INTERNAL MEDICINE SCENARIO

A 48-year-old female suffered a CVA affecting her entire left side and Broccas area of the brain-rendering her hemiplegic and aphasic. The patient resides in a local rehabilitation center for treatment of these sequelae. She is seen once a month by her rehabilitation physician for examination. The physician spent 90 minutes during a 30-day period reviewing continuing physical therapy, speech therapy, occupational therapy, and recreational therapy in a team setting. Treatment plans using the multidisciplinary team approach were updated during the month and physician orders revised as needed.

99313   Subsequent nursing facility care, level 3 (for examination)

99380   Physician supervision of a nursing facility patient (patient not present) requiring complex and multidisciplinary care modalities involving regular physician development and/or revision of care plans, review of subsequent reports of patient status, review of related laboratory and other studies, communication (including telephone calls) with other health care professionals involved in patient's care, integration of new information into the medical treatment plan and/or adjustment of medical therapy, within a calendar month; 30 minutes or more

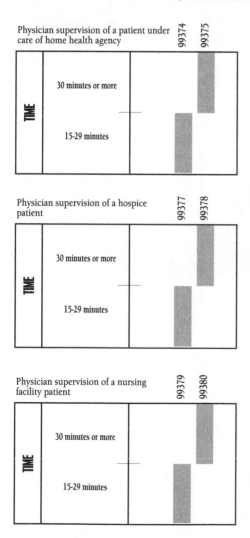

ICD•9 Diagnosis Code

Care Plan Oversight Services

Care plan oversight services identify physician supervision of a patient under the care of a home health agency, in a hospice, or in a nursing facility (if the patient is not present). The patient's condition requires recurrent supervision of therapy and complex or multidisciplinary care modalities. The codes for care plan oversight services are 99374–99380.

Preventive Medicine Services

Codes 99381–99397 report periodic preventive medicine examinations. Patients are categorized by new or established status, and by age. The services require a comprehensive history and examination, and include counseling, anticipatory guidance, and identification of patient risk factors. Laboratory, other diagnostic procedures, and immunizations should be reported additionally.

If problems or abnormalities are encountered that require additional work to perform key components of a problem-oriented E/M service, report separately with the appropriate office/outpatient code (99201–99215). Modifier -25 should be appended to identify a significant separately identifiable service.

FAMILY PRACTICE SCENARIO

A 70-year-old new patient presents at a multispecialty clinic for a routine history and physical with no complaints. A complete history and physical are performed as well as baseline lab work and a chest x-ray, both performed by the clinic laboratory.

99387	Initial preventive medicine evaluation and management of an individual including a comprehensive history, a comprehensive examination, counseling/anticipatory guidance/risk factor reduction interventions, and the ordering of appropriate laboratory/diagnostic procedures, new patient; 65 years and over
80050	General health panel
71020	Radiologic examination, chest, two views, frontal and lateral

New	Age	Established
99381	Under one year	99391
99382	1 through 4 years	99392
99383	5 through 11 years	99393
99384	12 through 17 years	99394
99385	18 through 39 years	99395
99386	40 through 64 years	99396
99387	65 years and older	99397

Preventive medicine evaluation and management of an individual including a comprehensive history, a comprehensive examination, counseling/anticipatory guidance/risk factor reduction interventions, and the ordering of appropriate laboratory/diagnostic procedures.

ICD•9 Diagnosis Code

MULTIPLE SPECIALTIES SCENARIO
Clinical Scenario

A 35-year-old male whose family history presents a high incidence of heart disease is counseled for 45 minutes in the factors and preventive measures, which include diet and exercise.

99403 Preventive medicine counseling and/or risk factor reduction intervention(s) provided to an individual (separate procedure); approximately 45 minutes

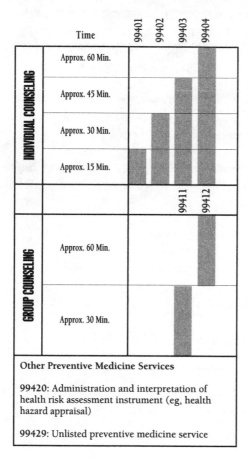

ICD•9 Diagnosis Code

Counseling and/or Risk Factor Reduction Intervention

Use 99401–99412 to report counseling provided to individuals at a separate encounter for issues such as family problems, diet and exercise, substance abuse, sexual practices, and so forth. Do not use these codes to report counseling and risk-factor-reduction services provided to patients with symptoms or illnesses. For patients with symptoms, use the appropriate office, hospital, or consultation codes.

The codes are divided into individual and group counseling, with time as the determining factor.

Code 99420 describes the administration and interpretation of health risk assessment instrument. This subcategory also has its own unlisted service code (99429).

Newborn Care

This series of codes (99431–99440) describes care provided to normal or high-risk newborns. The codes identify specific locations such as the hospital or birthing room, other than hospital or birthing room, and the office. Report the hospital discharge services of a newborn discharged on a date subsequent to admission with codes 99238 and 99239 when applicable.

These codes report newborn services. If an infant is readmitted to the hospital, use 99221–99233.

> **99431:** History and examination of normal newborn infant, initiation of diagnostic and treatment programs and preparation of hospital records. (code should also be used for birthing room deliveries)

> **99432:** Normal newborn care in other than hospital or birthing room setting, including physical examination of baby and conference(s) with parent(s)

> **99433:** Subsequent hospital care, for the evaluation and management of a normal newborn, per day

> **99435:** History and examination of normal newborn infant, including preparation of medical records (code should only be used for newborns assessed and discharged from the hospital or birthing room on the same date)

> **99436:** Attendance at delivery (when requested by delivering physician) and initial stabilization of newborn

> **99440:** Newborn resuscitation: provision of positive pressure ventilation and/or chest compressions in the presence of acute inadequate ventilation and/or cardiac output

Correct Code: 99431

PEDIATRICS/FAMILY PRACTICE SCENARIO

Initial examination and history of a healthy newborn delivered vaginally at the hospital birthing room, and scoring APGARs of 7 and 9. The newborn remained in the birthing room overnight with the mother before discharge.

ICD•9 Diagnosis Code

MULTIPLE SPECIALTIES

This group of codes (99450–99456) covers any purely evaluative services provided by a physician. Use these codes to report evaluations for life or disability insurance eligibility certificates and work-related medical disability. These services can be performed in the office or other setting, and no distinction is made between new or established patient.

These codes should not be used to indicate any active management of problems or conditions. If other E/M services and/or procedures are performed on the same date, report them with the appropriate E/M code in addition to the special evaluation code.

Code 99450 is a basic life or disability examination that includes: a medical history; height, weight, and blood pressure measurement; collecting blood and urine specimens; and filling out the necessary forms and reports.

Codes 99455 and 99456 are used for work-related or medical disability. Use 99455 for the treating physician and 99456 for other than the treating physician.

> **99450:** Basic life and/or disability examination that includes: measurement of height, weight, blood pressure, completion of a medical history following life insurance pro forma; collection of blood sample and/or urinalysis complying with "chain of custody" protocols; and completion of necessary documentation/ certificates.

> **99455:** Work related or medical disability examination by the treating physician that includes: completion of a medical history commensurate with the patient's condition; performance of an examination commensurate with the patient's condition; formulation of a diagnosis, assessment of capabilities and stability, and calculation of impairment; development of future medical treatment plan; and completion of necessary documentation/certificates and report.

> **99456:** Work related or medical disability examination by other than the treating physician that includes: completion of a medical history commensurate with the patient's condition; performance of an examination commensurate with the patient's condition; formulation of a diagnosis, assessment of capabilities and stability, and calculation of impairment; development of future medical treatment plan; and completion of necessary documentation/certificates and report.

Other E/M Services

> **99288:** Physician direction of emergency medical systems (EMS) emergency care, advanced life support

> **99499:** Unlisted evaluation and management service

Chapter Review

Several code subcategories in the E/M section are based on the patient's status as a new or established patient. The keys to selecting the correct level of E/M codes are the first three components of history, examination, and medical decision making. In most cases, all three components must be addressed in the documentation of the encounter. However, in established, subsequent, and follow-up categories, only two of the three must be met or exceeded for a given code level. All pertinent components of the codes must be documented. Physicians and staff members have developed numerous methods to document professional services and there is no single right way as long as all pertinent information is documented. The E/M section is broken down into subcategories by type of service. Review all guidelines in the E/M section of CPT annually. Also review the overview of these codes and the section including scenarios demonstrating how to match the clinical documentation to the proper codes.

KEY POINT

Correctly identifying the level of the three key components of most E/M codes is essential to selecting the correct code.

Review all E/M guidelines annually.

4 Anesthesia

Guidelines

Two organizations are responsible for developing anesthesia codes and guidelines. The American Medical Association (AMA) includes a section on anesthesia codes (00100-01999) in CPT immediately following the E/M section. In addition, CPT includes four codes (99100–99140) to report qualifying circumstances for anesthesia. The American Society of Anesthesiologists (ASA) publishes a Relative Value Guide (RVG) which contains codes from the anesthesia section of CPT but also includes: 1)codes to supplement those in the CPT anesthesia section and 2)codes from other sections of CPT for services frequently provided by anesthesiologists.

CPT and ASA guidelines are similar. Guidelines are as follows:

1. Both specify that reporting of anesthesia services is appropriate when provided by or under the medical supervision of a physician. The ASA further specifies that anesthesia services should be supervised by a physician anesthesiologist.

2. According to both sets of guidelines, anesthesia services include but are not limited to general, regional, supplementation of local anesthesia, and other supportive services required to afford the patient optimal anesthesia care. The ASA includes monitored anesthesia care in the service and also states that you report any professional anesthesia services as if an anesthetic was administered.

3. The ASA publication is a relative value guide. A relative value is a numeric ranking assigned to a procedure in relation to other procedures in terms of work and cost. Therefore, in addition to codes and descriptions, the ASA relative value guide provides information on the value of each anesthesia service. The ASA relative value guide is not a fee schedule, but only a guide intended to assist physicians in developing consistent and equitable fees for their services.

Organization of Anesthesia Codes

CPT

The anesthesia section of CPT is organized into 15 anatomical sites followed by two additional categories for radiological and other procedures. Codes are organized by type of procedure (open, closed, endoscopic, etc.), and each code relates to specific surgical procedures, though there is no one-to-one correspondence. One anesthesia code may be used to report several surgical procedures that share similar anesthesia requirements.

OBJECTIVES

Recognize the roles the AMA and ASA play in anesthesia coding

Learn the special circumstances surrounding anesthesia coding

Understand the standard formula based on units

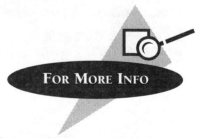

FOR MORE INFO

The two main resources available for coding anesthesia are listed below. Both are published and updated yearly:

- The **AMA**'s *Physicians' Current Procedural Terminology* (CPT)

- The **American Society of Anesthesiologists** (ASA) *Relative Value Guide* (RVG). Contact the ASA at: 520 N. Northwest Highway, Park Ridge, IL 60068-2573, (847) 825-5586

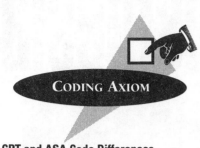

CODING AXIOM

CPT and ASA Code Differences

Following are ASA codes that do not appear in CPT:

00536
00550
00564
00636
00640
01112
01216
01905
01923
01924
01925
01926
01927
01928
01951
01952
01997 (No time is added to this code)
02000
02010
02020 (No time is added to this code)

Anesthesia codes in CPT which are not included in ASA RVG are as follows:

01900
01902
01904
01906
01908
01910
01912
01914
01916
01918

Example 1

01202	Anesthesia for arthroscopic procedures of hip joint

This procedure code would be selected to report anesthesia services related to the following surgical procedures:

29860	Arthroscopy, hip, diagnostic with or without synovial biopsy (separate procedure)
29861	Arthroscopy, hip, surgical; with removal of loose body or foreign body.
29862	with debridement/shaving of articular cartilage (chondroplasty), abrasion arthroplasty, and/or resection of labrum.
29863	with synovectomy

ASA Relative Value Guide

The codes in the main section of the ASA Relative Value Guide are the same as those in CPT with two exceptions: the ASA includes a few codes not found in CPT and excludes a few codes found in CPT. Codes in ASA RVG not found in CPT are designated with two asterisks (**) in front of the code. The codes are listed in the margin. The ASA RVG excludes only the CPT codes listed in the Radiology subsection and these are listed in the margin also.

In addition, some of the narrative descriptions used by the ASA differ slightly from those found in CPT. These are designated by one (*), three (***), or four (****) asterisks in front of the code. Explanations are provided at the bottom of the ASA RVG pages.

The ASA RVG also lists codes for other services frequently provided by anesthesiologists. These codes are CPT codes found in the Evaluation and Management, Medicine, and Surgery sections of CPT. The services include: pulmonary function testing, evaluation and management services, pain management and nerve blocks, and placement of venous catheters and monitoring devices. In all cases, the ASA provides a relative value designation for each code.

Reporting Anesthesia Services

Reporting anesthesia services differs from reporting other types of physician services. Reporting other physician services typically involves selecting the correct CPT code and submitting a specific fee for that CPT code. The fee is the same every time the service is provided. For example, a problem focused established patient exam and history is reported with code 99212 and the fee assigned to that procedure by a given physician is $30. The physician submits the fee of $30 every time he or she performs procedure 99212.

However, anesthesia billing is based on several variables specific to the particular anesthesia service. The fee submitted for a specific anesthesia code varies each time the code is reported.

The key terms described next are essential to the correct reporting of anesthesia services.

KEY TERMS

Basic Value or Base Unit. The basic value, also referred to as the base unit or relative value, has two components. One component reflects all usual services included in the anesthesia service. Usual services include: pre-operative and post-operative visits, administration of fluids and/or blood products incident to the procedure, and interpretation of non-invasive monitoring (ECG, temperature, blood pressure, oximetry, capnography, and mass spectrometry). The second component reflects the relative work or cost of the specific anesthesia service. Cost in this context refers to the physician's cost of doing business. For anesthesiologists , the majority of the cost goes to malpractice insurance. For example, the basic value for the anesthesia service related to a closed reduction of a radius fracture might be 3, as it has a relatively low level of work or cost. The basic value for an anesthesia service associated with an intrathoracic coronary artery bypass graft procedure might be 20, reflecting a high level of work or cost.

The ASA lists two exceptions to using the basic value listed in the Relative Value Guide. A **minimum basic value** of 5 is allowed for all procedures of the head, neck or shoulder girdle, requiring field avoidance. In addition, any procedure performed in any position other than lithotomy or supine has a **minimum basic value** of 5. If the anesthesia code associated with the surgical procedure carries a basic value greater than 5 the higher basic value is reported.

Base units for anesthesia listed in RVG are widely accepted across the United States by both physicians and payors. However, some payors, especially government agency payors, may use different relative value scales developed exclusively for their use. Other payors may use national relative value guides based on RVG, with some modification.

Time. Time is the actual time spent providing the anesthesia service. Time begins as the anesthesiologist prepares the patient for anesthesia care. Time ends when the personal attendance of the anesthesiologist is no longer required and the patient can be safely placed in post-anesthesia recovery under the supervision of nursing or other trained personnel.

Time is reported in units based on defined time increments. The most commonly used time increment is 15 minutes, with one unit being reported for each 15-minute increment. However, time units for anesthesia vary across the country. Both ASA and CPT suggest reporting time increments as customary in the geographic area.

The same holds for reporting fractions of time units. For example, a procedure requiring 65 minutes of anesthesia time, reported in 15-minute time increments, results in total time units of 4.33. In some areas, this is reported as the fractional amount 4.33; other areas might round to the nearest whole number 4; or another geographical area might allow reporting of another full unit for any fractional amount to 5.

For some anesthesia services time is not reported additionally. The ASA RVG designates a +TM after the base unit for procedures requiring time reported separately. Do not list time separately for procedures without the designation.

Physical Status Modifiers. Physical status modifiers reflect the patient's state of health. Individuals undergoing surgery may be healthy or may have varying degrees of systemic disease. A patient's health status affects the work related to providing the anesthesia service. CPT states that physical status modifiers reflect the level of complexity associated with the anesthesia service.

Physical status modifiers in CPT and ASA RVG are represented with the letter P followed by a single digit (e.g., -P1, -P2). ASA RVG lists the number of additional anesthesia units allowed with each physical status modifier to the right in the column titled "units."

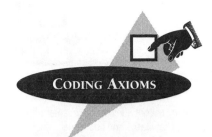

CODING AXIOMS

Medical records should clearly indicate when the patient is released by the anesthesiologist. To qualify for time, the anesthesiologist must be present continuously.

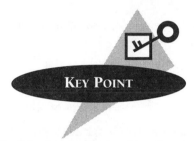

KEY POINT

The following are examples of how time units might be calculated:

Based on 15-minute Increments
Anesthesia provided from 8:00 a.m. to 10:08 a.m.

Time equals two hours and eight minutes, or 128 minutes

| Time | 128 | ÷ | 15-minute time increments |

| Total anesthesia time units billed | = | 8.53 units |

Based on 12-minute Increments
Anesthesia provided from 8:00 a.m. to 10:08 a.m.

Time equals two hours and eight minutes, or 128 minutes

| Time | 128 | ÷ | 12-minute time increments |

| Total anesthesia time units billed | = | 10.66 units |

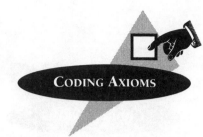

Many payors allow reimbursement for physical status and qualifying circumstances. List the applicable modifier or code (alone) on a separate line.

In actual coding and billing practice, modifier -51 is usually not considered applicable to anesthesia procedures for the following reasons:

1. Only the procedure with the highest basic unit value is reported, not a basic value for each service or code.

2. Time is not reported with a separate procedure code.

3. Physical status and qualifying circumstances are considered additional or "add on" procedures and are not subject to reduced reimbursement.

Check with the payor to determine guidelines for billing anesthesia.

Modifier	Description	Units
-P1	Normal healthy patient	0
-P2	Patient with mild systemic disease	0
-P3	Patient with severe systemic disease	1
-P4	Patient with severe systemic disease that is a constant threat to life	2
-P5	Moribund patient who is not expected to survive without the operation	3
-P6	A declared brain-dead patient whose organs are being removed for donor purposes	0

Qualifying Circumstances. Many anesthesia services are provided under particularly difficult circumstances depending on factors such as extraordinary condition of patient, notable operative conditions, and unusual risk factors. The information provided by both CPT and the ASA RVG includes a list of important qualifying circumstances that significantly impact the character of the anesthesia service provided. These procedures are not be reported alone but as additional procedure numbers to qualify an anesthesia procedure or service. The ASA provides modifying units which may be added to the basic unit values, as follows:

Code	Description	ASA RVG Units
99100	Anesthesia for patient of extreme age, under one year and over seventy	1
99116	Anesthesia complicated by utilization of total body hypothermia	5
99135	Anesthesia complicated by utilization of controlled hypotension	5
99140	Anesthesia complicated by emergency conditions (specify)	2

An emergency exists when a delay in treatment poses a significant increase in the threat to the patient's life or to a body part, as defined in both CPT and ASA RVG.

Conversion Factor. Anesthesia charges must be calculated by means of a conversion factor since the charges are not based on fixed amounts. A conversion factor is the dollar value associated with each unit of anesthesia. The dollar conversion factor is multiplied by the total number of anesthesia units for a given anesthesia service to arrive at the total charges for the anesthesia service.

The dollar conversion factor may vary significantly between geographical regions and to a lesser degree between physicians in a given geographic area. However, the standard formula to calculate total anesthesia units and anesthesia fees is basically the same both among regions and physicians as illustrated in the examples below.

Standard Formula

Now that the basic elements of the anesthesia service have been defined, total anesthesia units for a given anesthesia service can be determined. Using the total units and the conversion factor, the fee for a specific anesthesia service can then be calculated.

The total charge for a specific anesthesia service is calculated by means of the following formula:

Basic Value + Time Units + Modifying Units = Total Units

Total Units X Conversion Factor = Total Fee

Example 1

A closed reduction of a distal radius fracture is accomplished under general anesthesia. The patient is a healthy 10-year-old. The procedure is not performed on an emergency basis. The anesthesiologist reports procedure 01820 which has a basic value of 3. Total time for the procedure is 45 minutes. The anesthesiologist reports time units in 15 minute increments. The total units reported for the procedure are as follows:

Basic Value		3
Time Units (45 divided by 15)	+	3
Physical Status (P1)	+	0
Qualifying Circumstances (none)	+	0
Total Units	=	6

The anesthesiologist uses a conversion factor of $45 per unit of anesthesia.

Total Units		6
Conversion Factor	X	$45
Total Fee	=	$270

Example 2

An emergency appendectomy is performed on a 25-year-old patient with juvenile onset diabetes mellitus that is not well controlled. The anesthesiologist reports procedure 00840 which has a basic value of 6. Total time is 48 minutes. The anesthesiologist reports time units in 12 minute increments.

Basic Value		6
Time Units (48 divided by 12)	+	4
Physical Status (P3)	+	1
Qualifying Circumstances (emergency)	+	2
Total Units	=	13

The anesthesiologist uses a conversion factor of $30 per unit of anesthesia.

Total Units		13
Conversion Factor	X	$30
Total Fee	=	$390

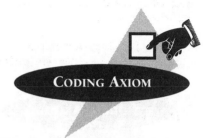

CODING AXIOM

This abbreviation describes the **standard anesthesia formula**:

B + T + M

(basic value + time + modifying circumstances)

A formula may also include **O** (other) for other allowed units charges.

Special Coding Situations

Multiple Procedures

When multiple surgical procedures are performed during a single anesthetic administration, the ASA recommends reporting only the anesthesia procedure with the highest unit value. In other words, only one basic value is assigned per single surgical session.

Additional Procedures

Services not included in the usual anesthesia services may be reported separately. These services include unusual forms of monitoring, prolonged physician services, and provision of additional anesthesia services such as post-operative pain management. These additional services are reported in terms of units with the appropriate CPT or ASA codes under the designation "other procedures." They are calculated as an additional variable in the standard formula.

Unusual monitoring. Unusual forms of monitoring anesthesia are reported by most anesthesiologists and many payors allow benefits beyond the basic anesthesia service. Codes 36488-36491 for insertion of a central venous catheter; 36620-36625 for insertion of an intra-arterial catheter, and 93503 Swan-Ganz insertion, represent unusual forms of monitoring that may be rendered by an anesthesiologist.

Prolonged physician services. Extended pre- or post-operative care provided to a patient whose condition requires services beyond the usual may be reported additionally. These services would be billed with prolonged service codes (99354-99359). (The current ASA RVG does not include these procedures, but lists the deleted CPT codes 99150-99151 instead. Most payors do not recognize these codes as valid and will require reporting with the new codes 99354-99359.)

Post-operative pain management. Normally post-operative pain management is provided or supervised by the surgeon by oral, intramuscular or intravenous medications. Post-operative pain management provided by the surgeon is included in the global fee for the surgical procedure. Some procedures and/or patients require more than the usual type of post-operative pain management, and this is frequently provided or supervised by an anesthesiologist. These services are additional procedures and are reported as follows:

Epidural or subarachnoid pain management is reported with procedure codes 62274-62279 for placement of the epidural or subarachnoid catheter which includes the initial day of pain management. Subsequent management is reported with 01996 and is reported per day.

Patient-controlled analgesia is reported with 01997 on a per day basis. Code 01997 is included only in the ASA Relative Value Guide not in CPT, but is recognized by most payors as a valid code for this anesthesia service.

Post-operative pain management services are not calculated based on time. These services are reported as a single, daily charge.

Monitored (Stand-By) Anesthesia

Monitored anesthesia care is defined in the ASA RVG as those instances when an anesthesiologist has been requested to provide specific services to a patient undergoing a planned procedure. The patient receives either local anesthesia or no anesthesia. However, the anesthesiologist is required to provide pre-operative assessment, to remain in attendance during the procedure to monitor the patient and to administer additional anesthetics should they be required, and to provide post-operative services as required.

Monitored care, as described above, is reported as is customary for any other anesthesia procedure. The procedure should be assigned the applicable anesthesia code with time and modifying units being added as is customary in the local area.

Obstetrical Anesthesia

The formula for reporting of epidural analgesia for labor and delivery may differ from the standard formula in some geographical areas. When epidural analgesia is administered, an anesthesiologist may attend to more than one patient. The anesthesiologist may insert the epidural catheter, start the continuous anesthetic, and leave the patient's bedside. The anesthesiologist periodically returns to check on the patient or to increase the amount of anesthetic while attending to other patients who are also receiving epidurals for vaginal deliveries. For this reason epidural analgesia for labor and delivery may be reimbursed at a reduced rate.

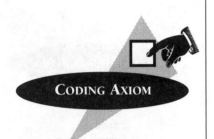

CODING AXIOM

Services not included in the usual anesthesia services may be reported separately. These services include:

- Unusual forms of monitoring

- Prolonged physician services

- Provision of additional anesthesia services

The following are some variations in reporting anesthesia services when the anesthesiologist is not required to be in constant attendance.

1. Basic value and modifying units are reported as usual. The first hour of anesthesia is reported at the usual rate, but subsequent hours are reported at a reduced rate. For example, total units for the first hour would be reported in full, but units for the second hour would be reported at 50 percent, and units for all subsequent hours at 25 percent. If 15-minute time increments were being used the first hour units would be reported as 4 units, the second hour as 2, and third and subsequent hours as 1 unit each.

2. A flat rate may be established and reported regardless of the actual epidural time. Basic value units are included in the flat rate. For example, the anesthesiologist may bill $500 for anesthesia services provided at every vaginal delivery. Modifying units may or may not be reported separately.

3. Basic value and modifying units are reported as usual. Actual time spent in attendance of the patient may be used and reported at the usual rate. For example, a patient who received epidural analgesia for four (4) hours, might have required the anesthesiologist's presence for only two (2) hours of the total time. If 15-minute time increments were used, the anesthesiologist would report 8 units.

These are examples of possible variations and should not be adopted without evaluating current practices in the geographic area. Payors should be queried as to their rules for reporting anesthesia services related to obstetrical care. A coding scenario later in this chapter further demonstrates obstetric coding.

Regional Anesthesia

Disagreement regarding the correct method of reporting regional IV anesthesia centers on code 01995 which has been assigned for regional IV administration of local anesthetic agent (upper or lower extremity). This procedure has no time units associated with it. In practice, anesthesiologists rarely report this service, and instead report regional anesthesia with the anesthesia code which describes the surgical procedure performed. For example regional anesthesia for repair of a tendon injury of the hand is reported with 01810 not 01995. Applicable time and modifying units are reported also.

If the anesthesiologist performs regional anesthesia with the usual pre- and post-operative care and monitors the patient throughout the procedure, the anesthesia code that describes the surgical procedure should be reported along with time and modifying units. However, if the anesthesiologist provides no service other than the initial administration of regional anesthetic, it may be appropriate to report code 01995 instead.

Unusual Anesthesia

CPT defines unusual anesthesia as follows:

-23 Unusual Anesthesia: Occasionally, a procedure, which usually requires either no anesthesia or local anesthesia, must be done under general anesthesia due to unusual circumstances. This circumstance may be reported by adding modifier -23 to the procedure code of the basic service or by use of the separate five-digit modifier code 09923.

Although it is generally inappropriate to report anesthesia with some E/M, medicine, surgery, and radiology codes, there are situations where medical necessity requires anesthesia (e.g. a baby,

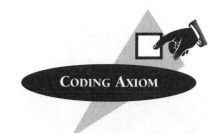

CODING AXIOM

Obstetrical anesthesia code narratives were changed in ASA RVG in 1998. CPT narratives for 1999 were not changed to reflect the changes in ASA RVG, however.

Compare the following:

CPT
00857 Continuous epidural analgesia, for labor and cesarean

ASA
00857 Neuroaxial analgesia/anesthesia for labor ending in cesarean section (This includes any repeat subarachnoid needle placement and drug injection and/or any necessary replacement of an epidural during labor)

CPT
00955 Continuous epidural analgesia, for labor and vaginal delivery

ASA
00955 Neuroaxial analgesia/anesthesia for labor ending in a vaginal delivery (This includes any repeat subarachnoid needle placement and drug injection and/or any necessary replacement of an epidural during labor)

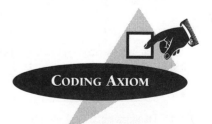

CODING AXIOM

The formula for reporting anesthesia services does not apply to chronic pain management services. These are distinct services that are not based on time, physical status, or qualifying circumstances.

small child, or hard-to-control patient needing dressings and/or debridement). Under these unusual circumstances, payors will usually allow the anesthesia charge. Submit an operative report and cover letter with the claim explaining the need for any unusual anesthesia.

Chronic Pain Management Services

Pre- and post-operative pain management is described under Additional Procedures. However, a different type of pain management service is provided to patients suffering chronic debilitating pain. Chronic pain management services are not anesthesia services. These are distinct services frequently performed by anesthesiologists who have additional training in pain management procedures. Pain management services are reported following the same rules as those for surgical procedures.

Pain management services include: initial and subsequent evaluation and management (E/M) services, trigger point injections, spine and spinal cord injections, and nerve blocks.

E/M services may be reported with outpatient/office codes 99201-99215 or outpatient consultation codes 99241-99245 depending on the nature of the E/M service. Guidelines for reporting E/M are covered in Chapter 3 of *Code It Right*.

Trigger point injections are reported with code 20550. More than one trigger point may be injected per treatment. Use modifier -51 appended to second and subsequent injections on the same date of service.

Codes 62274-62298 report spine and spinal cord injections.

Nerve blocks are reported with codes 64400-64530. Nerve blocks are defined as the introduction or injection of an anesthetic agent into a nerve or nerve branch.

Each code for pain management services should have a specific fee and the fee should be the same each time that specific code is reported. In other words, no adjustments are made based on time, physical status, or qualifying circumstances.

Special Report

A service that is rarely provided, unusual, variable, or new may require a special report to help the payor determine the medical appropriateness of the service. Pertinent information should include an adequate definition or description of the nature, extent, and need for the procedure; and the time, effort, and equipment necessary to provide the service.

Common Billing Errors

Incorrect ICD-9-CM or CPT coding is a frequent problem encountered in anesthesia reporting. The code(s) may be incorrect because they do not match the diagnosis or procedure reported by the surgeon. Claims must reflect the same diagnosis and procedure(s) by the anesthesiologist and surgeon, with the exception of listing a global surgery code when only part of the service is provided.

There are codes in the surgery section of CPT designated as "add on" codes. These add-on codes, however, are not used for coding anesthesia services.

For example, 11001 is an "add on" code. The primary procedure code is 11000* *Debridement of extensive eczematous or infected skin; up to 10 percent of body surface*. Note that 11001 should not be reported alone but always with or "in addition to" 11000* because its description states each additional 10 percent of the body surface. In this case, the appropriate CPT code for determining anesthesia base units and guidelines is 11000*.

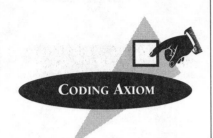

CODING AXIOM

The formula for reporting anesthesia services does not apply to chronic pain management services. These are distinct services that are not based on time, physical status, or qualifying circumstances.

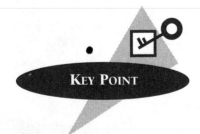

KEY POINT

Additional items which may be included in a **special report** are:

- complexity of symptoms
- final diagnosis
- pertinent physical findings
- diagnostic and therapeutic procedures
- concurrent problems
- follow-up care

Payor Requirements

While most payors recognize anesthesia codes 00100-01999, some payors do not and require the use of CPT codes from the surgery section (10040-69990) to report anesthesia services. This complicates the reporting of anesthesia services since it requires the anesthesiologist to understand surgery coding. Or, the surgeon and anesthesiologist must coordinate billing so that both assign the same surgical procedure code. To simplify this process, many anesthesiologists purchase software or publications with CPT anesthesia/surgery crosswalks in order to verify that the correct code has been selected.

DISCUSSION QUESTIONS

1. List the two main resources for coding anesthesia.

    _____

    _____

    _____

2. Explain the formula for calculating an anesthesia charge.

    _____

    _____

    _____

3. What are qualifying circumstances and how are they identified when coding?

    _____

    _____

    _____

4. Epidural analgesia for labor and vaginal delivery is often reported differently than other anesthesia services. Explain the rationale for variations in reporting this service.

    _____

    _____

    _____

5. Explain how reporting of chronic pain management services differ from other services provided by anesthesiologists.

    _____

    _____

    _____

Specialty-Specific Scenarios

The following scenarios are designed to help you make the leap from documentation to correct code choices. Some payors accept only surgery codes for anesthesia billing, so the scenarios in this section demonstrate the use of anesthesia codes and surgery codes.

OBJECTIVES

See the practical application of anesthesia coding

Identify the special circumstances and rules of specialties

OBSTETRICS SCENARIO

A female patient delivered a single, liveborn infant by cesarean section due to a breech presentation. The patient was under epidural analgesia. Code the ICD-9-CM diagnoses, CPT anesthesia, and surgery codes for the mother.

Anesthesia Codes

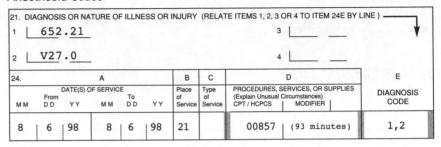

ICD-9-CM

652.21	Breech presentation without mention of version, delivered
V27.0	Outcome of delivery, single, liveborn

CPT

00857	Continuous epidural analgesia, for labor and cesarean section (CPT)

ASA

00857	Neuroaxial analgesia/anesthesia for labor ending in cesarean section (This includes any repeat subarachnoid needle placement and drug injection and/or any necessary replacement of an epidural during labor)

Surgery Codes

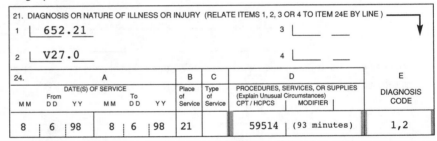

ICD-9-CM

652.21	Breech presentation without mention of version, delivered
V27.0	Outcome of delivery, single, liveborn

CPT

59514	Cesarean delivery only

MEDICAL SPECIALTIES-FAMILY PRACTICE SCENARIO

A patient had a normal, spontaneous, vaginal delivery of a single, liveborn infant while under epidural analgesia. Select the diagnosis, CPT anesthesia, and surgery codes for the mother.

Anesthesia Codes

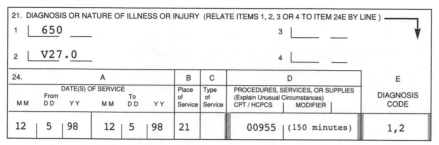

ICD-9-CM
650 Normal delivery
V27.0 Outcome of delivery, single liveborn

CPT
00955 Continuous epidural analgesia, for labor and vaginal delivery (CPT)

ASA
00955 Neuroaxial analgesia/anesthesia for labor ending in a vaginal delivery (This includes any repeat subarachnoid needle placement and drug injection and/or any necessary replacement of an epidural during labor)

Surgery Codes

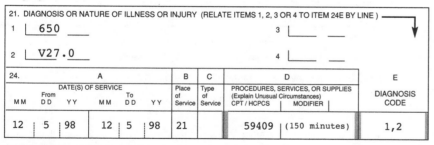

ICD-9-CM
650 Normal delivery
V27.0 Outcome of delivery, single liveborn

CPT
59409 Vaginal delivery only (with or without episiotomy and/or forceps)

There are cases when the anesthesiologist's procedure code does not match the surgeon's. Often, the obstetrician will use a global code for the antepartum, delivery, and postpartum care. Because the anesthesiologist attends only during delivery, his or her claim reports a code for only the delivery. The payor may require surgery codes instead of anesthesia codes to report anesthesia services.

Obstetrical anesthesia can be accomplished by epidural or general anesthesia. Calculation of time units for epidural analgesia for vaginal deliveries may vary from the standard formula. Consult professional organizations and payors to learn about coding practices specific to the local area.

When labor for a vaginal delivery fails and a cesarean is necessary, code only the procedure with the highest number of units. In this scenario it is the cesarean base units, not the base units for both procedures. Even though time units in some locations may be reduced for the vaginal epidural anesthetic, they are not reduced for a cesarean delivery when the anesthesiologist must be present continuously.

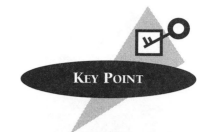

KEY POINT

Calculation of time units for epidural analgesia for vaginal deliveries may vary from the standard formula.

- Note that narrative descriptions for CPT and ASA differ for codes 00857 and 00955. ASA provides additional guidelines regarding replacement of the epidural and subarachnoid needle or catheter which are not included in CPT. Specifically, replacement is not reported separately.

RECONSTRUCTIVE SURGERY SCENARIO

A reconstructive surgeon requests that the anesthesiologist assume the care of the surgery patient for postoperative epidural pain management. The patient had a general anesthetic for a reimplantation of the right foot after a traumatic complete amputation. The injuries occurred when the patient was accidentally run over by machinery on his farm. Postoperative pain management requires placement of an epidural catheter for continuous injection of anesthetic. Daily pain management is provided for three additional days subsequent to the placement of the catheter. Code the ICD-9-CM diagnoses codes and the CPT anesthesia epidural pain management code.

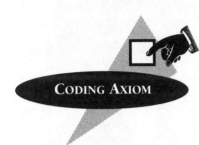

Consultations for pain management are not separately reported on the same day as placement of the catheter when provided as part of the daily management of epidural or subarachnoid drug administration.

Epidural Pain Management

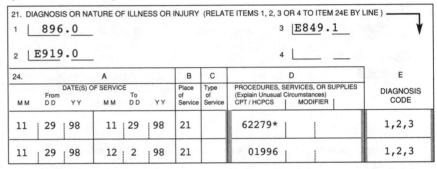

21. DIAGNOSIS OR NATURE OF ILLNESS OR INJURY (RELATE ITEMS 1, 2, 3 OR 4 TO ITEM 24E BY LINE)
1. 896.0   3. E849.1
2. E919.0   4.

24.	A					B	C	D		E
	DATE(S) OF SERVICE					Place of Service	Type of Service	PROCEDURES, SERVICES, OR SUPPLIES (Explain Unusual Circumstances)		DIAGNOSIS CODE
	MM	From DD	YY	MM	To DD	YY			CPT / HCPCS	MODIFIER	
	11	29	98	11	29	98	21		62279*		1,2,3
	11	29	98	12	2	98	21		01996		1,2,3

ICD-9-CM

896.0   Unilateral, traumatic amputation of foot

E919.0   Accident caused by agriculture machine

E849.1   Place of occurrence, farm

CPT

62279*   Injection of diagnostic or therapeutic anesthetic or antispasmodic substance (including narcotics); epidural, lumbar or caudal, continuous

01996   Daily management of epidural or subarachnoid drug administration (x 4)

Time is not a factor when reporting codes 62279* or 01996. Typically, the formula for payment calculation is the dollar conversion factor multiplied by the number of base units assigned to the code.

Code 62279 does not include daily management (01996), and should be reported separately if provided on the same date of service as placement of the catheter.

However, some payors will not allow payment for daily epidural pain management (01996) on the same day as the initial placement of the catheter, so check with indiviual payors. Replacement or repositioning of the catheter may be reported additionally though not all payors will allow additional payment.

Consultations for pain management are not separately reported on the same day as placement of the catheter or on the same day as daily management of epidural or subarachnoid drug administration.

ORTHOPEDIC SURGERY SCENARIO

A 35-year-old patient sustained an injury to his right hand while operating a hand power saw at work. The injury consisted of a complicated laceration involving a digital artery and nerve.

The patient was taken to the operating room where the arm was prepped and draped and regional anesthesia was administered by an anesthesiologist. The patient was monitored by the anesthesiologist throughout the procedure and received the usual pre- and postoperative care. The hand surgeon initially debrided nonviable tissue and performed a primary repair of the artery and nerve with the use of an operating microscope. It was necessary to further excise and undermine the wound edges to accomplish a complex closure of the 7.0 cm laceration. A sterile dressing and short arm splint were applied at the end of the procedure. Select the ICD-9-CM diagnoses and CPT anesthesia and surgery codes to report the anesthesia services performed by an anesthesiologist.

KEY POINT

Regional anesthesia is reported with the same codes and standard formula as general anesthesia when the anesthesiologist provides pre- and post-operative care and monitors the patient throughout the procedure. Code 01995 is reported for regional blocks only when the anesthesiologist administers the block but does not provide other pre-, post-, or intraoperative care.

Anesthesia Codes

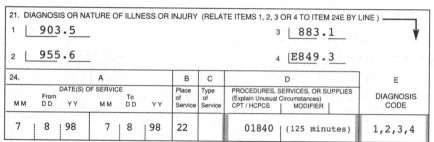

ICD-9-CM

903.5	Injury of blood vessel of upper extremity, digital blood vessels
955.6	Injury to peripheral nerve(s) of shoulder girdle and upper limb, digital nerve
883.1	Open wound of finger(s), complicated
E849.3	Place of occurrence, industrial place and premises

CPT

01840	Anesthesia for procedures on arteries of forearm, wrist, and hand; not otherwise specified

Surgery Codes

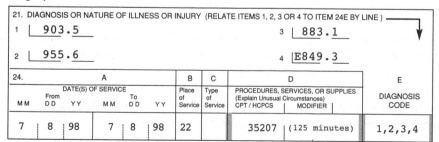

ICD-9-CM

903.5	Injury of blood vessel of upper extremity, digital blood vessels
955.6	Injury to peripheral nerve(s) of shoulder girdle and upper limb, digital nerve
883.1	Open wound of finger(s), complicated
E849.3	Place of occurrence, industrial place and premises

CPT

35207	Repair blood vessel, direct; hand, finger

E920.1 *Accident caused by powered hand tool*, is appropriate, also. However, only four spaces are provided on the HCFA-1500 for reporting diagnoses. Report the place of occurrence when only one space is available for an E code. Payors need this information for coordination of benefits (COB).

An anesthesiologist or a surgeon can provide regional anesthesia. If provided by an anesthesiologist, a CPT anesthesia code is reported. If provided by a surgeon, report the surgery CPT code with modifier -47 or 09947. Modifier -47 is never used as a modifier for anesthesia procedures 00100–01999.

The code with the highest basic value is reported for multiple surgical procedures. The coder must code all of the procedures to determine which code has the highest base unit value. Base values for all codes are not reported. In this scenario, the CPT codes are 35207, 64831, and 13132. Code 35207 is used in this scenario because it has the highest number of base units. Anesthesia codes related to this service include 01810 and 01840. Code 01840 is reported since it has the highest basic value.

NEUROSURGERY SCENARIO

A 40-year-old patient was brought to surgery for evaluation and removal of a mass of unknown nature in the thalamic region of the brain. After a stereotactic biopsy which showed a primary malignant neoplasm, a craniotomy was performed in a sitting position during the same operative session. The mass was visualized by an operating microscope and removed without difficulty. Code the ICD-9-CM diagnosis and CPT anesthesia and surgery codes used to report the anesthesia services.

Anesthesia Codes

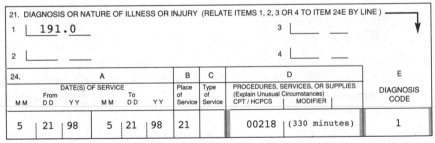

21. DIAGNOSIS OR NATURE OF ILLNESS OR INJURY (RELATE ITEMS 1, 2, 3 OR 4 TO ITEM 24E BY LINE)						
1. 191.0				3. ___ . ___		
2. ___ . ___				4. ___ . ___		

24. A	B	C	D	E
DATE(S) OF SERVICE	Place of Service	Type of Service	PROCEDURES, SERVICES, OR SUPPLIES (Explain Unusual Circumstances)	DIAGNOSIS CODE
From To MM DD YY MM DD YY			CPT / HCPCS MODIFIER	
5 21 98 5 21 98	21		00218 (330 minutes)	1

ICD-9-CM

191.0 Malignant neoplasm of cerebrum, except lobes and ventricles

CPT

00218 Anesthesia for intracranial procedures; procedures in sitting position

---

Surgery Codes

21. DIAGNOSIS OR NATURE OF ILLNESS OR INJURY (RELATE ITEMS 1, 2, 3 OR 4 TO ITEM 24E BY LINE)			
1 191.0		3	
2		4	

24.	A					B	C	D		E
	DATE(S) OF SERVICE					Place of Service	Type of Service	PROCEDURES, SERVICES, OR SUPPLIES (Explain Unusual Circumstances)		DIAGNOSIS CODE
	From			To				CPT / HCPCS	MODIFIER	
MM	DD	YY	MM	DD	YY					
5	21	98	5	21	98	21		61518	(330 minutes)	1

ICD-9-CM

191.0 Malignant neoplasm of cerebrum, except lobes and ventricles

CPT

61518 Craniectomy for excision of brain tumor, infratentorial or posterior fossa; except meningioma, cerebellopontine angle tumor, or midline tumor at base of skull

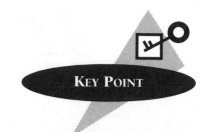

ASA RVG allows a minimum of five base units when the procedure is performed around the head, neck, or shoulder girdle and requires field avoidance or when the patient is in a position other than lithotomy or supine.

Report only the code with the highest base units. Time is reported as is customary in the local area. Physical status modifiers and qualifying circumstance do not apply to this anesthesia case. The scenario does not mention any unusual forms of monitoring, materials supplied by the physician, physical status, qualifying circumstances, or other services. The ASA RVG lists a minimum of five base units for field avoidance: when a procedure is performed around the head, neck, or shoulder girdle, or when the patient is positioned other than lithotomy or supine, even if the procedure performed has a lesser value. However, the anesthesia code 00218 has a higher basic value of 13 in ASA RVG, so the higher value (i.e., 13) is reported. For more information on ASA guidelines, consult the RVG.

GENERAL SURGERY SCENARIO

An 80-year-old woman with an acute bowel obstruction and severe systemic disease was taken to the OR where her surgeon resected two feet of necrotic proximal jejunum due to volvulus. Before he could reconnect the bowel, the patient became hemodynamically unstable due to heart failure. The case was terminated. The jejunum was closed with bowel clips and the patient was taken to the ICU. After 24 hours of aggressive medical management the patient was diagnosed with congestive heart failure. She was stabilized and taken back to the OR to complete the anastomosis of the jejunum. Code the ICD-9-CM diagnoses and CPT anesthesia and surgery codes that should be used to report the anesthesia services for the two separate dates.

KEY POINT

Most issues related to terminated procedures affect surgeon coding and not anesthesia coding. Information about discontinued procedures as they relate to the surgeon is covered in the surgery section.

Anesthesia Codes — First Surgery

21. DIAGNOSIS OR NATURE OF ILLNESS OR INJURY (RELATE ITEMS 1, 2, 3 OR 4 TO ITEM 24E BY LINE)		
1 │ 560.2	3 │ V64.1	
2 │ 997.1	4 │	

24.	A					B	C	D		E
	DATE(S) OF SERVICE					Place of Service	Type of Service	PROCEDURES, SERVICES, OR SUPPLIES (Explain Unusual Circumstances)		DIAGNOSIS CODE
	From			To				CPT / HCPCS	MODIFIER	
MM	DD	YY	MM	DD	YY					
6	30	98	6	30	98	21		00840	–P3 (125 minutes)	1,2,3
6	30	98	6	30	98	21		99100		1,2,3

ICD-9-CM

560.2   Intestinal obstruction without mention of hernia, volvulus

997.1   Cardiac complications, during or resulting from a procedure

V64.1   Surgical or other procedure not carried out because of contraindication

CPT

00840-P3   Anesthesia for intraperitoneal procedures in lower abdomen including laparoscopy; not otherwise specified; -P3 appended to 00840 — Patient with severe systemic disease

99100   Anesthesia for patient of extreme age, under one year and over seventy

Surgery Codes — First Surgery

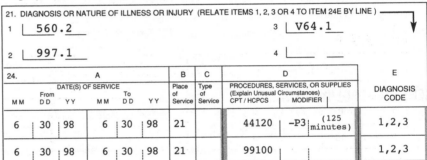

21. DIAGNOSIS OR NATURE OF ILLNESS OR INJURY (RELATE ITEMS 1, 2, 3 OR 4 TO ITEM 24E BY LINE)		
1 │ 560.2	3 │ V64.1	
2 │ 997.1	4 │	

24.	A					B	C	D		E
	DATE(S) OF SERVICE					Place of Service	Type of Service	PROCEDURES, SERVICES, OR SUPPLIES (Explain Unusual Circumstances)		DIAGNOSIS CODE
	From			To				CPT / HCPCS	MODIFIER	
MM	DD	YY	MM	DD	YY					
6	30	98	6	30	98	21		44120	–P3 (125 minutes)	1,2,3
6	30	98	6	30	98	21		99100		1,2,3

ICD-9-CM

560.2   Intestinal obstruction without mention of hernia, volvulus

997.1   Cardiac complications, during or resulting from a procedure

V64.1   Surgical or other procedure not carried out because of contraindication

CPT

44120-P3   Enterectomy, resection of small intestine; single resection and anastomosis — Patient with severe systemic disease

99100   Anesthesia for patient of extreme age, under one year and over seventy

Anesthesia Codes — Second Surgery

21. DIAGNOSIS OR NATURE OF ILLNESS OR INJURY (RELATE ITEMS 1, 2, 3 OR 4 TO ITEM 24E BY LINE)
1 ⎿ 863.39   3 ⎿___ __
2 ⎿ 428.0   4 ⎿___ __

24.	A					B	C	D		E
	DATE(S) OF SERVICE					Place of Service	Type of Service	PROCEDURES, SERVICES, OR SUPPLIES (Explain Unusual Circumstances)		DIAGNOSIS CODE
	From MM	DD	YY	To MM	DD YY			CPT / HCPCS	MODIFIER	
	7	1	98	7	1 98	21		00840	–P3 (140 minutes)	1,2
	7	1	98	7	1 98	21		99100		1,2

ICD-9-CM

863.39   Injury of small intestine with open wound into cavity

428.0   Congestive heart failure

CPT

00840-P3   Anesthesia for intraperitoneal procedures in lower abdomen including laparoscopy; not otherwise specified; -P3 appended to 00840 both surgeries — Patient with severe systemic disease

99100   Anesthesia for patient of extreme age, under one year and over seventy

Surgery Codes — Second Surgery

21. DIAGNOSIS OR NATURE OF ILLNESS OR INJURY (RELATE ITEMS 1, 2, 3 OR 4 TO ITEM 24E BY LINE)
1 ⎿ 863.39   3 ⎿___ __
2 ⎿ 428.0   4 ⎿___ __

24.	A					B	C	D		E
	DATE(S) OF SERVICE					Place of Service	Type of Service	PROCEDURES, SERVICES, OR SUPPLIES (Explain Unusual Circumstances)		DIAGNOSIS CODE
	From MM	DD	YY	To MM	DD YY			CPT / HCPCS	MODIFIER	
	7	1	98	7	1 98	21		44130	–P3 (140 minutes)	1,2
	7	1	98	7	1 98	21		99100		1,2

ICD-9-CM

863.39   Injury of small intestine with open wound into cavity

428.0   Congestive heart failure

CPT

44130-P3   Enteroenterostomy, anastomosis of intestine, with or without cutaneous enterostomy (separate procedure) — Patient with severe systemic disease

99100   Anesthesia for patient of extreme age, under one year and over seventy

The anesthesiologist reports the basic value, time, modifying circumstances, and any other reportable services for both days. The diagnosis for the second procedure reflects the reason for the current operative service, and is not the same as that reported for the first procedure. A special report should be sent explaining the nature, extent, and need for the procedure since the most appropriate diagnosis code 863.39 *Injury of small intestine with open wound into cavity*, does not fully reflect the circumstances related to this procedure.

KEY POINT

A special report should be sent with any service that is unusual, variable, or new.

Append modifier -23, Unusual anesthesia when a procedure which does not normally require a general anesthetic is performed with a general anesthetic.

ORAL AND MAXILLOFACIAL SURGERY SCENARIO

An oral maxillary surgeon requested general anesthesia for a child with active autism to facilitate drainage of an abscess from a dentoalveolar structure. Code the ICD-9-CM diagnoses and CPT procedure codes for the anesthesiologist.

Anesthesia Codes

21. DIAGNOSIS OR NATURE OF ILLNESS OR INJURY (RELATE ITEMS 1, 2, 3 OR 4 TO ITEM 24E BY LINE)						
1 ∟ 522.5				3 ∟		
2 ∟ 299.00				4 ∟		

24.	A				B	C	D		E
	DATE(S) OF SERVICE				Place of Service	Type of Service	PROCEDURES, SERVICES, OR SUPPLIES (Explain Unusual Circumstances)		DIAGNOSIS CODE
	From MM DD YY		To MM DD YY				CPT / HCPCS	MODIFIER	
	9 ¦ 26 ¦ 98		9 ¦ 26 ¦ 98		11		00170	–23 ¦ (55 minutes)	1,2

ICD-9-CM

522.5   Periapical abscess without sinus

299.00   Infantile autism, current or active state

CPT

00170-23   Anesthesia for intraoral procedures, including biopsy; not otherwise specified — Unusual anesthesia

Surgery Codes

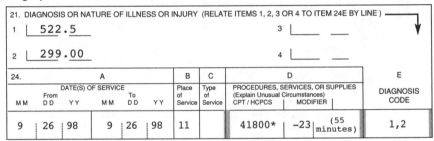

21. DIAGNOSIS OR NATURE OF ILLNESS OR INJURY (RELATE ITEMS 1, 2, 3 OR 4 TO ITEM 24E BY LINE)						
1 ∟ 522.5				3 ∟		
2 ∟ 299.00				4 ∟		

24.	A				B	C	D		E
	DATE(S) OF SERVICE				Place of Service	Type of Service	PROCEDURES, SERVICES, OR SUPPLIES (Explain Unusual Circumstances)		DIAGNOSIS CODE
	From MM DD YY		To MM DD YY				CPT / HCPCS	MODIFIER	
	9 ¦ 26 ¦ 98		9 ¦ 26 ¦ 98		11		41800*	–23 ¦ (55 minutes)	1,2

ICD-9-CM

522.5   Periapical abscess without sinus

299.00   Infantile autism, current or active state

CPT

41800*-23   Drainage of abscess, cyst, hematoma from dentoalveolar structures — Unusual anesthesia

Modifier -23 *Unusual anesthesia* specifies that occasionally, a procedure that usually requires no general anesthesia must be done under general anesthesia due to unusual circumstances. This circumstance may be reported by adding -23 to the procedure code or by reporting 09923.

Modifier -23 can be used with surgery codes since CPT does not specify to the contrary. An example of a modifier excluded from specific use is modifier -47. CPT states it should never be appended to the anesthesia codes.

GENERAL SURGERY SCENARIO

An emergency appendectomy is performed on an otherwise healthy 28-year-old male with appendicitis complicated by peritonitis. The anesthesiologist performed a venipuncture for administration of IV fluids. Code the ICD-9-CM diagnosis and CPT anesthesia and surgery procedures for the anesthesiologist.

Anesthesia Codes

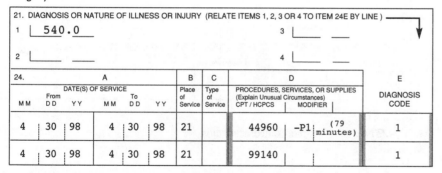

ICD-9-CM

540.0   Acute appendicitis with generalized peritonitis

CPT

00840-P1   Anesthesia for intraperitoneal procedures in lower abdomen including laparoscopy; not otherwise specified — A normal healthy patient

99140   Anesthesia complicated by emergency conditions

Surgery Codes

24. A DATE(S) OF SERVICE From MM DD YY / To MM DD YY	B Place of Service	C Type of Service	D PROCEDURES, SERVICES, OR SUPPLIES CPT/HCPCS	MODIFIER	E DIAGNOSIS CODE
4 30 98 / 4 30 98	21		44960	-P1 (79 minutes)	1
4 30 98 / 4 30 98	21		99140		1

Diagnosis 21: 1. 540.0

ICD-9-CM

540.0   Acute appendicitis with generalized peritonitis

CPT

44960-P1   Appendectomy; for ruptured appendix with abscess or generalized peritonitis — A normal healthy patient

99140   Anesthesia complicated by emergency conditions

Anesthesia guidelines state that anesthesia services include the usual preoperative and postoperative visits, the anesthesia care during the procedure, the administration of fluids and/or blood, and the usual monitoring services (e.g., ECG, temperature, blood pressure, oximetry, capnography, and mass spectrometry). Therefore, the venipuncture for administration of IV fluids is not reported separately.

KEY POINT

ASA and CPT narrative descriptions and codes differ for ventriculography procedures. The correct code when reporting ASA codes is 00214. The correct code when reporting CPT anesthesia codes is 01902. Consult individual payors when reporting this service.

RADIOLOGY SCENARIO

A 25-year-old patient with acquired hydrocephalus underwent a burr hole for a ventriculography. The patient was under anesthesia and the procedure was performed in the radiology department at a local hospital. The radiologist performed the injection of gas into the lateral ventricle through the burr hole and interpreted and reported the results of the ventriculogram. Identify the CPT codes reporting the services of the anesthesiologist.

Anesthesia Codes

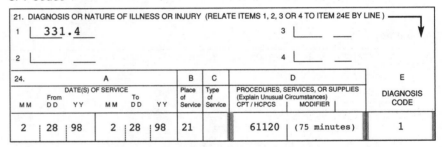

ICD-9-CM

331.4   Obstructive hydrocephalus

CPT

01902   Anesthesia for burr hole(s) for ventriculography

CPT Codes

21. DIAGNOSIS OR NATURE OF ILLNESS OR INJURY (RELATE ITEMS 1, 2, 3 OR 4 TO ITEM 24E BY LINE)					
1 ␣ 331.4			3 ␣ ␣		
2 ␣ ␣			4 ␣ ␣		

24.	A DATE(S) OF SERVICE		B Place of Service	C Type of Service	D PROCEDURES, SERVICES, OR SUPPLIES (Explain Unusual Circumstances) CPT / HCPCS MODIFIER	E DIAGNOSIS CODE
	From MM DD YY	To MM DD YY				
	2 ␣ 28 ␣ 98	2 ␣ 28 ␣ 98	21		61120 (75 minutes)	1

ICD-9-CM

331.4   Obstructive hydrocephalus

CPT

61120   Burr hole(s) for ventricular puncture (including injection of gas, contrast media, dye, or radioactive material)

Code 01902 is only listed in CPT and should be used for anesthesia for burr hole(s) for ventriculography. Code 00214 as described in CPT is used for anesthesia for intracranial procedures burr holes. However, CPT and ASA descriptions differ for code 00214. The ASA description states that it includes burr holes for ventriculography. The ASA does not list code 01902 in RVG. Therefore, code selection should be based on payor requirements. For payors using ASA codes, report 00214. For payors requiring CPT anesthesia codes, report 01902.

Advanced Coding Practice

CODING PRACTICE 1
An 82-year-old woman slipped on ice while crossing the street sustaining a femoral neck fracture. Open treatment of the fracture with prosthetic replacement was performed. The patient has adult onset diabetes (non-insulin dependent), which is not well controlled, as well as mild congestive heart failure. Code the anesthesia services (including physical status and qualifying circumstances) using both anesthesia codes and CPT surgery codes.

21. DIAGNOSIS OR NATURE OF ILLNESS OR INJURY (RELATE ITEMS 1, 2, 3 OR 4 TO ITEM 24E BY LINE)				
1		3		
2		4		

24. A DATE(S) OF SERVICE		B Place of Service	C Type of Service	D PROCEDURES, SERVICES, OR SUPPLIES (Explain Unusual Circumstances) CPT/HCPCS MODIFIER	E DIAGNOSIS CODE
From MM DD YY	To MM DD YY				

CODING PRACTICE 2

A 47-year-old woman was admitted for an outpatient laparoscopic procedure to treat chronic cholecystitis with cholelithiasis. Due to the patient's obesity, the surgeon was unable to perform the procedure laparoscopically and an open cholecystectomy with cholangiography was performed. The patient was admitted to the hospital as an inpatient. Code the anesthesia services (including physical status and qualifying circumstances) using both anesthesia codes and CPT surgery codes.

21. DIAGNOSIS OR NATURE OF ILLNESS OR INJURY (RELATE ITEMS 1, 2, 3 OR 4 TO ITEM 24E BY LINE)
1 ⎣___ ___   3 ⎣___ ___
2 ⎣___ ___   4 ⎣___ ___

24. A DATE(S) OF SERVICE						B Place of Service	C Type of Service	D PROCEDURES, SERVICES, OR SUPPLIES (Explain Unusual Circumstances) CPT/HCPCS MODIFIER	E DIAGNOSIS CODE
From MM DD YY			To MM DD YY						

Chapter Review

The differences in coding methodology, payor guidelines, and the combination of anesthesia and surgery codes used to report anesthesia services complicate anesthesia coding. To report anesthesia services accurately, it is necessary to understand the main terms, concepts, and logic behind anesthesia coding as well as the resources available for code selection. The two main resources available for coding anesthesia are the AMA's CPT and the ASA's RVG.

5 Surgery Services

Surgery Codes and Guidelines

The surgery section (10040-69979) is the largest section of CPT. It is divided into 17 subsections by body system (integumentary, endocrine), procedure site (mediastinum and diaphragm), or type of service (maternity care and delivery). The subsections are as follows:

Integumentary System
Musculoskeletal System
Respiratory System
Cardiovascular System
Hemic and Lymphatic Systems
Mediastinum and Diaphragm
Digestive System
Urinary System
Male Genital System
Intersex Surgery
Laparoscopy/Hysteroscopy
Female Genital System
Maternity Care and Delivery
Endocrine System
Nervous System
Eye and Ocular Adnexa
Auditory System

Guidelines which apply to all surgical codes are found at the beginning of the surgery section. In addition, guidelines or notes, specific to subsections, groups of codes and single codes are found throughout the surgery section. Guidelines, including terms and concepts, important to all surgical codes will be explained first. Then guidelines and notes specific to subsections or codes will be reviewed.

GENERAL GUIDELINES

Surgical procedures can generally be divided into two categories: diagnostic and therapeutic. Within those two broad categories, surgical procedures are either described as "package" services or "starred procedures." Understanding each of these terms and the special coding rules that apply to these different services is the key to correct coding.

OBJECTIVES

- **Define starred and packaged procedures, and the coding rules which apply to each**

- **Define diagnostic and therapeutic procedures, and the coding rules specific to each**

- **Identify minor procedures included in a surgical package**

- **Understand payor policies affecting the surgical package**

- **Learn to avoid unbundling or fragmentation in billing**

- **Identify the subsections with special instructions and learn how to apply these instructions to selected scenarios**

- **Learn to use modifiers to explain special circumstances affecting surgical care**

- **Identify the types of materials supplied by a physician that can be billed separately and how to bill for these materials**

CODING AXIOM

Although there may be a CPT code describing a procedure, payors are not obligated to reimburse a physician for that service. In other words, the fact that there is a code does not necessarily mean you will get paid.

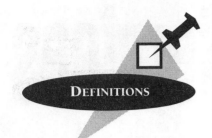

Surgical package defines the normal, uncomplicated performance of specific surgical services, with the assumption that on average, all surgical procedures of a given type are similar with respect to skill-level, duration, and length of normal uncomplicated follow-up care.

One form of **unbundling** or **fragmentation** is the process of breaking a surgical service into its multiple components, and reporting each component separately.

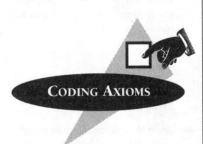

Normal postoperative care cannot be reported in addition to the surgical procedure. These follow-up days vary according to the payor and/or surgery. Medicare follow-up days differ by procedure, but will be assigned a standard follow-up period of 0, 10, or 90 days. A private payor may assign 0, 15, 45, or 90 days to a given procedure.

Examples of minor procedures considered by most payors to be part of the package for a primary surgical service include:

- Local infiltration of medication

- Closure of surgically created wounds, and minor debridement

- Lysis of moderate amounts of adhesions and fulguration of bleeding points

- Application of dressings and immobilizing splints

SURGICAL PACKAGE

The majority of the CPT surgical codes are "package" services; they include the actual surgical procedure, local infiltration, metacarpal and digital block or topical anesthesia (when used), and the normal, uncomplicated postoperative care. When a patient is seen for a routine follow-up postoperative visit within the normal follow-up period, use 99024 for normal uncomplicated postoperative care for documentation purposes only.

Services not defined in CPT as part of the surgical package include: preoperative care, care for postoperative complications, and care for unrelated conditions.

While preoperative care is not identified in CPT as included in the surgical package, many payors have strict guidelines related to reimbursement for preoperative services. Additional reimbursement for preoperative evaluation and management services is usually allowed prior to the decision for surgery or to establish the need for surgery. Reimbursement may be denied for any care provided after the decision for surgical intervention has been made.

However, some payors may identify a specific preoperative period (24 hours to 3 days), during which no additional reimbursement will be made for evaluation and management services. Because of these differing payor policies, it is important for individual providers to establish a policy related to the reporting of preoperative services. Patients should be made aware of this policy. Review contractual arrangements with payors to verify that your policy is not in violation of those contracts.

Postoperative complications are not included in the surgical package and should be reported separately. Postoperative complications include conditions such as wound dehiscence, infection, and bleeding. A diagnosis code should be assigned to reflect the nature of the complication when billing for services rendered to treat the complication.

Unrelated care is always coded. Report services unrelated to the operative problem, such as care for other diseases or injuries, with an appropriate inpatient or outpatient level of service modifier and a corresponding diagnostic code that identifies a problem other than the surgical diagnosis.

STARRED PROCEDURES

Certain relatively small surgical procedures are characterized by variable pre- and postoperative services. Because of these indefinite parameters, the usual package concept for surgical services cannot be applied. Such procedures are identified by a star (*) following the procedure code.

When a star follows a surgical procedure code, the service listed includes only the surgical procedure, not any associated pre- and postoperative services. Following is an example that illustrates a starred procedure, for an initial service, when the starred procedure constitutes the major service.

An 8-year-old boy steps on a piece of glass at home and is treated by a family practitioner. The medical record states, "Incision and removal of glass fragments in subcutaneous tissue, foot." The physician treats the patient in his office and uses his own surgical tray.

Starred Procedures

21. DIAGNOSIS OR NATURE OF ILLNESS OR INJURY (RELATE ITEMS 1, 2, 3 OR 4 TO ITEM 24E BY LINE)		
1. 892.0		3. E849.0
2. E920.8		4.

24. A DATE(S) OF SERVICE						B Place of Service	C Type of Service	D PROCEDURES, SERVICES, OR SUPPLIES (Explain Unusual Circumstances) CPT / HCPCS MODIFIER	E DIAGNOSIS CODE
From MM	DD	YY	To MM	DD	YY				
3	5	98	3	5	98	11		10120*	1,2,3
3	5	98	3	5	98	11		99025	1,2,3
3	5	98	3	5	98	11		A4550 *or*	1,2,3
3	5	98	3	5	98	11		99070	1,2,2

ICD-9-CM

892.0 Open wound of foot except toe(s) alone, without mention of complication

E920.8 Accident caused by other specified cutting and piercing instruments or objects

E849.0 Place of occurrence, home

CPT

10120* Incision and removal of foreign body, subcutaneous tissues; simple

99025 Initial (new patient) visit when starred (*) surgical procedure constitutes major service at that visit

A4550 Surgical tray

or

99070 Supplies and materials (except spectacles), provided by the physician over and above those usually included with the office visit or other services rendered (list drugs, trays, supplies, or materials provided)

Preoperative Services

Preoperative services are reported as follows:

- When a starred procedure is the major service provided to a new patient, procedure 99025 should be listed in lieu of the usual initial visit.

- When the starred procedure is performed along with other significant identifiable services, the appropriate evaluation and management visit should be reported in addition to the starred procedure.

- When a starred procedure is the major service provided to an established patient, only the starred procedure is reported.

- When the starred procedure requires hospitalization, an appropriate hospital visit should be reported in addition to the starred procedure.

Postoperative care is reported on a service-by-service basis.

Complications requiring additional service should be reported additionally. Identify all complications with the correct ICD-9-CM diagnosis code.

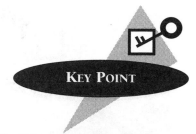

KEY POINT

The CPT **surgical package** concept excludes:

- Preoperative care

- Postoperative complications

- Care unrelated to the surgery

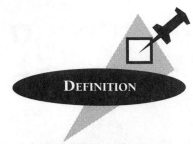

DEFINITION

Diagnostic services are performed to determine or establish a patient's diagnosis. For example, diagnostic arthroscopy may be performed to evaluate the need for a definitive procedure in the future or other treatment such as physical therapy.

Therapeutic services are performed for treatment of a specific condition. These services include performance of the procedure, various incidental elements, and normal, related follow-up care. (Unless the therapeutic service is a starred procedure).

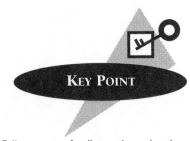

KEY POINT

Follow-up care for diagnostic services is for care of the postsurgical patient only, not care of the underlying problem.

Diagnostic Procedures

Diagnostic procedures are performed to evaluate the patient's complaints or symptoms. These procedures help the physician establish the nature of the patient's disease or condition so that definitive care can be provided. Diagnostic procedures include endoscopy, arthroscopy, injection procedures, and biopsies. Follow-up care for diagnostic procedures includes only care directly related to recovery from the diagnostic procedure itself. Care of the condition identified by the diagnostic procedures or other concomitant conditions are not included and may be listed separately.

The following illustrates reporting evaluation and management services not directly related to the diagnostic procedure.

A new patient presents with hoarseness for the past two weeks. An extended problem focused examination and history are performed. Because there is no history of upper respiratory infection, pain or irritation of the respiratory tract, a diagnostic laryngoscopy is performed. No cause is identified. The patient returns in two weeks for a scheduled follow-up. A second problem-focused exam is performed.

Diagnostic Services

21. DIAGNOSIS OR NATURE OF ILLNESS OR INJURY (RELATE ITEMS 1, 2, 3 OR 4 TO ITEM 24E BY LINE)						
1	784.49			3		
2				4		

24.	A		B	C	D	E
	DATE(S) OF SERVICE		Place of Service	Type of Service	PROCEDURES, SERVICES, OR SUPPLIES (Explain Unusual Circumstances) CPT / HCPCS MODIFIER	DIAGNOSIS CODE
	From MM DD YY	To MM DD YY				
	3 2 98	3 2 98	11		31505	1
	3 2 98	3 2 98	11		99202	1

ICD-9-CM

784.49   Other voice disturbance

CPT

31505   Laryngoscopy, indirect (separate procedure); diagnostic

99202   Office or other outpatient visit for the evaluation and management of a new patient, which requires these three key components: an expanded problem focused history; an expanded problem focused examination; and straightforward medical decision making. Counseling and/or coordination of care with other providers or agencies are provided consistent with the nature of the problem(s) and the patient's and/or family's needs. Usually, the presenting problem(s) are of low to moderate severity. Physicians typically spend 20 minutes face-to-face with the patient and/or family.

Therapeutic Services

Therapeutic services are performed for treatment of a specific diagnosis. These services include performance of the procedure, various incidental elements, and normal, related follow-up care, unless the therapeutic service is a starred procedure. See the guidelines for billing starred procedures in this chapter.

The following example illustrates reporting of evaluation and management services in conjunction with a therapeutic procedure.

The patient undergoes a direct laryngoscopy with excision of a benign neoplasm of the larynx. A routine postoperative follow-up exam is performed in the office four days later.

Therapeutic laryngoscopy was performed which includes follow-up services.

Therapeutic Services

21. DIAGNOSIS OR NATURE OF ILLNESS OR INJURY (RELATE ITEMS 1, 2, 3 OR 4 TO ITEM 24E BY LINE)		
1 212.1	3	
2 V67.0	4	

24.	A DATE(S) OF SERVICE						B Place of Service	C Type of Service	D PROCEDURES, SERVICES, OR SUPPLIES (Explain Unusual Circumstances) CPT / HCPCS MODIFIER		E DIAGNOSIS CODE
	From MM	DD	YY	To MM	DD	YY					
	2	5	98	2	5	98	22		31540		1
	2	9	98	2	9	98	11		99024		2,1

ICD-9-CM
> **212.1**   Benign neoplasm of larynx
> **V67.0**   Surgery follow-up examination

CPT
> **31540**   Laryngoscopy, direct, operative, with excision of tumor and/or stripping of vocal cords or epiglottis;
> **99024**   Postoperative follow-up visit, included in global service

The follow-up visit may be reported with code 99024; however 99024 has no dollar value associated with it. Code 99024 is used for record keeping. Payors do not reimburse for it.

FRAGMENTATION AND UNBUNDLING

Understanding unbundling and fragmentation can be accomplished by first defining the term, "bundle." A bundle is a defined set of items or services wrapped together in a group, bunch, or package. The items in the bundle can be related or unrelated, but all defined elements must be present to make a specific bundle. Consider a bundle that includes one dozen apples and oranges. Although at first it may seem that the apples and oranges are unrelated, they are both types of fruit and have been put together in a fruit bundle. Anyone purchasing this fruit bundle expects that all the apples and oranges are present (i.e., the buyer is purchasing the entire dozen). If, however, one of the apples is removed, and billed separately, in addition to paying the cost per dozen, the person buying the bundle is being charged twice for the apple.

Of course when it comes to coding, a bundle has nothing to do with apples and oranges. Instead, unbundling relates to CPT surgical codes and the global or package concept. Unbundling or fragmentation occurs primarily two ways.

First, unbundling occurs when minor integral services are reported separately or in addition to a major procedure. Unfortunately, since all minor components of a procedure may not be listed explicitly, it is sometimes difficult to determine which services are integral to a given procedure. One way to approach this is to ask what services are normally performed with a given procedure. A simple example is an excision of a skin lesion. To excise the skin lesion, an incision must be

DEFINITION

Bundled services are items or services wrapped together for reporting and reimbursement purposes. The items or services may be related or unrelated, but all defined elements must be present to make a specific bundle.

KEY POINT

The AMA has not developed a specific unbundling policy, but you can look in the following places for help in interpreting how to apply the CPT codes:

- Format of the terminology listed in the introduction

- Listed surgical procedures

- Separate procedures

- Subsection information in the surgery guidelines

made. An incision is always integral to an excision of a lesion and should not be billed separately. However, an incision is not described in the excision of skin lesion codes. It is implicit because it must be performed with every excision.

Second, unbundling occurs when a single procedure with two or more explicitly described components is broken into its component parts and reported with several CPT codes instead of the single CPT code for the combined service. A simple example of this type of unbundle can be illustrated with the procedure for a combined abdominal hysterectomy with colpo-urethrocystopexy. Because the two components of this procedure are frequently performed together, a combined code 58152 has been assigned to describe this service. However, it is also possible to perform each of the components separately (abdominal hysterectomy 58150 and colpo-urethrocystopexy 51840 or 51841). When the combined procedure is performed during a single surgical session, it must be reported with the bundled CPT code 58152. If it is reported with code 58150 in conjunction with 51840 or 58141, it is considered to be unbundled or fragmented.

Unbundling, whether intentional or not, is considered by payors to be a form of fraudulent or reckless billing. The rationale is simple. Unbundled services will frequently net more reimbursement than reporting the single bundled CPT code.

HCFA has adopted Correct Coding Initiative unbundling guidelines, an evolving list of codes that cannot be reported in combination with other codes for Medicare claims. CPT does not have a specific guideline for unbundling. Instead, payors and other interested parties have developed guidelines for bundled procedures from information that is listed in CPT. The four most common areas of CPT used for these interpretations are the format of the terminology listed in the introduction, listed surgical procedures, separate procedures, and subsection information in the surgery guidelines. Look at these four areas and how payors may interpret the guidelines. Keep in mind that while most payors will have many common rules and interpretations, they will have some rules specific to their company. Make an effort to understand these differences, requesting written documentation for rules which differ significantly from the norm.

Format of the Terminology

CPT guidelines state that some of the procedures are not printed in their entirety but refer back to a common portion of the procedure listed in a preceding entry. This space-saving format, previously described in Chapter 2 of *Code It Right*, means that many "indented" codes within a code range repeat some common portion of a procedure's description.

While some procedures presented in this indented form are mutually exclusive (i.e., cannot be billed together), others are not. For procedures which are not mutually exclusive, payors may make special allowances. Knowing which procedures are mutually exclusive, however, is the key to avoiding unbundles.

Example 1
Nasal/sinus endoscopy codes 31237-31240 contain common services that are demonstrated by the indented format. First, they include a diagnostic nasal/sinus endoscopy that is not explicitly described in the procedure narrative; and, second, they both include a surgical nasal/sinus endoscopy and approach of the same region. However, if the surgeon performs a nasal polypectomy (31237) in conjunction with a dacryocystorhinostomy (31239), would it be correct to report both procedures? This answer is "yes," because procedure 31237 for a nasal polypectomy does not normally include a dacryocystorhinostomy 31239. However, since these procedures do have services in common, payors may have different reimbursement rules. Payor options include:

- Allowing both procedures and paying the second procedure at a standard reduced rate of 50 percent

- Allowing both procedures and paying the second procedure at a reduced rate based on the work the two procedures have in common (i.e., the diagnostic endoscopy and the surgical endoscopy and approach)

- Allowing only the procedure with the highest allowable and appending modifier -22 indicate that the procedure was unusual or more difficult and reimbursing an additional 20 to 30 percent above the usual allowable for the single procedure to compensate for the increased difficulty

Example 2

Ethmoidectomy procedures 31200-31205 also have an indented format with the common portion being an ethmoidectomy. If an anterior and posterior intranasal ethmoidectomy is performed, would it be correct to report both the ethmoidectomy intranasal anterior (31200) and the ethmoidectomy intranasal total (31201)? The answer is "no." Procedure 31201 would be reported alone since a total ethmoidectomy includes excision of ethmoid tissue in both the anterior and posterior ethmoids. It is usual or necessary to perform an anterior ethmoidectomy as part of a total ethmoidectomy.

Listed Surgical Procedures

CPT guidelines state listed surgical procedures include the operation per se, local infiltration, metacarpal/digital block or topical anesthesia when used, and the normal, uncomplicated follow-up care. The concept is referred to as a "package" for surgical procedures. For example:

The physician performs a closed treatment of a phalangeal shaft fracture with manipulation after first performing a digital block.

Incorrect reporting

26725	Closed treatment of phalangeal shaft fracture, proximal or middle phalanx, finger or thumb; with manipulation, with or without skin or skeletal traction, each
64450*	Injection anesthetic agent; other peripheral nerve or branch

The injection procedure (64450*) cannot be reported separately because all listed surgical procedures include metacarpal or digital block. Therefore, the digital block is an integral part of the fracture treatment.

Correct reporting

26725	Closed treatment of phalangeal shaft fracture, proximal or middle phalanx, finger or thumb; with manipulation, with or without skin or skeletal traction, each

Separate Procedures

Separate procedures are services that are commonly carried out as an integral part of a larger service, and as such do not warrant separate identification. These services are noted in CPT with the parenthetical phrase (separate procedure). When this phrase appears before the semicolon, all indented descriptions that follow are covered by it.

Separate procedures are often improperly reported as related procedures. Related procedures are performed for the same diagnosis and within the same operative area. Reporting a separate

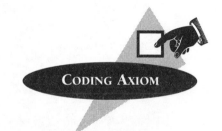

CODING AXIOM

Listed surgical procedures include(s) the operation per se, local infiltration, metacarpal/digital block or topical anesthesia when used, and the normal, uncomplicated follow-up care. This concept is referred to as a "package" for surgical procedures.

Because modifier -22 reports an unusual service it must be supported by documentation in the medical record. Additional documentation should accompany the claim when billing.

procedure in addition to the larger procedure to which it is related is improper. A separate procedure can be a component of, or incidental to, a larger, related procedure.

The following may be considered unbundling if reported separately when performed through the same incision during the same operative session:

43610	Excision, local; ulcer or benign tumor of stomach
49000-51	Exploratory laparotomy, exploratory celiotomy with or without biopsy(s) (separate procedure) — Multiple procedure

In this example, 49000 would be denied because a surgical opening (laparotomy) is necessary to enter the abdomen. The classification of separate procedure serves as a reminder to coders that the separate procedure is ordinarily a component of a larger procedure and should only be reported separately when it is performed alone or when it is performed as an unrelated or distinct procedural service. Most payors expect the above example to be reported as:

43610	Excision, local; ulcer or benign tumor of stomach

Payors interpret the rules and guidelines for separate procedures differently. Payors may base payment guidelines on definitions established by outside consultants or by their own internal sources. Some payors strictly interpret CPT while others may be more lenient in how they interpret separate procedure guidelines. The guideline "alone and for a specific purpose" may be interpreted to mean the procedure would not be performed with any other procedure. The guideline may also be interpreted to mean it may be performed with another procedure as long as it is not an integral part of the procedure.

The following may be considered unbundled:

59409	Vaginal delivery only (with or without episiotomy and/or forceps);
59430	Postpartum care only (separate procedure)

Suppose the physician performed the delivery but did not plan on seeing the patient for postpartum care. However, the patient came in for postpartum care when the claim for the delivery had already been submitted to the payor. The claim for the "postpartum care only" could be denied by the payor. The payor may weigh the fee for 59430 against the difference between the cost of 59409 and the fee for delivery including postpartum care (59410). If the difference in the amount was not more, the payor may reimburse for 59430. For accurate coding, the claim should have a corrected billing sent, reported as:

59410	Vaginal deliver only (with or without episiotomy and/or forceps); including postpartum care

Subsection Information
CPT guidelines state that several of the subheadings or subsections have special needs or instructions unique to that section. Where these are indicated (e.g., maternity care and delivery), special notes are presented preceding the procedural terminology listings. The notes refer to that subsection specifically. See CPT Surgery Guidelines for a complete list of subsections with special "Notes."

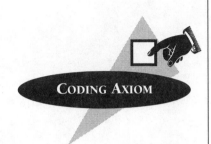

CODING AXIOM

When a procedure is designated as a "separate procedure" in CPT, but is performed with other unrelated or distinct services, append modifier -59 to the separate procedure code to indicate that it is a distinct and independent service.

According to the CPT guidelines, evaluation and management (E/M) codes should be reported for separately identifiable conditions. For example, a patient has diabetes and was seen for the management of the diabetes at different times during pregnancy.

59400	Routine obstetric care including antepartum care, vaginal delivery (with or without episiotomy, and/or forceps) and postpartum care
99214	Office or other outpatient visit for the evaluation and management of an established patient

However, the payor may deny the claim even when the ICD-9-CM code listed explained the complication of pregnancy if the E/M code is reported with the obstetric care. Report separate services as they happen unless instructed otherwise by the payor. Request prior authorization for these separate services so an authorization number for the separate services will be in the payor's claims system. If the claim is denied, speak to the utilization review or prior authorization nurse. Explain the problem and ask to submit the claim directly to them.

An example of a misinterpretation of this guideline by the provider and an unbundling of services would be the following:

A patient is seen for a routine glucose tolerance test at a regularly scheduled visit during the pregnancy and it is reported as:

99212	Office visit, problem focused history/exam
82951	Glucose; tolerance test, three specimens

Only the code for the lab test should be reported at this visit. The evaluation and management portion of this service would be considered part of the global service for obstetric care.

UNBUNDLE PREVENTION
Your office can take some easy steps to avoid problems with fragmentation or unbundling.

- Use a current CPT book as well as the current rules, regulations, and provider manuals for Medicare and for the private payors with whom you have a contractual arrangement.

- Educate everyone on CPT guidelines as well as the rules and regulations of your payors. Educational sessions should occur any time changes are made.

- When using a preprinted charge ticket or routing sheet, specify the exact CPT code and description. Always have an area on the charge ticket for the physician to indicate that a service should be coded by hand and code from the operative report or medical record. Many providers feel reimbursement is better by coding directly from the record or operative report.

- Date the charge ticket and update codes annually: in January for CPT and HCPCS; in October for ICD-9-CM.

- Create your charge tickets or routing sheets to avoid fragmented billing. Adding the abbreviation "SP" to separate procedure codes alerts the coder that a separate procedure should not be reported when related to, or integral to, a major procedure.

- Make sure physicians provide coders with complete documentation and concise information. Query the physician if documentation is not adequate to support the codes selected.

KEY POINT

Avoid the problems with unbundling:

- Use current CPT guidelines

- Specify CPT codes and descriptions when using preprinted charge tickets or routing sheets

- Design charge tickets or routing sheets to avoid fragmentation of services

- Use correct modifiers

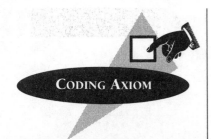

CODING AXIOM

Many insurers reimburse only for supplies that are excessive or extraordinarily expensive. Do not bill supplies that are customarily included in surgical packages, such as gauze, sponges, applicators, or steri-strips.

KEY POINT

Note that the highest dollar code is always sequenced first.

Codes 11200–11471 identify removal, shaving, or excisions of benign lesions. These codes include surgical removal of the following types of benign lesions: scars (cicatricial), skin tags, cysts, birthmarks, and integumentary inflammations.

Integumentary codes are based on the location and diameter of the largest lesion removed.

- Use the correct modifiers as appropriate to clarify or append circumstances that can arise within global package time periods.

As payors become increasingly proficient in interpreting CPT codes, coders must exercise caution when reporting integral procedures, even when benefits are allowed. Medicare and Medicaid closely monitor physicians' billing practices for possible abusive or fraudulent billing. Private payors also have mechanisms in place to scrutinize claims.

MATERIALS SUPPLIED BY A PHYSICIAN

Many payors reimburse only for supplies that are excessive or extraordinarily expensive. Do not report supplies that are customarily included in surgical packages, such as gauze, sponges, applicators, or Steri-strips. Surgical services do not include the supply of medications and sterile trays, which may be coded and billed separately. Applicable CPT codes are the following:

- 99070 for supplies, including reusable and disposable items. Specify the supply or type of medication, and the amount that was provided.
- 96545 for the provision of chemotherapy agent.
- 92330 and 92335 for ocular prostheses. Additional supplies relating to the eye (including contact lenses and spectacles) are identified with 92390–92396. HCPCS Level II codes also can report ocular prostheses. See Chapter 10 for more information on HCPCS codes.
- 78990 and 79900 for radiopharmaceutical(s), diagnostic or therapeutic, respectively.

Many payors prefer or require the use of HCPCS Level II codes for reporting supplies as they provide greater specificity. See Chapter 10 for HCPCS Level II codes that may be reported for supplies/equipment, such as glasses, wheelchairs, surgical trays, casting supplies, etc. To report injectable medications, also use HCPCS Level II J codes which specify the type of medication and amount used.

When reporting supplies, attach a statement to the claim form, informing the payor of the physician's cost, including a reasonable charge for handling and provide a description of the supply used.

Since many insurance companies do not reimburse supplies provided by physicians, monitor explanations of benefits to assure that charges for supplies were allowed and reimbursed by the payor. Monitoring also alerts you to payors who recognize HCPCS Level II codes or have an internal coding system for medicines and supplies. With the deletion of the narrative space following the code in the HCFA-1500 form, payors may be more likely to recognize or even require HCPCS Level II codes to avoid contacting the patient or provider for additional information.

SEQUENCING

The highest dollar code is always sequenced first when reporting multiple procedures. The second and subsequent codes are ordered and listed in decreasing dollar values with the correct modifier(s) appended. When reporting multiple procedures, do not reduce the amount of secondary codes. Let payors make the reduction according to their guidelines or contractual arrangements unless specifically instructed to do otherwise. The reason for reporting the full amount for secondary procedures is due to the likelihood of the claims processor applying another reduction to a code you have already reduced. However, if overpaid, reimburse the payor for the overpayment. Set a ceiling on nonactionable overpayments in policy or contracts (e.g. Up to $10 need not be refunded). Overpayments that are not returned to the payor may target an office for an audit.

DISCUSSION QUESTIONS

1. Define a separate procedure.

   _____

   _____

   _____

2. Why is it a problem to report a component of the surgical procedure separately with a global code?

   _____

   _____

   _____

3. Define a surgical package.

   _____

   _____

   _____

4. Give an example of fragmented billing.

   _____

   _____

   _____

Surgical Procedures

Several subsections of CPT contain guidelines, notes, definitions, and special instructions. Following is a list of some of the subsections:

- Removal of skin tags
- Shaving of epidermal/dermal lesions
- Excision of benign and malignant lesions
- Repair of wounds
- Adjacent tissue transfers
- Skin grafts and flaps
- Destruction of lesions
- Fracture care
- Cast and splint application
- Spine surgeries
- Pacemaker/defibrillator care
- Coronary artery bypass grafts
- Vascular catheterization/injection
- Gastrointestinal endoscopy
- Hernia repair
- Urodynamics
- Cystoscopy, urethroscopy and cystourethroscopy
- Laparoscopy and hysteroscopy
- Vulvectomy
- Maternity care and delivery
- Surgery of skull base

OBJECTIVES

Become familiar with the sections of surgical procedures and the guidelines of each

Recognize the special circumstances for coding surgery codes

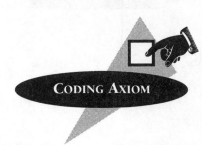

CODING AXIOM

Biopsy codes are arranged in the surgery section of CPT by the anatomic location of the biopsy site.

Code "excisional biopsies" that involve the removal of the entire lesion with codes that describe lesion excision.

Familiarize yourself with the surgical section of CPT, the procedures you are billing, and the guidelines for the section, category, subcategory or code you report. Following are some examples of surgical procedures and their guidelines.

General Coding Rules

BIOPSY SERVICES

Use biopsy codes to report the removal of a small amount of tissue to determine the extent of a disease or to determine or confirm a diagnosis. A single tissue sample may be lifted or picked out with forceps, or a portion of the lesion may be biopsied by incising the lesion and repairing the incision with sutures. Biopsy codes are appropriate for needle aspiration, incisional biopsy, and partial excision, as well as for scraping, curetting, and using a skin punch. Examples include:

21920	Biopsy, soft tissue of back or flank; superficial
24065	Biopsy, soft tissue of upper arm or elbow area; superficial
44025	Colotomy, for exploration, biopsy(s), or foreign body removal
58100*	Endometrial sampling (biopsy) with or without endocervical sampling (biopsy), without cervical dilation, any method (separate procedure)
67810*	Biopsy of eyelid

Use integumentary codes when the biopsy is of skin and subcutaneous tissue only. A biopsy code is reported when tissue is sampled; an excision code is reported when all suspect tissue is removed. If the biopsy and excision occur during the same surgical session, only the excision is reported. If the biopsy is performed on a different date, it is reported separately.

The following case study illustrates reporting for biopsy and excision services performed during separate operative sessions. A 32-year-old female with a lump in her breast was referred to a general surgeon for an incisional breast biopsy and treatment. A biopsy confirmed the lump was malignant, and a modified radical mastectomy including pectoralis minor muscle and axillary lymph nodes was performed several days later.

Biopsy Services Performed on a Different Date

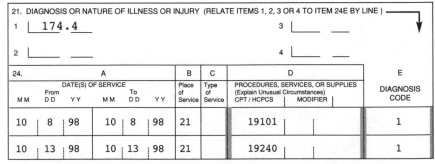

ICD-9-CM

174.4	Malignant neoplasm of female breast, upper-outer quadrant

CPT

19101	Biopsy of breast; incisional
19240	Mastectomy, modified radical, including axillary lymph nodes, with or without pectoralis minor muscle, but excluding pectoralis major muscle

Do not report both a biopsy and a lesion excision of the same anatomic location that occurs during the same surgical session. If a sample is removed (a biopsy), and evaluation of a frozen section indicates the need for excision of additional tissue during the same operative session, report only the greater of the two procedures. In this case report the excision of the lesion. It is permissible and accurate, however, to code both a biopsy and a later excision of the same lesion, provided the procedures are done during separate surgical sessions.

The following case study illustrates reporting a surgical procedure that includes incidental biopsy services. A 40-year-old with hyperparathyroidism undergoes a biopsy of adjacent cervical nodes. Based on the results of the biopsy, the physician performs a parathyroidectomy.

Incidental Biopsy Services

21. DIAGNOSIS OR NATURE OF ILLNESS OR INJURY (RELATE ITEMS 1, 2, 3 OR 4 TO ITEM 24E BY LINE)			
1	252.0	3	
2		4	

24.	A						B	C	D	E
	DATE(S) OF SERVICE						Place of Service	Type of Service	PROCEDURES, SERVICES, OR SUPPLIES (Explain Unusual Circumstances) CPT / HCPCS MODIFIER	DIAGNOSIS CODE
	From MM DD YY			To MM DD YY						
	3	19	98	3	19	98	21		60500	1

ICD-9-CM

252.0   Hyperparathyroidism

CPT

60500   Parathyroidectomy or exploration of parathyroid(s);

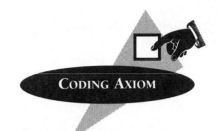

LASER SURGERY

Many insurance companies consider laser use a technical function that does not significantly change the desired outcome of a primary procedure. This is demonstrated by a change in terminology for many CPT codes. The words "destruction by any method" identify the result, not the method. When laser use significantly alters procedure performance, use codes that specifically identify laser in the description. Refer to the surgical destruction subsection of the surgery guidelines in CPT.

Codes 17000–17286 specify the destruction of lesions by any method, including laser, cryosurgery, or electrosurgery. The method of destruction is usually not a consideration in coding.

17000*   Destruction by any method, including laser, with or without surgical curettement, all benign or premalignant lesions (eg, actinic keratoses) other than skin tags or cutaneous vascular proliferative lesions, including local anesthesia; first lesion

INTEGUMENTARY SYSTEM

Removal of Skin Tags (11200-11201)

Removal of skin tags may be accomplished by any single or combination of the following techniques: scissoring, sharp excision, ligature, strangulation, electrosurgical destruction. Administration of local anesthesia and any chemical or electrocautery is included.

Shaving of Epidermal Lesions (11300-11313)

Shaving is the removal of epidermal or dermal skin lesions without a full-thickness dermal excision by use of a transverse incision or horizontal slicing technique. Administration of local anesthesia and any chemical or electrocautery is included.

Excision Benign and Malignant Lesions (11400-11646)

Excision is defined as a full-thickness removal of lesion including simple closure of the wound. Excision codes are selected on the basis of the type of lesion (benign or malignant), anatomic site, and lesion diameter. Benign lesions include those described as cicatricial, fibrous, inflammatory, congenital and cystic as well as any other lesion that is noninvasive or nonmalignant. Malignant lesions are typically invasive or have the potential to metastasize and include lesions such as basal cell carcinomas and melanomas of the skin.

Benign Lesion

21. DIAGNOSIS OR NATURE OF ILLNESS OR INJURY (RELATE ITEMS 1, 2, 3 OR 4 TO ITEM 24E BY LINE)							
1 ∟ 216.5				3 ∟			
2 ∟				4 ∟			

24. A DATE(S) OF SERVICE			B Place of Service	C Type of Service	D PROCEDURES, SERVICES, OR SUPPLIES (Explain Unusual Circumstances)	E DIAGNOSIS CODE
From MM DD YY	To MM DD YY				CPT / HCPCS | MODIFIER	
4 ¦ 6 ¦ 98	4 ¦ 6 ¦ 98		22		11403 ¦ ¦	1

ICD-9-CM

216.5   Benign neoplasm of skin of trunk, except scrotum

CPT

11403   Excision, benign lesion, except skin tag (unless listed elsewhere), trunk, arms or legs; lesion diameter 2.1 to 3.0 cm

Excision codes for malignant lesions are assigned according to the largest diameter of the lesion excised. Simple closure is included. When the excision of a malignancy results in a defect requiring complex closure, the closure of the defect (using intermediate or complex repair) is reported separately. Codes for adjacent tissue transfer or rearrangement include lesion excision. Lesion excision is not separately reportable with codes 14000–14350.

Wound Repair (12001–13300)

Repair is the surgical closure of a wound. The wound may be a result of injury/trauma or it may be a surgically created defect. Repairs can be any of the following:

- Stand alone procedures
- Separately reportable services when performed with certain other procedures as in the case of excisions requiring intermediate or complex repair
- An integral part of a more complex procedure and not separately reportable

Repairs are divided into three categories: simple, intermediate, and complex. They are further described by anatomic site and wound size.

Simple repair is performed when the wound is superficial, e.g., involving partial or full-thickness damage to the skin and/or subcutaneous tissues. There is no significant involvement of deeper structures and only simple, one layer, primary suturing is required. This procedure includes local anesthetic and chemical or electrocauterization of wounds not closed.

Simple Closure scenario

This example reviews simple repair reporting. While in a public park, an 8-year-old was bitten by a dog and received a 5 cm wound on the forearm. He was treated by his family physician in the physician's office on an emergency basis and was given a tetanus toxoid booster. The physician repaired the laceration with simple closure.

Wound Repair

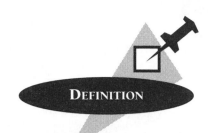

DEFINITION

Wound repair is described by anatomic site and wound size. Repairs are divided into three categories:

- Simple
- Intermediate
- Complex

21. DIAGNOSIS OR NATURE OF ILLNESS OR INJURY (RELATE ITEMS 1, 2, 3 OR 4 TO ITEM 24E BY LINE)			
1. 881.00		3. E849.4	
2. E906.0		4.	

24.	A DATE(S) OF SERVICE						B Place of Service	C Type of Service	D PROCEDURES, SERVICES, OR SUPPLIES (Explain Unusual Circumstances) CPT / HCPCS	MODIFIER	E DIAGNOSIS CODE
	From MM	DD	YY	To MM	DD	YY					
	2	25	98	2	25	98	11		12002*		1,2,3
	2	25	98	2	25	98	11		99058		1,2,3
	2	25	98	2	25	98	11		90703		1,2,3
	2	25	98	2	25	98	11		90471		1,2,3

ICD-9-CM

881.00	Open wound of forearm, without mention of complication
E906.0	Injury caused by dog bite
E849.4	Place of occurrence, place for recreation and sport

CPT

12002*	Simple repair of superficial wounds of scalp, neck, axillae, external genitalia, trunk, and/or extremities (including hands and feet); 2.6 cm to 7.5 cm
99058	Office services provided on an emergency basis
90703	Tetanus toxoid absorbed, for intramuscular or jet injection use
90471	Immunization administration (includes percutaneous, intradermal, subcutaneous, intramuscular and jet injections and/or intranasal or oral administration); single or combination vaccine/toxoid

Intermediate repair is performed for wounds and lacerations in which one or more of the deeper layers of subcutaneous tissue and non-muscle fascia are repaired in addition to the skin and subcutaneous tissue. Single-layer closure can also be coded as an intermediate repair if the wound is heavily contaminated and requires extensive cleaning or removal of particulate matter.

Complex repair includes repair of wounds requiring more than layered closure. Wounds coded from this category include those requiring revision, debridement, extensive undermining, and placement of stents or retention sutures. Complex repairs also include those requiring creation of a defect (e.g., extending excision) and special preparation of the site.

The following rules should be followed when reporting repairs:

1. Measure the length of the repaired wound or wounds and report in centimeters.

2. Add together the lengths of multiple wounds in the same classification and report as a single item.

For example, a simple repair of a 2 cm scalp wound and a simple repair of a 1.5 cm wound of the forearm would be reported with a single code.

12002   Simple repair of superficial wounds of scalp, neck, axillae, external genitalia, trunk and/or extremities (including hands and feet); 2.6 cm to 7.5 cm

This procedure is coded with a single procedure code because both wounds are classified as simple and both are in the same group of simple repairs (12001–12007). Total length of the two wounds is 3.5 cm so 12002 is reported.

3. Wounds in more than one classification should be listed separately with the more complicated service listed as the primary procedure and the less complicated listed as the secondary procedure with modifier -51 appended.

    Example, code a simple repair of a 2 cm laceration of the scalp and an intermediate repair of a 2.5 cm laceration of the cheek.

    12051   Layer closure of wounds of face, ears, eyelids, nose, lips and/or mucous membranes; 2.5 cm or less

    12001-51 Simple repair of superficial wounds of scalp, neck, axillae, external genitalia, trunk and/or extremities (including hands and feet); 2.5 cm or less

4. Decontamination and/or debridement is considered integral to wound repair except when gross contamination requires prolonged cleansing or when appreciable amounts of devitalized contaminated tissue must be removed.

5. Repair of nerves, blood vessels, and tendons should be reported under the appropriate system. Repair of associated skin wounds is considered integral to the repair of nerves, blood vessels, and tendons and is not reported separately unless the wound repair qualifies as complex. In these instances report the complex repair with modifier -51 appended.

6. Simple exploration of nerves, blood vessels, and tendons exposed in an open wound is considered integral to the repair and should not be reported separately.

7. Wounds requiring exploration, enlargement, extension, dissection, removal of foreign body, and/or ligation or coagulation of minor blood vessels of subcutaneous tissue, muscle fascia, or muscle should be reported with 20100–20103 as indicated.

ADJACENT TISSUE TRANSFER/REARRANGEMENT (14000–14350)

Adjacent tissue transfer or rearrangement is defined by anatomic site and size of defect. Adjacent tissue transfers include excision of the defect or lesion so excision codes should not be reported additionally. Terms used to describe transfer or rearrangement procedures include: Z-plasty, W-plasty, V-Y-plasty, rotation flap, advancement flap, double pedicle flap. When applied to primary traumatic wound closure, the configuration listed must be developed by the surgeon to accomplish the repair. Transfer and rearrangement codes should not be applied when traumatic wounds incidentally result in these configurations.

Tissue transfer or rearrangement codes describe moving normal tissue from the donor site to the recipient site. The donor site is adjacent or next to the affected area, allowing the tissue to remain attached to its original location and blood supply, ensuring survival of the graft.

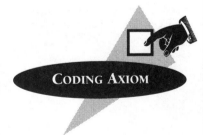

CODING AXIOM

Adjacent tissue transfer and rearrangement includes excision of the defect or lesion.

The following case study illustrates reporting of the excision of a congenital nevus when an adjacent tissue transfer is used to close the defect. A patient presents with a 4.0 cm congenital nevus of the shoulder. Because of the size of the lesion, adjacent tissue is used to close the defect.

21. DIAGNOSIS OR NATURE OF ILLNESS OR INJURY (RELATE ITEMS 1, 2, 3 OR 4 TO ITEM 24E BY LINE)				
1 216.6			3	
2			4	

24.	A				B	C	D		E
	DATE(S) OF SERVICE				Place of Service	Type of Service	PROCEDURES, SERVICES, OR SUPPLIES (Explain Unusual Circumstances)		DIAGNOSIS CODE
	From		To						
	MM DD YY		MM DD YY				CPT / HCPCS MODIFIER		
	1 4 98		1 4 98		22		14000	–77	1

ICD-9-CM

216.6   Benign neoplasm of skin of upper limb, including shoulder

CPT

14000-77   Adjacent tissue transfer or rearrangement, trunk; defect 10 sq cm or less — Repeat procedure by another physician

FLAPS AND GRAFTS (15000-15770)

Flaps and grafts are procedures which involve moving normal tissue (skin, skin and deep tissues, muscle, composite tissue) from one site to another. The site where the tissue originates is referred to as the donor site, while the site where the tissue is being relocated is referred to as the recipient site. Surgical preparation of the recipeint site should be reported separately with codes 15000–15001. Flap and grafts codes are divided into three sections.

Free skin grafts are defined by size, location of the defect (recipient site), and type of graft (pinch, split-thickness, full-thickness). Free skin grafts should be reported separately as a secondary procedure when done in conjunction with other procedures. Examples of procedures which might require skin grafts at the time of the primary procedure include: musculoskeletal deep tumor removal, neck dissection, radical mastectomy, and orbitectomy.

Flaps of skin and deep tissues are defined by type of graft (direct, tube, delayed, intermediate, muscle, myocutaneous, fasciocutaneous) and site. The site listed is the recipient site when the flap is being attached to the final site. However, when the flap is being formed for delayed transfer, the site refers to the donor site. Any extensive immobilization with casts or other devices is considered an additional procedure and should be reported separately. Repairs of the donor site with skin grafts or local flaps are reportable separately.

Other flaps and grafts include island pedicle, free muscle skin or fascial flaps requiring micovascular anastamosis, and composite grafts.

Example: After suffering a degloving injury to a portion of his ring finger while working on his car transmission at home, an 18-year-old male underwent a cross finger pedicle flap from his long finger. Immobilization was accomplished with a plaster short arm splint.

DEFINITION

Flaps of skin and deep tissues are defined by site and the type of graft, such as:

- Direct
- Tube
- Delayed
- Intermediate
- Muscle
- Myocutaneous
- Fasciocutaneous

Free skin grafts are reported based on percent of body area for infants and children, but are reported per 100 sq cm for adults. Percentages apply only to children under the age of 10.

21. DIAGNOSIS OR NATURE OF ILLNESS OR INJURY (RELATE ITEMS 1, 2, 3 OR 4 TO ITEM 24E BY LINE)			
1 | 881.00		3 |E849.0	
2 | E919.6		4 |___ ___	

24.	A								B	C	D			E
	DATE(S) OF SERVICE								Place	Type	PROCEDURES, SERVICES, OR SUPPLIES			DIAGNOSIS
	From				To				of	of	(Explain Unusual Circumstances)			CODE
	MM	DD	YY	MM	DD	YY			Service	Service	CPT / HCPCS	MODIFIER		
	2	20	98	2	20	98			22		15580			1,2,3

ICD-9-CM

883.0   Open wound of finger(s) without mention of complication

E919.6   Accident caused by transmission machinery

E849.0   Place of occurrence, home

CPT

15580   Cross finger flap, including free graft to donor site

DESTRUCTION OF LESIONS (17000-17360)

Destruction is defined as the ablation of benign, premalignant, or malignant tissue by any of the following methods used alone or in combination: electrosurgery, cryosurgery, laser, and chemical treatment. Lesions include condylomata, papillomata, molluscum contagiosum, herpetic lesions, warts, milia, actinic keratosis, or other benign, premalignant or malignant lesions. Destruction includes administration of local anesthesia. Codes from this section should not be used when a more specific destruction code is listed under the specific anatomic site. For example, code 40820 should be used for destruction of lesions of the vestibule of the mouth.

Moh's micrographic surgery is listed in the destruction subsection. This is a special technique used to treat complex or ill-defined skin cancer and requires a single physician to provide two distinct services. The first service is surgical and involves the destruction of the lesion by a combination of chemosurgery and excision. The second service is that of a pathologist and includes mapping, color coding of specimens, microscopic examination of specimens, and complete histopathologic preparation.

FRACTURE CARE

CPT codes for fracture management are found in the musculoskeletal subsection. These codes are package services and include percutaneous pinning and open or closed treatment of the fracture, application and removal of the initial cast or splint, and normal, uncomplicated follow-up care.

Guidelines at the beginning of this subsection define terms unique to fracture care. The instructional notes for the musculoskeletal subsection state that the terms "closed treatment," "open treatment," and "percutaneous skeletal fixation" have been carefully chosen to accurately reflect current orthopedic procedural treatments.

This example illustrates reporting of closed treatment of a fracture. A 54-year-old man fell from a ladder while hanging decorations at a dance hall. The patient was seen by the emergency department physician for closed treatment with manipulation of a fracture of the distal end of the radius.

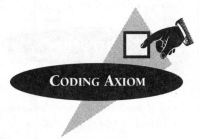

CODING AXIOM

Destruction of malignant lesions is reported based on site and diameter of the lesion.

Destruction of benign or premalignant lesions (except cutaneous vascular proliferative) are not site or size specific.

Closed Treatment of Fracture

21. DIAGNOSIS OR NATURE OF ILLNESS OR INJURY (RELATE ITEMS 1, 2, 3 OR 4 TO ITEM 24E BY LINE)		
1. ∟ 813.52	3. ∟E849.6	
2. ∟E881.0	4. ∟___	

24.	A						B	C	D		E
	DATE(S) OF SERVICE						Place of Service	Type of Service	PROCEDURES, SERVICES, OR SUPPLIES (Explain Unusual Circumstances)		DIAGNOSIS CODE
	From MM DD YY			To MM DD YY					CPT / HCPCS	MODIFIER	
	3 5 98			3 5 98			23		25605		1,2,3

ICD-9-CM
813.52   Other fractures of distal end of radius (alone)
E881.0   Fall from ladder
E849.6   Place of occurrence, public building

CPT
25605   Closed treatment of distal radial fracture (eg, Colles or Smith type) or epiphyseal separation, with or without fracture of ulnar styloid; with manipulation

Internal and External Fixation
Two types of fixation — internal and external — are described in CPT. Internal skeletal fixation involves wires, pins, screws, and/or plates placed through or within the fractured area to stabilize and immobilize the injury. This procedure is generally accomplished through an incision over the fracture site. It is commonly described as an open reduction with internal fixation (ORIF). Internal fixation may also be accomplished by percutaneous technique. Deep internal devices are usually left in place even after the fracture has healed. If the hardware is removed, report codes 20670* or 20680. Use modifier -78 *return to the operating room for a related procedure* or modifier -58 *staged or related procedure by the same physician during the postoperative period*, if removal is performed during the initial hospital care or during the postoperative follow-up period. If the removal is performed after the postoperative follow-up period, use 20670* or 20680. The ICD-9-CM code is assigned according to the reason for the removal (e.g., pain, infection). The codes describing internal fixation are interspersed throughout the fracture care codes.

External fixation (20690–20694) is hardware passing through bone and skin and held rigid by cross-braces outside the body. External fixation is always removed after the fracture has healed and removal usually is considered part of the global service. However, if required to remain in place beyond the usual postoperative period, its removal should be reported (20694).

Application of Casts and Strapping
Codes found in the application of casts and strapping section (29000–29799) should be reported separately when:

- The cast application or strapping is a replacement procedure used during or after the period of follow-up care

- The cast application or strapping is an initial service performed **without** restorative treatment or procedures to stabilize or protect a fracture, injury, or dislocation and/or to afford comfort to a patient

- An initial casting or strapping when no other treatment or procedure is performed or will be performed by the same physician

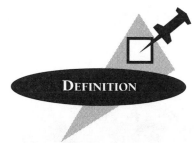

DEFINITION

Internal fixation involves wires, pins, screws, and/or plates placed through or within the fractured area to stabilize and immobilize the injury.

External fixation is hardware passing through bone and skin and held rigid by cross-braces outside the body.

Closed treatment describes a fracture site that is not surgically opened. There are three methods of closed treatment of fractures: without manipulation, with manipulation, and with or without traction.

Open treatment describes a fracture site that is opened surgically for visualization and possible internal fixation.

Manipulation describes the attempted reduction or restoration of a fracture of joint dislocation to its normal anatomic alignment by the application of manually applied forces.

Skeletal traction is the application of a force to a limb segment through a wire, pin, screw, or clamp attached to bone.

Skin traction is the application of a force to a limb using felt or strapping applied directly to the skin only.

Percutaneous skeletal fixation describes fracture treatment that is neither open nor closed. In this procedure, the fracture fragments are not visualized but fixation (e.g., pins) is placed across the fracture site, usually under x-ray imaging.

• A physician performs the initial application of a cast or strapping subsequent to another physician having performed a restorative treatment or procedure

A physician who applies the initial cast, strap, or splint and also assumes all of the subsequent fracture, dislocation, or injury care cannot use the application of casts and strapping codes as an initial service. The first cast, splint, or strap application is included in the treatment of the fracture and/or dislocation codes. In the following example, no fracture occurs, so the cast application is reported.

A patient falls on the steps at home and sprains his wrist. His family physician sees the patient in the office and checks the patient for other injuries to the head, neck and hip. The physician diagnoses a radiocarpal joint sprain and applies a short-arm cast in the office to immobilize the wrist.

Cast Application

21. DIAGNOSIS OR NATURE OF ILLNESS OR INJURY (RELATE ITEMS 1, 2, 3 OR 4 TO ITEM 24E BY LINE)

| 1 | 842.02 | 3 | E849.0 |
| 2 | E880.9 | 4 | |

24.	A					B	C	D		E
	DATE(S) OF SERVICE					Place of Service	Type of Service	PROCEDURES, SERVICES, OR SUPPLIES (Explain Unusual Circumstances)		DIAGNOSIS CODE
	From			To				CPT / HCPCS	MODIFIER	
MM	DD	YY	MM	DD	YY					
3	15	98	3	15	98	11		99213	–25	1
3	15	98	3	15	98	11		29075		1,2,3
3	15	98	3	15	98	11		99070		1,2,3
								OR		
3	15	98	3	15	98	11		A4590		1,2,3

ICD-9-CM

842.02	Sprain and strain of radiocarpal (joint) (ligament) of wrist
E880.9	Accidental fall on or from other stairs or steps
E849.0	Place of occurrence, home

CPT

99213-25	Office or other outpatient visit for the evaluation and management of an established patient, which requires at least two of these three key components: an expanded problem focused history; an expanded problem focused examination; medical decision making of low complexity. Counseling and coordination of care with other providers or agencies are provided consistent with the nature of the problem(s) and the patient's and/or family's needs. Usually, the presenting problem(s) are of low to moderate severity. Physicians typically spend 15 minutes face-to-face with the patient and/or family — Significant, separately identifiable E/M service by the same physician on the same day of the procedure or other service.
29075	Application; elbow to finger (short arm)
99070	Supplies and materials (except spectacles), provided by the physician over and above those usually included with the office visit or other services rendered (list drugs, trays, supplies, or materials provided)
OR	
A4590	Special casting material (e.g., fiberglass)

CODING AXIOM

Initial cast application is included in the treatment of fractures and dislocations, and should not be reported separately. However, it is appropriate to report casting supplies used for the initial cast application, see 99070, A4580, A4590.

ARTHROSCOPIC SURGICAL PROCEDURES

The codes and guidelines for arthroscopic procedures begin with an instructional note stating surgical arthroscopy always includes a diagnostic arthroscopy. When a diagnostic arthroscopy of the temporomandibular joint (TMJ) is performed without a definitive surgical procedure, the following code applies:

29800   Arthroscopy, temporomandibular joint, diagnostic, with or without synovial biopsy (separate procedure)

However, when a surgical arthroscopy is performed in conjunction with the diagnostic arthroscopy, it would be reported as follows:

29804   Arthroscopy temporomandibular joint, surgical

Do not report 29800 separately as it is part of 29804.

CPT also states that when arthroscopy is performed with an arthrotomy, modifier -51 or 09951 should be reported. In this case, do not report the primary and secondary procedures with a single code. Instead, report both codes, listing first the service with the highest value. List the secondary procedures (performed during the same operative session) as subsequent line items with their assigned fees and append modifier -51 to indicate a multiple procedure.

29877   Arthroscopy, knee, surgical; debridement/shaving of articular cartilage (chondroplasty)
27425-51   Lateral retinacular release (any method) – Multiple procedure

SPINAL SURGERY

Procedure codes for reporting spine surgeries are found in two sections of CPT. Fracture/dislocation, spinal fusion/instrumentation, and treatment of scoliosis/kyphosis are reported with codes from the musculoskeletal section (22100-22999). Procedures of the spine with spinal cord involvement are reported with codes from the nervous system section (62268-63746). It is not unusual for procedures to require both a procedure from the musculoskeletal section (arthrodesis, instrumentation) with a procedure from the nervous system section (laminectomy, hemilaminectomy, diskectomy), and it is appropriate to report both procedures separately.

Arthrodesis is a joint fusion and spinal arthrodesis is reported with 22548-22632. These codes are assigned based on technique (anterior/anterolateral, posterior/posterolateral, or lateral). Codes 22548-22558, 22590-22612, 22630 are for single interspace arthrodesis — two adjacent vertebral segments. When the surgery is performed on more than one interspace, each additional interspace is reported with 22585, 22614, or 22632. These procedures are considered "add on" services and are not reported with modifier -51.

Procedures for scoliosis and kyphosis (22800-22819) also include arthrodesis procedures. The arthrodesis procedures in this section differ since they involve multiple vertebral segments, and the code is assigned based on the number of segments treated.

Spinal instrumentation (22840-22855) involves placement of rods, hooks, and/or wires to stabilize the fusion or fracture. Instrumentation codes are assigned based on the type of instrumentation (segmental, non-segmental), the approach (anterior, posterior) and the number of vertebral segments involved. Instrumentation codes are exempt from modifier -51 and are reported in addition to the definitive procedure.

Diskectomy is the excision of intervertebral disk material.

Laminectomy is the removal of the entire lamina on both sides, inclusive of the spinous process.

Hemilaminectomy is the excision of the right or left lamina.

Laminotomy is the process to create a hole in the lamina to achieve the required result.

Bone allografts and autografts should be reported separately with codes 20930-20938. These codes are also modifier -51 exempt and are reported in addition to the definitive procedure. Only one code from this section can be reported per operative session.

Procedures of the spine with spinal cord are found in the nervous system section (62268-63746) and include: diskectomy, laminectomy, hemilaminectomy, and laminotomy.

Diskectomy is the excision of intervertebral disk material. Codes 63075–63078 are specific to this surgery; however, many other codes from this section of the nervous system include diskectomies as a component of the procedure. Laminectomy is the removal of the entire lamina on both sides, inclusive of the spinous process. Hemilaminectomy is the excision of the right or left lamina, the posterior bony covering of the spinal cord. Laminotomy is the process of creating a hole in the lamina to achieve the required result, for example, excising a herniated intervertebral disk.

CARDIOVASCULAR SYSTEM
Pacemaker/Defibrillator Care (33200-33249)
Pacemaker and defibrillator systems include a pulse generator which contains electronics and a battery and one or more electrodes (leads). The pulse generator is placed in a subcutaneous pocket. Electrodes are inserted through a vein (transvenous) or on the surface of the heart (epicardial).

Pacemaker systems are either single or dual chamber systems. In a single chamber system a single electrode is placed in either the atrium or ventricle. In a dual chamber system two electrodes are placed, one into the atrium and one into the ventricle.

Repositioning or replacement procedures performed during the first 14 days after the initial insertion or reportable replacement are included in the code for the initial procedure and should not be reported separately. Repositioning and replacement procedures performed after 14 days are considered new, not repeat, services and modifiers -76 and -77 should not be used.

Replacement of a pulse generator requires assignment of two codes, one for the removal and another for the insertion.

Coronary Artery Bypass Grafts (33510-33536)
Coronary artery bypass grafts (CABG) are coded by type of graft. Venous grafting alone is reported with 33510-33516. Arterial grafting alone is reported with 33533-33545. Combined arterial-venous grafting is reported with 33517-33523 in combination with 33533-33535. Codes 33517-33523 cannot be reported alone.

Procurement of vein and artery grafts is included in CABG procedures and should not be reported separately. If the graft procurement is performed by a second surgeon, those services should be reported as assistant surgeon services with modifier -80 appended to the applicable CABG code(s).

Vascular Catheterization/Injection (36000-36299)
Vascular catheterization/injection services include local anesthesia, introduction of needle or catheter, injection of contrast media, and use of power injections. Since these are diagnostic procedures, only the pre-injection and post-injection care directly related to the procedure is included. Catheters, drugs, and contrast media should be reported separately.

Selective vascular catheterization codes include introduction and all lesser order vessels catheterized used in the approach. Selective catheterization of the right middle cerebral artery includes the introduction and placement catheterization of the right common and internal carotid arteries. Only code 36217 for the third order branch would be reported. Additional second or third order vessels supplied by the same first order branch are reported with "add on" procedure codes 36012, 36218, and 36248.

These procedures are reported by vascular family and, as such, any procedure performed on more than one vascular family is reported separately using the conventions described above. Bilateral procedures are reported as separate vascular families.

These procedures are some of the most difficult for payors to adjudicate. It is important to identify involved vessels with the correct ICD-9-CM diagnosis codes and that these diagnosis codes are attached to the correct procedure codes. You may want to submit a procedure report with every claim for payor clarification.

DIGESTIVE SYSTEM

Gastrointestinal Endoscopy

Gastrointestinal endoscopy codes are reported by site and are listed as follows: esophagus (43200-43228), upper gastrointestinal (43234-43259), other small intestine or stomal (44360-44394), large intestine (45300-45385), and endoscopic retrograde cholangiopancreatography (ERCP) (43260-43272).

Endoscopic procedures may be diagnostic or surgical. The procedure is considered diagnostic when performed to visualize an abnormality or determine the extent of disease. When anything more than visualization is performed, the procedure is considered to be a surgical procedure. A surgical endoscopy always includes a diagnostic endoscopy.

For example, if the patient is to have a diagnostic flexible sigmoidoscopy with biopsy of a lesion during the same surgical session, the diagnostic portion of the procedure (45330) would not be reported separately. Only the surgical portion of the procedure (45331) would be reported.

Diagnostic endoscopic procedures can be reported with open or incisional procedures.

For example, a colonoscopy with removal of tumor (45384) was planned. However, upon visualization of the lesion it was determined that the tumor was too large to treat endoscopically. An open (incisional) partial colectomy with anastomosis was performed, which should be reported as follows:

44140	Colectomy, partial; with anastomosis
45378-51	Colonoscopy, flexible, proximal to splenic flexure; diagnostic with or without collection of specimen(s), by brushing/washing, with or without colon decompression (separate procedure)

Hernia Repair (49495-49611)

Hernia repair codes are categorized primarily by type of hernia (inguinal, femoral, incisional/ventral, epigastric, umbilical, spigelian). Some hernias are further categorized based on whether there has been a previous hernia repair (initial, recurrent). Additional variables include patient age and clinical presentation (reducible, strangulated/incarcerated).

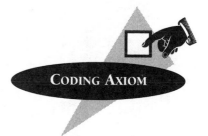

CODING AXIOM

Hernia repair codes are categorized primarily by type of hernia (inguinal, femoral, incision/ventral, epigastric, umbilical, spigelian). Some hernias are further categorized based on whether there has been a previous hernia repair (initial, recurrent).

Implantation of mesh or prosthesis may be performed with hernia repairs. However, the implantation should be reported separately only when used for repair of incisional and ventral hernias (49560-49566). When used for repair of other types of hernias, it is not considered a separately reportable procedure.

Repair of strangulated organs or structures should be reported in addition to the hernia repair. Structures most often involved include intestine (44120), testicles (54520), and ovaries (58940).

URINARY SYSTEM

Urodynamics (51725-51797)

Urodynamics is a diagnostic service performed to evaluate the storage of urine and urine flow through the urinary tract. All procedures in this section represent complete procedures (both the professional and technical components). Physicians reporting these services as complete procedures are expected to supply all instruments/equipment, supplies, and technician services. A physician performing only the operation of the equipment and interpretation of the report should report only the professional component by appending modifier -26 to the procedure codes.

Cystoscopy, Urethroscopy, and Cystourethroscopy (52000-52700)

Cystoscopy, urethroscopy, and cystourethroscopy are listed so that the main procedure can be identified without listing all minor related procedures performed. For example, a cystourethroscopy with dilation of a urethral stricture (52281) includes calibration, meatotomy, and the injection procedure for cystography which are all explicitly described in the procedure.

Secondary endoscopic procedures performed on the same site which are not explicitly included and involve significant additional time and work may be reported either of two ways. CPT instructions state that the secondary procedure should not be reported additionally, but reported instead by modifier -22 appended to the primary procedure. However, many physicians do report secondary procedures with a separate code and append modifier -51. When billing for the secondary procedure either with modifier -22 or with the actual procedure code, verify that it can be justified based on the additional time and work required. Documentation may need to be submitted with the claim.

Many procedures on the ureter require placement of a temporary stent. Placement and removal of temporary stents are not reported separately. However, placement of more permanent, self-retaining, indwelling stents (52332) should be reported with the code for the primary procedure. For example, a cystourethroscopy with removal of ureteral calculus and placement of indwelling double-J type stent would be reported as follows:

52320	Cystourethroscopy (including ureteral catheterization); with removal of ureteral calculus
52332-51	Cystourethroscopy, with insertion of indwelling ureteral stent (eg, Gibbons or double-J type)

LAPAROSCOPY/HYSTEROSCOPY (56300-56399)

Laparoscopic procedures are accomplished via an endoscope inserted through a small incision in the abdomen. Until recent years, this type of procedure was used most frequently to perform minor procedures on the female reproductive tract. Now, however, laparoscopy is used to perform many procedures on both males and females, including major procedures such as cholecystectomy, splenectomy, and intestinal resection.

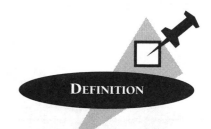

Laparoscopy and hysteroscopy may utilize many methods to accomplish the desired result, including hot cautery, CO_2 laser, ND-YAG laser, and pelvioscopy. The CPT code is the same regardless of the technique used.

Like other endoscopic procedures, laparoscopy and hysteroscopy are listed to easily identify the main procedure without reporting all minor related procedures performed at the same time. The example given in CPT involves fulguration of the oviducts (56301) with lysis of adhesions and fulguration of bleeding points. In this example, fulguration of bleeding points does not have a separate procedure code, but is inherent to procedure 56301. However, lysis of adhesions is described by two CPT codes, 56304 for salpingolysis/ovariolysis or 56310 for enterolysis. Note that both of the procedures are designated as separate procedures. They are not normally billed with another definitive procedure at the same site during the same surgical session.

As with other coding rules, there are exceptions. The key to deciding whether the lysis of adhesions should be billed separately hinges on the additional time and work involved. Do not be tempted to over report services, especially services involving adhesiolysis. Report secondary procedures when the time and work justify additional compensation as illustrated by the following example:

A removal of the left ovary is complicated by dense adhesions of the left fallopian tube and ovary to the bowel requiring extensive dissection. In addition, dense adhesions are encountered between the bowel and omentum requiring extensive dissection. Adhesiolysis requires additional operative time of more than one hour. In this case, the additional work may be reported in either of two ways. A report of the procedure should be submitted with the claim regardless of which method of reporting is selected.

The laparoscopy with removal of adnexal structures (oophorectomy) could be reported with modifier -22.

56307-22   Laparoscopy, surgical; with removal of adnexal structures (partial or total oophorectomy and/or salpingectomy) (service provided greater than that usually required for the listed procedure)

The other option is to report both the oophorectomy and adhesiolysis. Only one adhesiolysis code should be reported. Since all adhesions involve the bowel, code 56310 would be the most appropriate.

56307   Laparoscopy, surgical; with removal of adnexal structures (partial or total oophorectomy and/or salpingectomy)

56310-51   Laparoscopy, surgical; enterolysis (freeing of intestinal adhesion) (separate procedure)

FEMALE GENITAL SYSTEM
Vulvectomy (56620-56640)
Vulvectomy procedures are described by several terms that have specific definitions in CPT. The following definitions would be employed when selecting a vulvectomy code:

- Simple - Removal of skin and superficial subcutaneous tissues
- Radical - Removal of skin and deep subcutaneous tissues
- Partial - Removal of less than 80 percent of the vulvar area
- Complete - Removal of 80 percent or more of the vulvar area

ND-YAG laser is the acronym for neodymium yttrium aluminum garnet, a type of laser that has been used in the treatment of tumors.

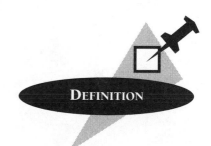

A **vulvectomy** is the excision of the vulva. Aseptic technique is used for urethral and catheter care. Sitz baths are discouraged because infections are easily acquired.

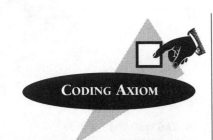

The guideline to maternity care states that normal care includes monthly visits up to 28 week gestation, biweekly visits to 36 week gestation, and weekly visits from week 36 until delivery. Additional visits for other medical or surgical intervention should be reported with the appropriate evaluation and management codes.

MATERNITY CARE AND DELIVERY

Maternity care is outlined in the maternity care and delivery section. The codes for normal, uncomplicated care to the maternity patient (59400, 59510, 59610, 59618) include antepartum care, delivery, and postpartum care by the same physician.

Antepartum care includes the initial and routine subsequent history and physical exams, patient's weight, blood pressure, fetal heart tones, and routine urinalysis.

Delivery includes admission to the hospital, including the admitting history and exam, the management of uncomplicated labor, and either a vaginal or cesarean delivery.

Postpartum care includes the inpatient hospital care and any office visits following vaginal or cesarean delivery.

Six relatively new, delivery codes deserve some additional explanation. These codes report delivery after a previous cesarean delivery when an attempt is made to accomplish the delivery vaginally, also referred to as a VBAC. Codes 59610–59614 report a successful vaginal delivery after a previous cesarean delivery (VBAC). Codes 59618–59622 are reported if a vaginal birth attempt is unsuccessful and another cesarean delivery is carried out. These codes for global care are reported on claims following the delivery.

When different physicians provide components of the total obstetric service, report the services separately using the codes designated for each component. Codes 59425 and 59426 identify a different physician providing four or more antepartum care visits. Use the appropriate E/M codes when a different physician provides one to three antepartum care visits. Use 59409, 59514, 59612, or 59620 when the physician performs vaginal or cesarean delivery only. Use 59410, 59515, 59614, or 59622 when the physician performs vaginal or cesarean delivery with postpartum care.

Services unrelated to the pregnancy should be reported with Evaluation and Management codes or the procedure codes for the service. For example, a patient seen for a sore throat with a throat culture should have both the throat culture and E/M service reported separately. Clearly identify the reasons for the services as pharyngitis, not pregnancy.

Services directly related to the pregnancy, but not included in the global service, should be reported separately. Examples include ultrasound examination of pregnant uterus (76805–76816), glucose tolerance test (82951–82953), and pap smear (88150).

High-Risk Maternity Care/Complications of Pregnancy

The guideline to maternity care states that normal care includes monthly visits up to 28 weeks gestation, biweekly visits to 36 weeks gestation, and weekly visits until delivery. For the patient at risk who is seen more frequently or for other medical/surgical intervention, code the additional services with a code representing the appropriate level of E/M service. The documentation must reflect the necessity of these visits as well as any additional laboratory or radiologic tests performed.

When the physician monitors the patient for a prolonged period, document the time spent in actual attendance and use prolonged services codes as appropriate. Codes 99356 and 99357 describe maternal-fetal monitoring, which is reported in addition to the delivery. Always include documentation to substantiate medical necessity.

NERVOUS SYSTEM

Surgery of Skull Base (61580-61616)

Neurosurgical procedures of lesions involving the skull base often require the skills of several surgeons of different surgical specialties. These procedures have been broken into their component parts, categorized by the approach, definitive procedure, and repair/reconstruction of surgical defects following the definitive procedure.

The approach is defined as the portion of the procedure necessary to obtain adequate exposure of the lesion. It is described by anatomical area involved which includes: anterior, middle, or posterior cranial fossa; brain stem; and upper spinal cord.

The definitive portion includes: biopsy, excision, resection or repair of the lesion, and primary closure of the dura, mucous membrane and skin.

Repair/reconstruction is reported separately only when extensive dural grafting, cranioplasty, myocutaneous flaps, or extensive skin grafts are employed to close the surgical defect.

When different surgeons perform the component parts of skull base procedures, each reports only the code for the specific portion the physician has performed.

If one surgeon performs both the approach and definitive procedure, both codes should be reported, appending modifier -51 to the secondary procedure(s).

CHRONIC PAIN MANAGEMENT SERVICES (20550, 62274-62298, 64400-64530)

Chronic pain management services and reporting guidelines are included in Chapter 4 - Anesthesia, since pain management services are frequently performed by an anesthesiologist with special training in pain management procedures.

Surgical Coding Methodology

Use a step-by-step approach for determining the correct codes for surgical procedures. Correct coding will generally minimize claim rejection. Turnaround time in processing may decrease, which could increase cash flow and lessen the likelihood of appeals, denials, and audits. Always use the most recent versions of CPT, ICD-9-CM, and HCPCS Level II for accurate coding. Checking each claim submitted against the guidelines listed below will help improve coding accuracy.

1. Read the surgery guidelines at the beginning of the surgery section.

2. Locate the code in the index that most accurately describes the procedure(s) performed.

3. Read the descriptive nomenclature of the code carefully, and read any information before and after the code that might give directions. Make sure your documentation and/or operative report justifies the use of the code.

4. Page back as necessary to the subheading for the code and read any notes or directions for the section that apply to the code.

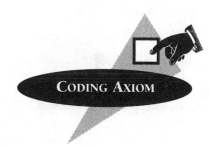

CODING AXIOM

Use a step-by-step approach for determining the correct codes for surgical procedures. Correct coding will generally minimize claim rejection. Always use the most recent versions of CPT, ICD-9-CM, and HCPCS Level II codes.

5. Watch for notes or *see* references that apply to the code you wish to use. Does a note specify the code cannot be used with another code? Does it send you to another area for a more correct code? Does it explain additional procedures that may be billed with the code?

6. Consider the code and what is included in it. Do not unbundle, but do not miss the opportunity to code additional procedures not included in the code.

7. Enter the code correctly on the claim form, always listing the most revenue-intensive code first.

8. When more than one code is used, apply the correct modifiers from the list of modifiers in Chapter 2 of *Code It Right* that apply to second and additional codes. Except when reporting modifier -52 or -53, never reduce the fee for codes appended with modifiers. Let the payor make any necessary adjustments.

9. On the HCFA-1500 claim form, apply the correct diagnostic codes and indicate next to the CPT code in the correct box every diagnosis that applies to the surgery or procedure.

10. Follow any contractual arrangements you may have with the payor.

Do not rely on a computerized coding system to give you the correct code. While computer systems are meant to speed up coding, they are not meant to replace CPT or other coding books. The most sophisticated coding programs are incapable of consistently applying the correct codes and rules.

If the code has been deleted or a note below the code sends you to another code, always look it up — an older reference may not have been deleted. Look at other codes in that section. You may find a code that more accurately describes the procedure performed.

Look for key phrases in the operative report and within the code description that can help you determine the correct code (e.g., with or without, includes, separate procedure, eponym, single, unilateral, bilateral, excludes, primary, secondary, in addition, open, closed, etc.).

DISCUSSION QUESTIONS

1. Biopsy codes are appropriate for reporting what type of surgical services?

2. Is the method of destruction a consideration in reporting laparoscopic procedures? Explain.

3. When is closure of the operative wound included in the surgical service of lesion excision?

4. How do you assign excision codes for malignant lesions?

    _____

    _____

    _____

5. Tissue transfer or rearrangement codes (14000–14350) describe moving normal tissue. The tissue from the donor site is moved to what other type of site?

    _____

    _____

    _____

6. Explain the difference between open and closed treatment in fracture care.

    _____

    _____

    _____

7. Why is diagnostic arthroscopy always included with surgical arthroscopy?

    _____

    _____

8. How should you report complications of labor and delivery?

    _____

    _____

    _____

9. Define medical necessity. Why must medical necessity be documented, for example, in maternity situations requiring maternal-fetal monitoring?

    _____

    _____

    _____

10. Surgical coding methodology is an involved process that is vital to appropriate reimbursement and to avoid claims auditing. Cite steps you can take to improve coding accuracy and how these steps can be incorporated into your office.

    _____

    _____

    _____

Specialty-Specific Scenarios

OBSTETRICS AND GYNECOLOGY SCENARIO – INPATIENT

The patient delivered vaginally November 1, and an emergency curettage was performed November 3 for postpartum hemorrhage due to retained placental fragments.

Gynecology

21. DIAGNOSIS OR NATURE OF ILLNESS OR INJURY (RELATE ITEMS 1, 2, 3 OR 4 TO ITEM 24E BY LINE)							
1. 666.22				3.			
2. V27.0				4.			

24.	A						B	C	D		E
	DATE(S) OF SERVICE						Place of Service	Type of Service	PROCEDURES, SERVICES, OR SUPPLIES (Explain Unusual Circumstances)		DIAGNOSIS CODE
	From MM	DD	YY	To MM	DD	YY			CPT / HCPCS	MODIFIER	
	11	1	98	11	1	98	21		59400		2
	11	3	98	11	3	98	21		59160	–78	1

ICD-9-CM

666.22 Delayed and secondary postpartum hemorrhage

V27.0 Single liveborn

CPT

59400 Routine obstetric care including antepartum care, vaginal delivery (with or without episiotomy, and/or forceps) and postpartum care

59160-78 Curettage, postpartum — Return to the operating room for related procedure during the postoperative period

The fifth digit 2 specifies to the payor that the patient was delivered during this admission with a postpartum complication. Although the delivery was uncomplicated, do not code 650. Code 650 specifically states that it cannot be used with any other code in the range 630–676.

DERMATOLOGY SCENARIO – OUTPATIENT

A 23-year-old man has a suspicious 0.5 cm lesion, on his shoulder. The dermatologist excises the lesion in his office. A microscopic pathology report showing a squamous cell carcinoma with positive borders is sent to the patient's family physician. The family physician refers the patient again to the dermatologist who re-excises the site (previous wound size 1.0 cm including skin margins) who performs a simple primary closure of the wound.

Dermatology

21. DIAGNOSIS OR NATURE OF ILLNESS OR INJURY (RELATE ITEMS 1, 2, 3 OR 4 TO ITEM 24E BY LINE)

1. | 173.6

2. |

3. |

4. |

24.	A DATE(S) OF SERVICE						B Place of Service	C Type of Service	D PROCEDURES, SERVICES, OR SUPPLIES (Explain Unusual Circumstances)		E DIAGNOSIS CODE
	From MM	DD	YY	To MM	DD	YY			CPT / HCPCS	MODIFIER	
	2	17	98	2	17	98	11		11600		1
	2	19	98	2	19	98	11		11601	–58	1

ICD-9-CM

173.6   Other malignant neoplasm of skin of upper limb, including shoulder

CPT

11600   Excision, malignant lesion, trunk, arms, or legs; lesion diameter 0.5 cm or less

11601-58   Excision, malignant lesion, trunk, arms, or legs; lesion diameter 0.6 to 1.0 cm — Staged or related procedure or service by the same physician during the postoperative period

Reporting a malignant skin lesion excision can be tricky. The size of the lesion is used to report a primary excision. Simple closure is included in the code description. If a lesion is re-excised due to positive borders or recurrence in a scar, the size of the old incision is used in coding. Medically, the entire wound is considered malignant if any of the tumor is left behind.

Whenever possible, coders should not submit claims for excision or biopsy until the pathology report is available. Coding the excision of a malignancy as a benign lesion results in reduced reimbursement. Coding benign lesions as malignancies results in labeling the patient as a cancer risk. See Chapter 1 for outpatient and inpatient ICD-9-CM coding of neoplasms.

NEUROSURGERY SCENARIO – INPATIENT

A 71-year-old female presents with acromegaly and multiple medical problems associated with the disease. A MRI scan shows a large pituitary macroadenoma and surgery is elected. The patient undergoes a microscopic trans-sphenoidal pituitary adenectomy with insertion of a lumbar subarachnoid drain.

The right thigh is opened and a muscle and fascia plug is taken from the fascia lata. The graft is placed in the sella. The floor of the sella is reconstructed with a piece of bone and covered with Gelfoam and fat. The wound is closed and dressed and the lumbar drain is removed.

Neurosurgery

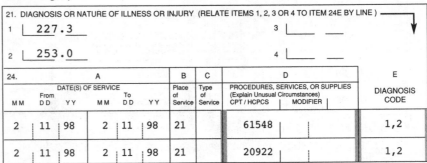

ICD-9-CM

227.3	Benign neoplasm of pituitary gland and craniopharyngeal duct (pouch)
253.0	Acromegaly and gigantism

CPT

61548	Hypophysectomy or excision of pituitary tumor, transnasal or transseptal approach, nonstereotactic
20922	Fascia lata graft; by incision and area exposure, complex or sheet

Grafts from outside the operative area should be reported separately. Documentation should identify the donor site, the size of graft, and type of graft used. Placement of drains, closures, and dressings are incidental to the surgical procedures. Even though this procedure is described as microscopic, procedure 69990 *Use of operating microscope,* is not reported separately. There is a specific note related to procedure 61548 stating 69990 cannot be reported additionally.

INTERNAL MEDICINE SCENARIO – OUTPATIENT

A 44-year-old woman with a history of breast cancer complains of shortness of breath to her internist. Her visit includes an expanded problem focused history, a detailed exam, and low complexity decision making. A chest x-ray in the office shows a small pleural effusion on the right lung. The physician performs a thoracentesis, draws off the fluid, and sends it for cytology and chemistry analysis.

Internal Medicine

21. DIAGNOSIS OR NATURE OF ILLNESS OR INJURY (RELATE ITEMS 1, 2, 3 OR 4 TO ITEM 24E BY LINE)		
1. 511.9	3.
2. V10.3	4.

24.	A DATE(S) OF SERVICE						B Place of Service	C Type of Service	D PROCEDURES, SERVICES, OR SUPPLIES (Explain Unusual Circumstances)		E DIAGNOSIS CODE
	From MM	DD	YY	To MM	DD	YY			CPT / HCPCS	MODIFIER	
	3	31	98	3	31	98	11		32000*		1,2
	3	31	98	3	31	98	11		71020		1,2
	3	31	98	3	31	98	11		99213		1,2

ICD-9-CM

511.9	Unspecified pleural effusion
V10.3	Personal history of malignant neoplasm of breast

CPT

32000*	Thoracentesis, puncture of pleural cavity for aspiration, initial or subsequent
71020	Radiologic examination, chest, two views, frontal and lateral;
99213	Office or other outpatient visit for the evaluation and management of an established patient, which requires at least two of these three key components: an expanded problem focused history; an expanded problem focused examination; medical decision making of low complexity. Counseling and coordination of care with other providers or agencies are provided consistent with the nature of the problem(s) and the patient's and/or family's needs. Usually, the presenting problem(s) are of low to moderate severity. Physicians typically spend 15 minutes face-to-face with the patient and/or family

Starred procedures fall outside the global surgery concept. They do not include pre- or post-operative care. When a level of service is performed with a starred procedure, it is reported separately. If a new patient is seen for the sole purpose of the starred procedure, e.g. paring of a benign lesion by a dermatologist, report 99025 *Initial (new patient) visit when starred (*) surgical procedure constitutes major service at that visit.* If an established patient is seen for the sole purpose of a starred procedure, e.g. arthrocentesis, report only the procedure and not an E/M code.

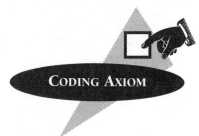

CODING AXIOM

Starred procedures fall outside the global surgery concept. They do not include preoperative or postoperative care. When a level of service is performed with a starred procedure, it is reported separately.

GENERAL SURGERY CODING SCENARIO

A general surgeon attempts a laparoscopic cholecystectomy on a 44-year-old woman suffering from acute cholecystitis with gallstones but no obstruction. Because of an unusual anatomic variation, however, the physician aborts the laparoscopic procedure after the diagnostic peritoneoscopy and completes the cholecystectomy via an open laparotomy.

General Surgery

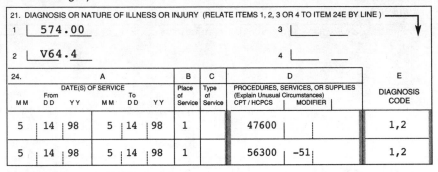

ICD-9-CM

574.00	Calculus of gallbladder with acute cholecystitis, without mention of obstruction
V64.4	Laparoscopic surgical procedure converted to open procedure

CPT

47600	Cholecystectomy;
56300-51	Laparoscopy (peritoneoscopy), diagnostic; (separate procedure) — Multiple procedure

The physician made the decision to abort the procedure via laparoscope, and complete the procedure as an open cholecystectomy. A cover letter and operative report should be submitted with the claim to provide the payor with answers to questions regarding the peritoneoscopy.

OTORHINOLARYNGOLOGY CODING SCENARIO – INPATIENT

A 26-year-old female with amenorrhea and galactorrhea is referred by her gynecologist to the neurosurgeon for further workup. MRI and endocrine studies reveal a microadenoma of the pituitary. Surgery is elected and the patient undergoes exposure by the otorhinolaryngologist. Transnasal excision of a pituitary tumor is performed by the neurosurgeon.

Neurosurgeon

21. DIAGNOSIS OR NATURE OF ILLNESS OR INJURY (RELATE ITEMS 1, 2, 3 OR 4 TO ITEM 24E BY LINE)
1   227.3   3
2   4

24. A DATE(S) OF SERVICE						B Place of Service	C Type of Service	D PROCEDURES, SERVICES, OR SUPPLIES (Explain Unusual Circumstances) CPT / HCPCS MODIFIER	E DIAGNOSIS CODE
From MM	DD	YY	To MM	DD	YY				
6	8	98	6	8	98	1		61548 -62	1
								Cosurgery charge 25% of total added	
								Neurosurgeon's responsibility for excision of tumor & follow-up 70% of total	

Otolaryngologist

21. DIAGNOSIS OR NATURE OF ILLNESS OR INJURY (RELATE ITEMS 1, 2, 3 OR 4 TO ITEM 24E BY LINE)
1   227.3   3
2   4

24. A DATE(S) OF SERVICE						B Place of Service	C Type of Service	D PROCEDURES, SERVICES, OR SUPPLIES (Explain Unusual Circumstances) CPT / HCPCS MODIFIER	E DIAGNOSIS CODE
From MM	DD	YY	To MM	DD	YY				
6	8	98	6	8	98	1		61548 -62	1
								Cosurgery charge 25% of total added	
								Otolaryngologist's responsibility for incision & exposure 30% of total	

ICD-9-CM

227.3   Benign neoplasm of pituitary gland and craniopharyngeal duct (pouch)

CPT

61548-62   Hypophysectomy or excision of pituitary tumor, transnasal or transseptal approach, nonstereotactic — Two surgeons

Single shared cosurgery is a solitary procedure with at least two separate, but integrated parts requiring two or more surgeons. The physicians are responsible for only their portions. In this case, each performed separate parts of a single procedure. The normal surgical fee may be increased by a reasonable percentage to accommodate the cosurgery circumstance. State the division of the surgical fee and extra charge for the cosurgery increase on each surgeon's claim. The claim forms for both physicians should be submitted together with a cover letter and copies of the operative reports.

CODING AXIOM

Single shared cosurgery is a solitary procedure with at least two separate but integrated parts requiring two or more surgeons. The physicians are responsible for only their portions.

OPHTHALMOLOGY SCENARIO –OUTPATIENT

The ophthalmologist repairs two horizontal muscles for alternating esotropia, and a lid retraction repair at an outpatient hospital surgical suite. The following is an example of the multiple procedures modifier -51. The billing would be submitted as follows:

Ophthalmology

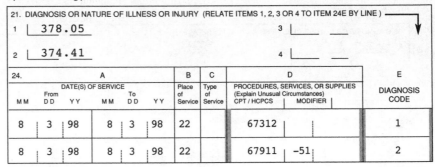

ICD-9-CM

378.05	Alternating esotropia
374.41	Lid retraction or lag

CPT

67312	Strabismus surgery, recession or resection procedure; two horizontal muscles
67911-51	Correction of lid retraction — Multiple procedure

INTERVENTIONAL RADIOLOGY SCENARIO – OUTPATIENT

A 64-year-old patient presents with severe headaches and blackouts. Previous EEG and CT scans are negative. An interventional radiologist performs bilateral common carotid and left vertebral artery (cerebral) angiography. A retrograde right femoral approach is used. Selective catheterization of the right common carotid artery, the left common carotid artery, and subsequently the left vertebral artery is performed. In addition, photographic subtractions are obtained of the AP view on the vertebral run. The radiologist's interpretation concludes the patient has cerebral atherosclerosis.

Radiology

21. DIAGNOSIS OR NATURE OF ILLNESS OR INJURY (RELATE ITEMS 1, 2, 3 OR 4 TO ITEM 24E BY LINE)		
1	437.0	3
2		4

24.	A DATE(S) OF SERVICE						B Place of Service	C Type of Service	D PROCEDURES, SERVICES, OR SUPPLIES (Explain Unusual Circumstances)		E DIAGNOSIS CODE
	From MM	DD	YY	To MM	DD	YY			CPT / HCPCS	MODIFIER	
1	28	98	1	28	98	22		36216	–RT	1
1	29	98	1	29	98	22		36216	–LT –51	1
1	29	98	1	29	98	22		36215	–LT –51	1
1	28	98	1	28	98	22		75680	–26	1
1	28	98	1	28	98	22		75685	–26	1
1	29	98	1	29	98	22		76350	–26	1

ICD-9-CM

437.0   Cerebral atherosclerosis

CPT

36216-RT   Selective catheter placement, arterial system; initial second order thoracic or brachiocephalic branch, within a vascular family — Right side (HCPCS modifier)

36216-LT-51   Selective catheter placement, arterial system; initial second order thoracic or brachiocephalic branch, within a vascular family — Left side (HCPCS modifier) — Multiple procedure

36215-LT-51   Selective catheter placement, arterial system; each first order thoracic or brachiocephalic branch, within a vascular family — Left side (HCPCS modifier) — Multiple procedure

75680-26   Angiography, carotid, cervical, bilateral, radiological supervision and interpretation — Professional component

75685-26   Angiography, vertebral, cervical, and/or intracranial, radiological supervision and interpretation — Professional component

76350-26   Subtraction in conjunction with contrast studies — Professional component

The key to component billing versus unbundling is to identify the highest order catheterization within a vascular family that includes all lesser order and nonselective catheterizations. Remember, bilateral studies are reported as separate vascular families. The left common carotid artery branches off the aorta, so it is a first order branch (36215). The right common carotid branches off the brachio-cephalic artery and is a second order vessel (36216). The left vertebral artery branches off the subclavian artery and is also a second order vessel (36216). Each of these vessels belong to different vascular families so they are all reported separately.

Report 75680-26 for the bilateral carotid angiography and 75685-26 for the vertebral angiography.

Subtraction is reported according to the number of separate masks prepared from the contrast studies.

KEY POINTS

Remember when selecting CPT surgical codes:

- Read surgical code descriptions carefully

- Modifiers may have a significant impact on reimbursement

- Avoid unbundling and fragmenting

- Surgical procedures may be either diagnostic or therapeutic

- Use a step-by-step approach for determining correct codes

Advanced Coding Practice

CODING PRACTICE 1

A 42-year-old woman with a long history of back pain treated conservatively is admitted to the hospital for surgery of herniated lumbar disks because of progressive radiculopathy of the right leg. An MRI obtained one week prior to admission had demonstrated herniation at the L4-5 and L5-S1 interspaces. A hemilaminectomy with decompression of nerve root(s), including excision of herniated disks is performed at each level. A posterior interbody arthrodesis is performed at each level. Morselized bone obtained from the iliac crest is grafted into the surgical site. Code physician services provided during this inpatient hospitalization.

21. DIAGNOSIS OR NATURE OF ILLNESS OR INJURY (RELATE ITEMS 1, 2, 3 OR 4 TO ITEM 24E BY LINE)						
1 ⌊_ _⌋				3 ⌊_ _⌋		
2 ⌊_ _⌋				4 ⌊_ _⌋		

24.	A		B	C	D	E
	DATE(S) OF SERVICE		Place of Service	Type of Service	PROCEDURES, SERVICES, OR SUPPLIES (Explain Unusual Circumstances)	DIAGNOSIS CODE
M M	From D D Y Y	To M M D D Y Y			CPT / HCPCS MODIFIER	

CODING PRACTICE 2

A 79-year-old male with a dual chamber pacemaker used to treat bradycardia caused by Wenckebach type atrioventricular block is admitted for change of the battery in his pacemaker. An electronic analysis at the cardiologist's office indicates that the battery is malfunctioning and needs to be replaced. The battery has been in place for several years and has functioned without problems until recently. The procedure is performed on an outpatient basis at the hospital. Code the physician services provided during the outpatient surgery.

21. DIAGNOSIS OR NATURE OF ILLNESS OR INJURY (RELATE ITEMS 1, 2, 3 OR 4 TO ITEM 24E BY LINE)				
1		3		
2		4		

24. A DATE(S) OF SERVICE						B Place of Service	C Type of Service	D PROCEDURES, SERVICES, OR SUPPLIES (Explain Unusual Circumstances)		E DIAGNOSIS CODE
From MM DD YY			To MM DD YY					CPT / HCPCS	MODIFIER	

Chapter Review

To select CPT surgical codes that accurately reflect the service performed, read surgical code descriptions carefully and remember that modifiers may have a significant impact on reimbursement. The practice of coding incidental services separately from a major surgical procedure is called unbundling or fragmenting and should be avoided. Surgical procedures may be either diagnostic or therapeutic. In addition, they may be classified as a "package" or starred services. Different coding rules apply to these different types of procedures. Diagnostic services are performed to determine or establish a patient's diagnosis. When a star (*) follows a surgical code, the service listed includes only the surgical procedure, no associated pre- and postoperative services. Use a step-by-step approach for determining the correct codes for surgical procedures. The surgical section of CPT contains guidelines specific to the section, subsection, category, subcategory, or code. Familiarize yourself with these guidelines and be aware of the special coding circumstances for each subsection.

6 Radiology Services

Radiology Codes and Guidelines

Perhaps no area of medicine integrates technological advancement faster than radiology. The specialty regularly employs imaging, diagnostic, and therapeutic technologies developed only a few decades ago. Consequently, the radiology section (70010–79999) is under constant review to reflect current standards of service.

Radiological procedures are divided into four subsections in CPT: diagnostic radiology, including computerized tomography (CT), magnetic resonance imaging (MRI), and interventional radiology procedures; diagnostic ultrasound; radiation oncology; and diagnostic and therapeutic nuclear medicine. Codes are ordered according to anatomic site (head, chest, abdomen), and body system (gastrointestinal, aorta, and arteries). The subject listings in the radiological services section may be reported when a physician either performs or supervises the services.

Procedures are described by type of service (modality), specific body site, and are followed by additional information regarding the use of contrast material and the complexity of the procedure.

CPT provides guidelines for radiology codes at the beginning of each radiology section. Notes clarify the use of codes within the subsections. Code categories, subcategories, and parenthetical phrases also may be presented. The guidelines are arranged similar to other sections of CPT and are unique to the individual code, category, subcategory, or range of codes.

Procedures frequently performed by radiologists may be found outside the radiology section, such as Noninvasive Vascular Diagnostic Studies (93875–93990) covered in Chapter 8. Services involving the invasive or interventional component of interventional radiology services are found in the surgery section. These include percutaneous biopsies, injection procedures, and transcatheter procedures which are discussed in this chapter.

OBJECTIVES

- **Become familiar with the four subsections of radiology**

- **Recognize the importance of documentation**

- **Determine the difference between the technical and professional components in radiology procedures**

- **Distinguish the components of interventional radiology**

- **Know when to report modifiers and x-ray consultations**

- **Identify common radiology terms**

TECHNICAL AND PROFESSIONAL COMPONENTS
Radiology procedures are comprised of two components: technical and professional. The technical component includes the provision of the equipment, supplies, technical personnel, and costs attendant to the performance of the procedure other than the professional services. The professional component encompasses the physician's work in providing the service, including supervision, interpretation, and report of the procedure. Education, malpractice insurance, and other expenses incident to maintaining a practice are also part of the professional component.

A common division for reimbursement of routine diagnostic procedures is 60 percent for the technical component and 40 percent for the professional component.

Technical component includes the provision of the equipment, supplies, technical personnel, and costs attendant to the performance of the procedure other than the professional services.

Professional component encompasses all of the physician's work in providing the service, including interpretation and report of the procedure.

Coding radiology services has been difficult due to the technical component inherent to this area of medicine. The sophisticated and expensive equipment required for radiology services has been owned by hospitals and large facilities. Hospitals reported the use of the equipment, the specially trained personnel, and related costs associated with the technical component. The advent of freestanding medical facilities including physician offices capable of offering imaging services, catheterizations, and other diagnostic and therapeutic radiology services poses a challenge in securing reimbursement for both components. As the standard coding reference, CPT reports the physician component of services rather than the technical. Coders will not find a modifier in CPT to reflect technical services. HCPCS Level II provides the modifier -TC specifically for reporting the technical component. And even though CPT now lists some HCPCS Level II modifiers, -TC has not been included in CPT 1999.

While the problem with reporting these services has not been solved, most payors now accept modifier -TC for the technical component. In addition, payors have developed fee schedules reflecting each component separately and many also have a fee reflecting a global reimbursement rate for the service provided. Reimbursement for each component performed requires the use of the correct modifiers.

Unless instructed otherwise by payors, the professional component should be reported with modifier -26, the technical component with modifier -TC. The global service (technical and professional) can be reported either once without a modifier, or two times, once with the modifier -TC and once with the modifier -26.

Technical Component
The following case study is an example of technical component reporting. When a radiological examination is performed at a hospital or other facility where a radiologist is employed and reports his or her services separately, the hospital or other facility reports the technical component.

An elderly patient trips on a sidewalk and the treating physician suspects a fracture of the scaphoid in the patient's left wrist. The physician refers her to the outpatient radiology department of a nearby hospital for diagnostic x-rays. Three radiologic views of the wrist are required.

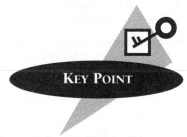

Free-standing medical facilities securing reimbursement
Reimbursement may be difficult to secure until payers and claims processors recognize which freestanding facilities in their area are capable of providing both the technical and professional components of a service. If claims are denied for the technical component, contact the utilization or provider relations manager and ask to have a note placed in the claims system stating a complete service should be reimbursed.

21. DIAGNOSIS OR NATURE OF ILLNESS OR INJURY (RELATE ITEMS 1, 2, 3 OR 4 TO ITEM 24E BY LINE)							
1 ⌊ 814.01					3 ⌊___ ___		
2 ⌊ E885 ___					4 ⌊___ ___		

24.	A		B	C	D		E
	DATE(S) OF SERVICE		Place of Service	Type of Service	PROCEDURES, SERVICES, OR SUPPLIES (Explain Unusual Circumstances)		DIAGNOSIS CODE
MM DD YY (From)	MM DD YY (To)				CPT / HCPCS	MODIFIER	
4 12 98	4 12 98		71		73110	–TC	1,2

ICD-9-CM

814.01   Closed fracture of navicular (scaphoid) of wrist

E885   Fall on same level from slipping, tripping, or stumbling

CPT

73110-TC   Radiologic examination, wrist; complete, minimum of three views
Technical component modifier

This example employs the HCPCS Level II modifier -TC best understood by payors handling Medicare and Medicaid claims. Billing private third-party payors varies. See Chapter 10 for information regarding HCPCS codes and modifiers.

Professional Component
A physician who reads films after another party has performed the technical component (such as a hospital) reports only the professional component which requires adding modifier -26 to the CPT code. This signals payors to expect the other party to report the technical portion. The following example illustrates reporting the professional component for a unilateral hip x-ray.

A young house painter sustains a right femoral neck fracture in a fall from a ladder. A single-view x-ray is required. The radiologist reads the film and reports his interpretation separately.

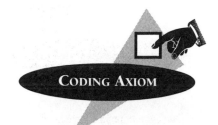

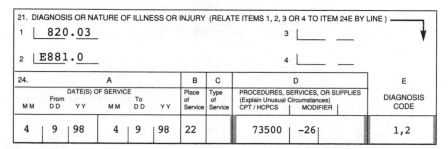

ICD-9-CM

820.03 Transcervical closed fracture of base of neck of femur

E881.0 Fall from ladder

CPT

73500-26 Radiologic examination, hip, unilateral; one view — Professional component modifier

Global Service
A global service may be reported when one physician provides both components of the radiology procedure, such as owning the equipment, employing the technologist, and providing a written interpretation of the examination. The following case study is an example of global service reporting.

A 10-year-old girl falls from her bicycle, breaking the shaft of her right radius. Two views of her forearm are taken (A/P and lateral) and interpreted at the orthopedic clinic.

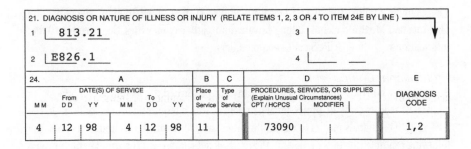

21. DIAGNOSIS OR NATURE OF ILLNESS OR INJURY (RELATE ITEMS 1, 2, 3 OR 4 TO ITEM 24E BY LINE)

1. | 813.21   3 |
2. | E826.1   4 |

24.	A						B	C	D		E
	DATE(S) OF SERVICE						Place of Service	Type of Service	PROCEDURES, SERVICES, OR SUPPLIES (Explain Unusual Circumstances)		DIAGNOSIS CODE
	From			To					CPT / HCPCS	MODIFIER	
MM	DD	YY	MM	DD	YY						
4	12	98	4	12	98		11		73090		1,2

ICD-9-CM

813.21   Closed fracture of shaft of radius (alone)

E826.1   Road vehicle accident, pedal cyclist

CPT

73090   Radiologic examination; forearm, anteroposterior and lateral views

— OR —

21. DIAGNOSIS OR NATURE OF ILLNESS OR INJURY (RELATE ITEMS 1, 2, 3 OR 4 TO ITEM 24E BY LINE)

1. | 813.21   3 |
2. | E826.1   4 |

24.	A						B	C	D		E
	DATE(S) OF SERVICE						Place of Service	Type of Service	PROCEDURES, SERVICES, OR SUPPLIES (Explain Unusual Circumstances)		DIAGNOSIS CODE
	From			To					CPT / HCPCS	MODIFIER	
MM	DD	YY	MM	DD	YY						
4	12	98	4	12	98		11		73090	–26	1,2
4	12	98	4	12	98		11		73090	–TC	1,2

ICD-9-CM

813.21   Closed fracture of shaft of radius (alone)

E826.1   Road vehicle accident, pedal cyclist

CPT

73090-26   Radiologic examination; forearm, anteroposterior and lateral views — Professional Component

73090-TC   Radiologic examination; forearm, anteroposterior and lateral views — Technical Component

Types of Radiology Services

As stated earlier, the Radiology section of CPT is divided into four subsections. These are:

Diagnostic Radiology
Diagnostic Ultrasound
Radiation Oncology
Nuclear Medicine

DIAGNOSTIC RADIOLOGY

Procedures in Diagnostic Radiology section establish a diagnosis or follow the progression or remission of a disease process. However, also included in this section are procedures that are therapeutic in nature. These therapeutic procedures are often referred to as interventional or invasive radiology services. Codes in this chapter of CPT report the radiological supervision and interpretation of these interventional and invasive procedures.

Diagnostic radiology uses different modalities, including x-rays, fluoroscopy, CT, and MRI. Procedures in the diagnostic radiology section are ordered by anatomic site. They are then described by type of service (modality), specific body site, number of views, and use of contrast materials.

Services described in CPT as a "radiological examination" refer to plain films of specific sites. Other terms used to describe plain films include standard or conventional films. Services employing other modalities and/or additional techniques are described by the modality or technique, such as radiography with fluoroscopy, computerized axial tomography, or magnetic resonance imaging. Some terms related to these modalities are described in the margin. Recent and more commonly used modalities are described below.

Computerized axial tomography (CT or CAT scan) is a type of imaging that employs basic tomographic technique enhanced by computer imaging. Computer enhancement synthesizes the images obtained from different directions in a given plane, effectively reconstructing a cross-sectional plane of the body.

Magnetic Resonance Imaging (MRI) involves the appliation of an external magnetic field that forces a uniform alignment of hydrogen atom nuclei in the soft tissue. The nuclei emit radiofrequency signals that are converted into sets of tomographic images and displayed on a computer screen for three-dimensional visualization of the soft tissue structure.

Views describe the patient's position in relation to the camera. A code may specify a position, as in 71010 which describes a single frontal view of the chest. Other codes do not specify a position, but designate the number of views, as in 73610 which specifies a minimum of three views of the ankle. Terms related to the views are defined in the margin.

Procedures performed with contrast matieral often do not specify the type of contrast, as in 74160 which reports computerized axial tomography of the abdomen with contrast. However, other codes are more specific. Radiologic examination of the colon using barium enema contrast is reported with 74270. An air contrast with specific high density barium is reported with 74280.

The radiological supervision and interpretation of many interventional and invasive procedures are reported with codes from Diagnostic Radiology. Interventional/invasive codes may be used to report procedures diagnostic in nature, such as fluoroscopic localization for percutaneous renal biopsy 76003. Or, the codes may be used to report therapeutic procedures, such as radiologic supervision and interpretation of transcatheter embolization 75894.

DIAGNOSTIC ULTRASOUND
Procedures in Diagnostic Ultrasound are organized by anatomic site. However, when the ultrasound is part of an interventional radiology procedure for localization purposes, the procedure is listed under *Ultrasonic Guidance Procedures*.

Codes for ultrasounds performed for diagnostic purposes are selected based on the technique or type of study (A-mode, B-scan), the extent of the study (limited, complete, follow-up), and additional services performed with certain ultrasounds (intraocular lens power calculation).

DEFINITIONS

Radiology Glossary
Radiology contains terms unique to those codes. The following list contains those most frequently applied:

Anteroposterior (AP): Front to back.

Anteroposterior and Lateral: Two projections are included in this examination: front to back and side.

Cineradiography: Movies by x-ray.

Contrast Material: Radiopaque material that is placed into the body to visualize a system or body structure. Terms include: non-ionic and low osmolar contrast media (LOCM), ionic and high osmolar contrast media (HOCM), barium, and gadolinium.

Decubitus (DEC): Patient lying on the side.

Frontal: Face forward.

Lateral (LAT): Side view.

Modality: A form of imaging. This includes x-ray, fluoroscopy, ultrasound, nuclear medicine, duplex Doppler, CT, and MRI.

Oblique (OBL): Slanted view of the object being x-rayed.

Posteroanterior (PA): Back to front.

Real-time: Immediate imaging, usually in movement.

Stent: Tube to provide support in a body cavity or lumen.

Subtraction: Removal of an overlying structure to better visualize the structure in question. This is done by imposing one x-ray in a series on top of another.

Tomogram: Specialized type of x-ray imaging that provides slices through a body structure to obliterate overlying structures. This is commonly performed for studies on the kidneys or the temporomandibular joint.

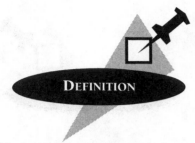

DEFINITION

Ultrasound studies visualize deep body structures by recording the echoes of ultrasonic waves that are directed into the body tissues.

Technique

A-mode (a-scan) — ultrasonic scanning procedure providing one-dimensional measurement.

M-mode — ultrasonic scanning procedure that measures the amplitude and velocity of moving echo-producing structures to allow one-dimensional viewing.

B-scan — two-dimensional ultrasonic scanning procedure providing a two-dimensional display.

Real-time — two-dimensional scanning procedure that displays both structure and movement in time.

Doppler — ultrasonic scanning procedure that measures the velocity of moving objects and often applied in the study of blood flow.

Extent

Complete — complete procedure that implies a scan of the entire body area.

Limited — limited procedure that involves scanning a single organ, quadrant, or completing a partial examination.

Follow-up/Repeat — implies performing a limited study on an area previously scanned.

Ultrasound procedures may be found in other sections of CPT. For example, echocardiography procedures are in the *Medicine Section* under *Cardiovascular Services*. Color mapping in conjunction with fetal echocardiography (76825–76826) is reported with 93325 in the Medicine Section. Duplex scans and Doppler studies of the Vascular system are found in the Medicine Section under the heading *Noninvasive Vascular Diagnostic Studies*. These services are described in Chapter 8.

RADIATION ONCOLOGY

Radiation oncology is a therapeutic method as opposed to a diagnostic service. The radiologist manages and prescribes treatment for patients who have malignant neoplasms responsive to radiation therapy.

Radiation oncology involves the following services: consultation, clinical treatment, planning, medical radiation physics, and treatment delivery and management.

Consultation codes from the Evaluation and Management (E/M) section of CPT report consultations conducted by radiation oncologists and the E/M guidelines must be followed when applying these codes. Office/outpatient consultations are reported with codes 99241–99245; codes 99251–99263 are reported for inpatient consultations.

Clinical treatment planning consists of two services, planning and simulation to determine the best course of treatment. Planning is reported with codes 77261–77263, depending on the extent or complexity of the process. Simulation is reported with codes 77280–77295, depending on the extent or complexity of the service.

- Report 77261 for simple planning that requires assessment of a single treatment area. No interpretation of special tests is required. The treatment site can be encompasssed in a single port or simple parallel opposed ports with simple or no blocking.

- Report 77262 for an intermediate level of planning that requires interpretation of tests performed for tumor localization. The radiation oncologist may need to assess two separate treatment areas or protect sensitive organs.

- Report 77263 for the interpretation of complex testing procedures, including CT and MR localization and/or special laboratory tests. Planning requires complex blocks and/or custom shielding blocks for the protection of sensitive normal structures. Tangential ports may be required. Three or more areas may require treatment. In addition, complex treatment planning often involves a combination of modalities such as brachytherapy, hyperthermia, chemotherapy and surgery.

Simulation sets the treatment portals to specific treatment volumes. Simulation should be reported only once per time of set-up procedure.

- Simple simulation (77280) involves a single port or single pair of parallel ports on a single treatment area.

- Intermediate simulation (77285) involves three or more ports directed at a single treatment area. It also is required when two separate treatment areas are involved.

- Complex simulation (77290) involves a combination of multiple treatment areas, complex blocking rotation or arc therapy, multiple modalities, and use of contrast materials.

- Three-dimensional simulation (77295) involves computer-generated three-dimensional reconstruction of the tumor and surrounding critical structures.

Medical radiation physics involves dosimetry calculation, the design and construction of treatment devices, and special services as defined below:

- Dosimetry calculation is the process the physician uses to select the proper energy and modality to be used for each portal.

- Design and construction involves fabricating devices for the blocks. The physician must be involved in the design, selection, and placement of the devices and must document the involvement.

- Special services include hyperthermia or brachytherapy in combination with basic radiation therapy.

Treatment delivery and management (77401–77799) involves the delivery of radiation therapy and care of the patient during the course of therapy. While the treatments may be delivered by nonphysician personnel, the physician is responsible for checking and documenting the accuracy of the treatment. In addition, the physician responds to any adverse reactions to treatment and monitors the effects of the treatment on the tumor and surrounding tissues. Ongoing patient examinations are part of this service and not reported separately.

NUCLEAR MEDICINE

Nuclear medicine relies on radium or other radioelements for either diagnostic imaging or radiopharmaceutical therapy. Radiopharmaceutical therapy destroys diseased tissues, usually malignant neoplasms, using radioelements. This subsection is organized first by the nature of the procedure, diagnostic or therapeutic. The diagnostic codes are organized by body system. Procedures are further defined by the extent or complexity of the service.

DEFINITION

Interventional radiology involves an invasive component (such as a biopsy or injection) and a radiological component.

Component coding standardizes the reporting of interventional radiological services. Component coding allows a physician, regardless of specialty, to identify and report those aspects of the service the physician provided, whether the procedural component, the radiological component, or both.

Procedures in nuclear medicine are independent services. Diagnostic work-up or follow-up care is reported separately, except when specifically noted as included in the service. These services do not include the provision of radium or other radioelements. Report 78990 for diagnostic radiopharmaceuticals and 79900 for therapeutic radiopharmaceuticals.

Example
A patient with a previously diagnosed prostatic adenocarcinoma, treated with radiation therapy, complains of right hip pain. Because of the advanced state of the prostatic cancer at the time of diagnosis, the physician suspects metastasis to the acetabulum and/or femur. A nuclear bone scan performed at a freestanding facility confirms metastases to both areas.

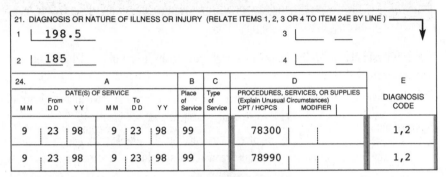

ICD-9-CM

198.5	Secondary malignant neoplasm of bone and bone marrow
185	Malignant neoplasm of prostate

CPT

78300	Bone and/or joint imaging; limited area
78990	Provision of diagnostic radiopharmaceutical(s)

— OR —

21. DIAGNOSIS OR NATURE OF ILLNESS OR INJURY (RELATE ITEMS 1, 2, 3 OR 4 TO ITEM 24E BY LINE)			
1	198.5	3	
2	185	4	

24.	A DATE(S) OF SERVICE							B Place of Service	C Type of Service	D PROCEDURES, SERVICES, OR SUPPLIES (Explain Unusual Circumstances)		E DIAGNOSIS CODE
	From MM DD YY			To MM DD YY					CPT / HCPCS	MODIFIER	
	9	23	98	9	23	98	99		78300	−26	1,2
	9	23	98	9	23	98	99		78300	−TC	1,2
	9	23	98	9	23	98	99		78990		1,2

ICD-9-CM

198.5	Secondary malignant neoplasm of bone and bone marrow
185	Malignant neoplasm of prostate

CPT

78300-26	Bone and/or joint imaging; limited area (professional component)
78300-TC	Bone and/or joint imaging; limited area (technical component)
78990	Provision of diagnostic radiopharmaceutical(s)

Both the professional and technical components should be reported since the procedure was performed at a freestanding facility. Report the service according to the payors requirements, either by reporting the code once without a modifier to designate a global service or by reporting the code twice, once with modifier -26 for the professional service and once with modifier -TC for the technical component. The provision of the radiopharmaceutical is reported separately.

Report both the secondary and primary malignant neoplasms. The secondary malignant neoplasm is sequenced first since the procedure was performed to diagnose the metastatic disease.

Special Coding Situations

INTERVENTIONAL RADIOLOGY

Interventional Radiology services involve both an invasive component (such as a biopsy or injection) and a radiological component (radiological supervision and interpretation of the procedure). The invasive component, which may be either a diagnostic or therapeutic service, is reported with codes from the surgery section. Examples of the invasive component include: injection procedure for shoulder arthrography (23350), percutaneous renal biopsy (50200*), and transcatheter occlusion of a vascular malformation (61624–61626). The radiology component for supervision and interpretation is reported with codes from the Diagnostic Radiology and Diagnostic Ultrasound subsections. In the Diagnostic Radiology subsection, codes are found throughout. However, the Diagnostic Ultrasound subsection organizes interventional services under the heading Ultrasonic Guidance Procedures. For example, the radiology component for shoulder arthrography is reported with 73040-26; the radiology component for the renal biopsy with 76003-26, 76360-26, or 76942-26 depending on modality; and the radiology component for the transcatheter occlusion/embolization with 75894-26.

Component coding was developed for services that can be performed by a single physician, usually an interventional radiologist, or by two physicians, a surgeon and a radiologist. Whether performed by one or two physicians, an interventional radiology procedure must be documented as thoroughly as a surgical procedure.

When a invasive procedure is performed by two physicians, each physician documents the portion of the service he or she provided and references the other's involvement in the written report. Each physician reports only the CPT code for the portion of the service the respective physician provided.

One Physician
Shoulder arthrography is performed by a hospital-based radiologist who provides both the injection service and the supervision and interpretation.

23350	Injection procedure for shoulder arthrography
73040-26	Radiologic examination, shoulder, arthrography, radiological supervision and interpretation — Professional component modifier

Two Physicians
Shoulder arthrography is performed in an outpatient hospital setting by an orthopedic surgeon and a radiologist. The radiologist directs the fluoroscopy to guide placement of the needle by the orthopedic surgeon, who subsequently injects air and contrast material into the joint space. The radiologist documents the flow of contrast on spot-films as the orthopedic surgeon manipulates

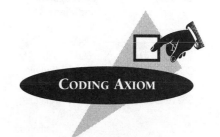

Coding Axiom

The invasive procedure and the radiological study are generally performed by the same physician, but not always. Whether performed by one or two physicians, an interventional radiology procedure should be documented as thoroughly as a surgical procedure.

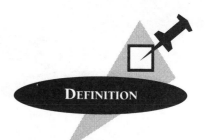

Definition

Nuclear medicine involves radioactive elements for either diagnostic imaging or radiopharmaceutical imaging. A radioactive element, such as uranium, spontaneously emits energetic particles by the disintegration of the nuclei.

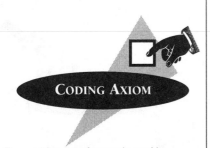

the joint in varying positions. Final interpretation and report of the images is performed by the radiologist.

Orthopedic Surgeon
23350   Injection procedure for shoulder arthrography

Radiologist
73040-26   Radiologic examination, shoulder, arthrography, radiological supervision and interpretation — Professional component modifier

Surgery codes were added to CPT as it became apparent that existing codes did not address the needs of interventionalists. Coders will find some interventional radiology codes that match one-to-one with corresponding codes in surgery. Other interventional radiology codes may work with many surgery codes. Parenthetical guidelines in CPT help direct coders to the appropriate surgery codes.

NONINVASIVE VASCULAR DIAGNOSTIC STUDIES

A description of noninvasive vascular diagnostic services (93875–93990) is included in Chapter 8, Medicine Services. They are mentioned here since radiologists frequently perfom them also.

Vascular study procedures are comprised of the following services: patient care required during performance of the study, supervision of the study, written interpretation of study results, a hard copy of output, and analysis of all data.

MODIFIERS

As in other specialties, modifiers in radiology denote circumstances that affect the performance of services and procedures. Radiologists most frequently apply -26, which reports the physician (professional) component of a service separately from the technical portion. Other modifiers for radiology include, but are not limited to:

-22   Unusual procedural services
-52   Reduced services
-59   Distinct procedural service
-76   Repeat procedure by same physician
-77   Repeat procedure by another physician

X-RAY CONSULTATIONS

Code 76140 *Consultation on x-ray examination made elsewhere, written report* is used by a physician who provides a second interpretation and report on a radiologic procedure. The previous interpretation is usually from a source outside of the physician's practice and is provided at the request of another physician. Both written reports must be maintained as part of the patient's medical record. The initial report and the consultation must document the specific procedure reviewed and the complexity of the procedure, such as the number of views.

Do not report 76140 for outside films that are reviewed in conjunction with evaluation and management services. The medical decision making component of E/M codes includes "amount and/or complexity of data to be reviewed."

Documenting Radiology Services

Payors scrutinize radiology services for medical necessity. As a result, payment may be denied for radiological services not shown to be medically necessary. Diagnostic coding is critical in establishing medical necessity, even though the radiologist may not have the information necessary to assign a definitive diagnosis. For example, many radiological services are performed to rule out a particular problem. Tests that are normal effectively rule out the suspected condition but the radiologist must be provided enough information about the patient's clinical history to justify medical necessity. In instances of a rule-out diagnosis, the radiologist should receive information from the physician, regarding the patient's symptoms, signs, or complaints.

In general, the patient's physician orders the study and a radiologist performs and/or interprets the procedure. The radiologist sends a report to the referring physician who includes it in the overall assessment of the patient. For coding and reimbursement purposes, the radiologist's portion of the service is reported as a complete procedure or as the professional component of the study. The ordering physician evaluates the results of the study for consideration in the medical decision making but does not file a claim for any portion of the radiological study.

Requesting Physician Responsibilities

The emphasis on medical necessity of radiological services demands that the radiologist know the reason for the exam. The physician requesting the study must provide this information. Even routine radiological studies, such as x-rays for preoperative clearance or for family history, must be medically necessary.

The physician should sign or initial the radiologist's report as evidence the information was reviewed and considered in medical decision making. While the actual film may be stored elsewhere, a written report should be incorporated into the patient's medical record to prove the study was medically necessary.

Radiologist Responsibilities

Radiologists must complete a written report for every service where a claim is filed. The specific name or title of the study must appear on the report; for example, "Chest x-ray, PA and lateral."

In addition to reporting the number and type of views taken, reports also must indicate any other circumstances that may affect the exam such as, a patient's state of fasting for a bowel study.

In addition to a report and the circumstances affecting the exam, documentation should also include:

- Quality of the study (clear or blurry)
- Pertinent positive findings (abnormal)
- Pertinent negative findings (normal)
- Other aspects of the film such as incidental findings in other areas
- Radiologist's impression and diagnosis
- Recommendations for further studies or treatment
- Signature

Radiology reports are almost universally transcribed. For that reason, precautions must be taken to keep the patient's record current. Whenever possible, apply the rules for dictated operative

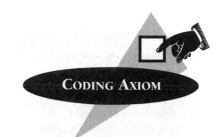

Coding Axiom

Payment is often denied for radiological services not shown to be medically necessary. Diagnostic coding is critical in establishing medical necessity.

Responsibilities
When documenting radiological services, there are two aspects to consider: the attending (requesting) physician's responsibilities and the radiologist's responsibilities. Coders must understand these responsibilities and know who to contact for further information for assigning diagnosis or procedure codes.

Date of Service
To eliminate any confusion that may arise during an audit, the date in the heading of the dictated report must reflect the date of service rather than the date of dictation.

Key elements to document
The following list identifies types of radiology services and the key elements that should be documented to support the complexity of the procedure and to accurately code the service provided:

Diagnostic procedures
- number of views
- limited or complete
- unilateral or bilateral

Ultrasonic procedures and noninvasive vascular diagnostic studies (NVDS)
- complete, limited, or follow-up
- unilateral or bilateral
- with or without duplex scan

Nuclear medicine procedures
- type and amount of radionuclide
- limited, multiple area, or whole body
- single or multiple determination
- with or without flow
- qualitative or quantitative

Computed tomography (CT)
- with or without contrast media (type and amount)
- multiplanar scanning and/or reconstruction

Magnetic resonance imaging (MRI)
- with or without contrast media (type and amount)
- number of sequences

reports to radiology reports. For example, a handwritten summary of the study should be placed in the chart until the transcription is available. The radiologist should read the transcription for accuracy and sign it before it is sent to the ordering physician or placed permanently in the patient's record. Coders must make code assignments based on the completed, signed and transcribed report.

Dictated reports should include the number and type of views taken, whether the study required a contrast medium, and the type and amount of contrast medium or radionuclide. This information plus other pertinent documentation is necessary to support CPT code selection and eliminate any extra time that could be necessary for verification.

Document all additional views beyond the usual number. Report with modifier -22 (unusual procedural services) added to the CPT code which may qualify the service for higher reimbursement.

Although the ordering physician must indicate the medical necessity, the radiologist must also indicate the reason in the report. The complexity of the study dictates the depth of the radiology statement.

Results from radiological studies done for urgent, acute problems, must be communicated verbally by the radiologist to the physician as soon as they are available. In these cases, the outcome of the study is often crucial to the physician's diagnosis and treatment. These conversations must be documented in the patient record.

Second Readings
The requesting physician may interpret a radiological study following the radiologist's interpretation. A second interpretation cannot be billed as it is part of the overall patient assessment.

If the physician disagrees with the radiologist's findings, it should not be recorded in the patient chart. The physician should discuss any differences of opinion with the radiologist and if a change in interpretation is made, a final corrected statement should be made in the chart. A brief note stating the reason for the change should be included. This clarifies the final diagnostic interpretation of the service which simplifies the process of assigning accurate codes.

Additional Studies
Findings from a routine x-ray exam may warrant further studies. For example, a radiologist may elect to do tomograms on a patient whose chest x-ray revealed a mass. The documentation must indicate that the existence of the mass establishes the medical necessity for further studies. In such a situation, the radiologist usually is not required to check with the ordering physician before proceeding with additional studies. However, the service may require prior authorization from the payor, depending on the payor's guidelines.

Steps for Accurate Coding and Documentation
The following procedures should be followed for complete and accurate coding and documentation:

1. Obtain sufficient history from the ordering physician to assign an accurate diagnosis code.
2. Document the exam in sufficient detail to allow complete and accurate procedure coding.
3. If the report is dictated, review the transcribed report for accuracy. Correct any error on the transcribed report and return to the transcriptionist to generate new and corrected hard copy.

DISCUSSION QUESTIONS

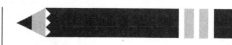

1. What is the difference between the technical and professional components?

    _____

    _____

    _____

2. Which key elements should be documented in a radiology report? Why?

    _____

    _____

    _____

3. What is modifier -26 used for and why is it most frequently reported by radiologists?

    _____

    _____

    _____

4. What two components make up interventional radiology?

    _____

    _____

    _____

5. What are the major divisions in CPT for radiology services?

    _____

    _____

    _____

OBJECTIVES

- See the practical application of CPT radiology coding

- Identify the special circumstances and rules of specialties

Specialty-Specific Scenarios

The following scenarios are designed by specialty to help you make the leap from documentation to correct code choices.

UROLOGY SCENARIO

A patient presents to a urology clinic with a history of chronic calculus in the pelvis of the kidney. He has a history of allergies and has had a reaction to ionic contrast in the past. He is sent to a local hospital as an outpatient and is injected with a bolus 100 cc of nonionic contrast material and an intravenous pylogram (IVP) is performed. Because the left calyx and ureter were not visible, a limited ultrasound is performed.

Professional Component

21. DIAGNOSIS OR NATURE OF ILLNESS OR INJURY (RELATE ITEMS 1, 2, 3 OR 4 TO ITEM 24E BY LINE)
1. 592.0   3.
2. V15.0   4.

24. A DATE(S) OF SERVICE						B Place of Service	C Type of Service	D PROCEDURES, SERVICES, OR SUPPLIES (Explain Unusual Circumstances)		E DIAGNOSIS CODE
MM	From DD	YY	MM	To DD	YY			CPT / HCPCS	MODIFIER	
6	8	98	6	8	98	22		76775	–26	1,2
6	8	98	6	8	98	22		74410	–26	1,2

ICD-9-CM

592.0   Calculus of kidney

V15.0   Personal history of allergy, other than to medicinal agents

CPT

76775-26   Echography, retroperitoneal (eg, renal, aorta, nodes), B-scan and/or real time with image documentation; limited — Professional component modifier

74410-26   Urography, infusion, drip technique and/or bolus technique — Professional component modifier

Nonionic contrast material is reported in addition to any study when it is medically necessary. To be deemed medically necessary, Medicare requires accompanying documentation of medical necessity. Report with HCPCS level II codes A4644, A4645, or A4646 rather than 99070.

An IVP with tomograms should be reported with 74415. There are individual CPT codes for intravenous versus a bolus infusion for hypertensive study. Ultrasound with an IVP should reflect the limited nature of the study as well as the fact that it is in the retroperitoneum.

NEUROLOGY SCENARIO

A 64-year-old patient presents with severe headaches and blackouts. Previous EEG and CT scan were negative. The neurologist inserts a catheter to perform an arch study using a retrograde right femoral approach. The study reveals tortuous and partially occluded precerebral vessels. The diagnosis is listed as arteriosclerosis of multiple bilateral precerebral vessels.

Neurology

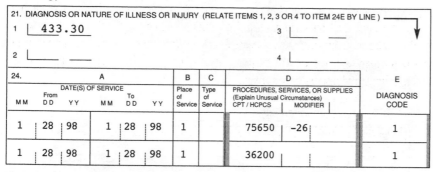

ICD-9-CM

433.30   Occlusion and stenosis of multiple and bilateral precerebral arteries without mention of cerebral infarction

CPT

75650-26   Angiography, cervicocerebral, catheter, including vessel origin, radiological supervision and interpretation — Professional component modifier

36200   Introduction of catheter, aorta

This interventional radiology service was performed by a single physician. Therefore, the physician reports both the catheterization, 36200, and the radiological supervision and interpretation, 75650-26.

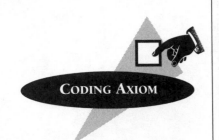

ORTHOPEDIC SCENARIO

A patient presents to the emergency room with a minimally displaced fracture of the lower end of the ulna and radius. The fracture was sustained when the patient fell five feet from a mountain and landed on a cliff ledge. X-rays are obtained by the hospital. The patient and the x-rays are transferred to the orthopedist's office, where the patient is seen on an emergency basis. The patient's arm is prepped, the fracture site injected with xylocaine and the fracture easily reduced. Postreduction x-rays taken by the physician's staff demonstrate good alignment of the bones. A long-arm fiberglass cast is applied and the patient is instructed to return in one week. Code procedures performed in the orthopedist's office.

Orthopedics

21. DIAGNOSIS OR NATURE OF ILLNESS OR INJURY (RELATE ITEMS 1, 2, 3 OR 4 TO ITEM 24E BY LINE)		
1. 813.44	3. E849.8	
2. E884.1	4.	

24.	A DATE(S) OF SERVICE						B Place of Service	C Type of Service	D PROCEDURES, SERVICES, OR SUPPLIES (Explain Unusual Circumstances)		E DIAGNOSIS CODE
	From MM DD YY			To MM DD YY					CPT / HCPCS	MODIFIER	
	4	21	98	4	21	98	3		25565		1,2,3
	4	21	98	4	21	98	3		73090		1,2,3
	4	21	98	4	21	98	3		99058		1,2,3
	4	21	98	4	21	98	3		99070		1,2,3
									OR		
	4	21	98	4	21	98	3		A4590		1,2,3

ICD-9-CM

813.44   Fracture of radius with ulna, lower end

E884.1   Fall from cliff

E849.8   Place of occurrence, other specified places

CPT

25565   Closed treatment of radial and ulnar shaft fractures; with manipulation

73090   Radiologic examination; forearm, anteroposterior and lateral views (global service)

99058   Office services provided on an emergency basis

99070   Supplies and materials (except spectacles), provided by the physician over and above those usually included with the office visit or other services rendered (list drugs, trays, supplies, or materials provided)

or

HCPCS

A4590   Special casting material (e.g., fiberglass)

No modifier is appended to code 73090 for the post reduction x-rays since the physician provided both the technical and professional components.

Code 99058 identifies office services provided on an emergency basis and does not include the actual medical or surgical service performed.

Casting of the fracture is included in the treatment of fractures. However, casting supplies should be reported separately. Use either CPT code 99070 or HCPCS code A4590, not both.

Only the post reduction x-rays are reported by the orthopedist. The hospital-based radiologist will report services provided at that facility.

MEDICAL SPECIALTIES SCENARIO-EMERGENCY ROOM PHYSICIAN

A patient is evaluated in the ED for an acute rigid abdomen of the right lower quadrant. The ED physician orders a supine, upright, and decubitus and a PA chest, which are read by a radiologist.

Medical Specialties

21. DIAGNOSIS OR NATURE OF ILLNESS OR INJURY (RELATE ITEMS 1, 2, 3 OR 4 TO ITEM 24E BY LINE)							
1	789.43			3			
2				4			

24.	A					B	C	D		E
	DATE(S) OF SERVICE					Place of Service	Type of Service	PROCEDURES, SERVICES, OR SUPPLIES (Explain Unusual Circumstances)		DIAGNOSIS CODE
	From			To						
	MM	DD	YY	MM	DD	YY			CPT / HCPCS	MODIFIER	
	3	14	98	3	14	98	23		74022	–26	1

ICD-9-CM

789.43   Abdominal rigidity, right lower quadrant

CPT

74022-26   Radiologic examination, abdomen: complete acute abdomen series, including supine, erect, and/or decubitus views, upright PA chest — Professional component

It is common, but incorrect, to report a one-view, chest x-ray with an x-ray series of the abdomen or ribs. However, careful review of the CPT description confirms that a PA chest is included in 74022.

GENERAL SURGERY SCENARIO

A 14-year-old male with abdominal pain is referred to a general surgeon in a multispecialty clinic by a family practitioner. Because the pain presents a confusing picture, the surgeon orders a complete acute abdomen series. The x-rays are performed at the clinic and reviewed by the surgeon. The final diagnosis is abdominal pain due to foreign body in stomach, with possible perforation. Code the CPT radiological exam for the physician and the ICD•9 diagnosis code.

General Surgery

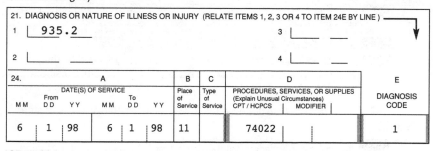

21. DIAGNOSIS OR NATURE OF ILLNESS OR INJURY (RELATE ITEMS 1, 2, 3 OR 4 TO ITEM 24E BY LINE)							
1	935.2			3			
2				4			

24.	A					B	C	D		E
	DATE(S) OF SERVICE					Place of Service	Type of Service	PROCEDURES, SERVICES, OR SUPPLIES (Explain Unusual Circumstances)		DIAGNOSIS CODE
	From			To						
	MM	DD	YY	MM	DD	YY			CPT / HCPCS	MODIFIER	
	6	1	98	6	1	98	11		74022		1

ICD-9-CM

935.2   Foreign body in stomach

CPT

74022   Radiologic examination, abdomen: complete acute abdomen series, including supine, erect, and/or decubitus views, upright PA chest

The surgeon may report both components of the radiologic exam because the x-rays are performed at the clinic and interpreted by the surgeon there. The listing of a service in a specific section of CPT does not restrict its use to a specialty. In outpatient coding, the foreign body is the definitive diagnosis and abdominal pain is not reported because it is due to the foreign body. Rule-out, possible, probable, or suspected conditions are not reported.

OPHTHALMOLOGY SCENARIO

An ophthalmologist performs an A-scan ultrasound with intraocular lens power calculation. The diagnosis is immature cataract not yet affecting vision.

Ophthalmology

21. DIAGNOSIS OR NATURE OF ILLNESS OR INJURY (RELATE ITEMS 1, 2, 3 OR 4 TO ITEM 24E BY LINE)				
1. 366.12			3.	
2.			4.	

24.	A						B	C	D		E
	DATE(S) OF SERVICE						Place of Service	Type of Service	PROCEDURES, SERVICES, OR SUPPLIES (Explain Unusual Circumstances)		DIAGNOSIS CODE
	From			To					CPT / HCPCS	MODIFIER	
	MM	DD	YY	MM	DD	YY					
	8	23	98	8	23	98	11		76519		1

ICD-9-CM

366.12   Incipient senile cataract

CPT

76519   Ophthalmic biometry by ultrasound echography, A-scan; with intraocular lens power calculation

The ophthalmologist performs both the professional and technical components of this procedure, so the global service is reported.

NUCLEAR MEDICINE SERVICES

A patient with Grave's disease elects radiopharmaceutical therapy, thyroid suppression, for treatment of the disease. This procedure is performed on an outpatient basis at an acute care facility. The radiologist performs an initial evaluation and supervises the initial procedure. Code the radiologist's services.

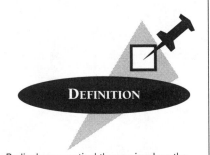

DEFINITION

Radiopharmaceutical therapy involves the use of a radioactive drug for therapeutic services.

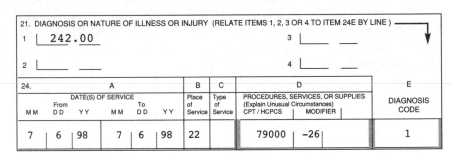

21. DIAGNOSIS OR NATURE OF ILLNESS OR INJURY (RELATE ITEMS 1, 2, 3 OR 4 TO ITEM 24E BY LINE)				
1. 242.00			3.	
2.			4.	

24.	A						B	C	D		E
	DATE(S) OF SERVICE						Place of Service	Type of Service	PROCEDURES, SERVICES, OR SUPPLIES (Explain Unusual Circumstances)		DIAGNOSIS CODE
	From			To					CPT / HCPCS	MODIFIER	
	MM	DD	YY	MM	DD	YY					
	7	6	98	7	6	98	22		79000	–26	1

ICD-9-CM

242.00   Toxic diffuse goiter, without mention of thyrotoxic crisis or storm

CPT

79000-26   Radiopharmaceutical therapy, hyperthyroidism; initial, including evaluation of patient — Professional component

Most nuclear medicine services are reported independent of the initial evaluation and follow-up care. However, 79000 includes the initial evaluation of the patient, so an evaluation and management service should not be reported separately.

OB/GYN SCENARIO

A 42-year-old woman presents for a baseline screening mammogram at the request of her OB-GYN. Her only risk factor is first pregnancy after the age of 30. Two views of each breast are taken and reviewed immediately by the radiologist. Microcalcifications are identified in the upper outer quadrant of the left breast and additional magnification views of that area are obtained after receiving authorization from the payor. Additional views are inconclusive and the patient is told to return in 6 months for follow-up studies.

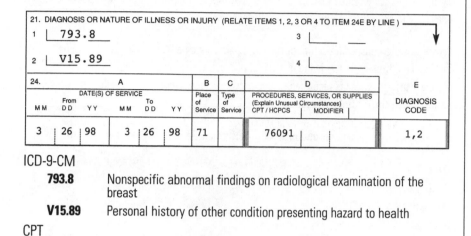

ICD-9-CM

793.8 Nonspecific abnormal findings on radiological examination of the breast

V15.89 Personal history of other condition presenting hazard to health

CPT

76091 Mammography; bilateral

Even though this patient was initially referred for a screening mammogram, additional views were required because of the identification of microcalcifications. Because a bilateral diagnostic mammogram includes two views of each breast and additional films as necessary, only the bilateral mammogram procedure is reported.

Additional views are inconclusive, and therefore, no definitive diagnosis can be made. The code for nonspecific abnormal findings is reported. The V-code for personal history of other condition presenting hazard to health (first pregnancy after age 30), should also be reported to identify a risk factor and may help to justify any additional work-up.

Advanced Coding Practice

CODING PRACTICE 1

A 58-year-old white male is referred to a cardiologist for complaints of precordial chest pain. After obtaining a comprehensive history, and performing a complete cardiovascular examination, a stress ECG is obtained but is inconclusive. Other previously performed lab and x-ray tests are significant for an elevated LDL to HDL ratio and this is complicated by the patient's moderate obesity. The patient is at a moderate risk for complications.

Because of the nonspecific nature of the chest pain as well as the inconclusive findings on stress ECG, a Thallium stress test is requested and performed the next day. Significant atherosclerotic coronary artery disease is identified in the inferior/posterior coronary vessels. This procedure is performed in the cardiologist's office.

Code all pertinent diagnoses and procedure performed on both day one and day two.

Day 1

Diagnoses

Procedures

Day 2

Diagnoses

Procedures

CODING PRACTICE 2

A 59-year-old female with adult onset, noninsulin dependent diabetes under good control presents with complaints of weight loss. The patient states that she has not been able to eat because eating causes severe pain in the periumbilical area. She had previously been prescribed nitroglycerin for coronary angina and states that this also seems to alleviate her abdominal pain. The patient is referred for Doppler ultrasound of the abdominal arteries.

A duplex scan of the abdominal area, including the celiac axis and superior mesenteric artery shows reduced blood flow in these areas. The procedure is performed at a free standing facility. A diagnosis of chronic mesenteric vascular insufficiency due to arteriosclerosis is made. The patient is referred to an interventional radiologist for mesenteric arteriography to determine the severity of the obstruction.

The interventional radiologist performs both the injection procedure and radiological supervision and interpretation related to the arteriography. An arterial catheter is introduced into the femoral artery and threaded into the abdominal aorta. The catheter is first threaded into the superior mesenteric artery and arteriograms are obtained. Arteriograms are also obtained of the celiac artery. The procedure is performed as an outpatient procedure at a hospital. Code only the interventional radiologist services.

Initial visit

Diagnoses

Procedures

Duplex scan

Diagnoses

Procedures

Interventional radiology

Diagnoses

Procedures

Coding answers related to the Coding Practice problems are found at the end of the book.

21. DIAGNOSIS OR NATURE OF ILLNESS OR INJURY (RELATE ITEMS 1, 2, 3 OR 4 TO ITEM 24E BY LINE)						
1			3			
2			4			

24.	A				B	C	D		E
	DATE(S) OF SERVICE				Place of Service	Type of Service	PROCEDURES, SERVICES, OR SUPPLIES (Explain Unusual Circumstances)		DIAGNOSIS CODE
	From MM DD YY		To MM DD YY				CPT / HCPCS	MODIFIER	

There are two aspects to consider when documenting radiological services:

- Technical component includes provision of equipment, supplies, technical personnel, and costs attendant to the performance of the procedure

- Professional component encompasses all of the physician work in providing the service

Chapter Review

CPT coding and nomenclature in the radiology section (70010–79999) are under constant review in an effort to reflect current standards of service. These services are divided according to two components: technical and professional. The technical component includes the provision of the equipment, supplies, technical personnel, and costs attendant to the performance of the procedure other than the professional services. The professional component encompasses all of the physician's work in providing the service, including interpretation and report of the procedure.

The modifier most frequently used by radiologists is -26, which reports the physician (professional) component of a service separately from the technical portion. But before assigning any code or component, carefully study the guidelines found in the radiology sections of CPT. Also, make sure documentation meets payor requirements for medical necessity or payment may be denied.

7 Pathology & Laboratory

Pathology and Laboratory Subsections

The pathology and laboratory (80049–89399) section of CPT is divided into 14 subsections. Subsections are as follows:

- Organ or Disease Oriented Panels
- Drug Testing
- Therapeutic Drug Assays
- Evocative/Suppression Testing
- Consultations (Clinical Pathology)
- Urinalysis
- Chemistry
- Hematology/Coagulation
- Immunology
- Transfusion Medicine
- Microbiology
- Anatomic Pathology
- Surgical Pathology
- Other Procedures

Guidelines that clarify how pathology and laboratory codes should be used are found at the beginning of the section and in notes, and parenthetical phrases throughout the section. The guidelines are in the same arrangement as the other sections of CPT and unique to the section, subsection, subheading, range of codes, or to an individual code.

Inpatient coders are not required to code pathology or laboratory tests since they are not necessary in the assignment of DRGs (Diagnosis Related Groups which are discussed in Chapter 9). However, pathology and laboratory codes are itemized on chargemasters for reporting services and supplies to patients.

Outpatient coders frequently code pathology and laboratory tests. Coding instructions include listing each laboratory procedure separately, unless it is part of a panel. Never use modifier -51 for multiple procedures in pathology or laboratory coding.

Many lab tests can be performed by different methods. To choose the correct code, carefully review code descriptions as well as any notes. When in doubt, request information from the physician or laboratory for clarification, or consult an authoritative reference.

OBJECTIVES

Understand the methodology used for reporting pathology and laboratory codes

Recognize the difference between the professional and technical components

Learn the special instructions in the code subsections

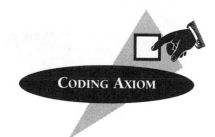

CODING AXIOM

Inpatient coders seldom code pathology or laboratory tests since they are not necessary in the assignment of DRGs. Outpatient coders, on the other hand, frequently must code pathology and laboratory tests.

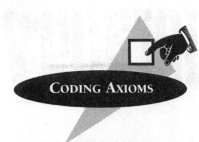

In many instances, identification of the method is key to appropriate coding and reimbursement for pathology and laboratory.

There is no mechanism in CPT for reporting lab procedures performed on a stat basis. Physician documentation with an order for immediate or "stat" testing must be included in the medical record.

Panel codes should only be reported when all tests included in the panel are performed. Performance of additional tests not included in the panel should be reported separately.

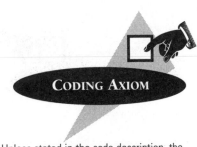

CODING AXIOM

Unless stated in the code description, the therapeutic drug assays and chemistry subsections list codes for quantitative tests only.

Watch for tests that are included in panels. A thyroid panel code (80091) should not be reported with 84436 *Thyroxine, total* or 84479 *triiodothyronine* (T3); because CPT guidelines specify that a thyroid panel includes those two tests.

Codes for reporting automated multichannel test (80002–80019) have been deleted. To report services previously reported with codes 80002–80019, see Organ or Disease Oriented Panels (80049–80092).

Correct diagnostic coding is extremely important in pathology and laboratory test reimbursement. Many payors will exclude payment if a diagnosis code does not match the list of diagnoses a payor has assigned to a particular test.

Pathology and laboratory services are provided by the physician or by technologists under the supervision of a physician. The majority of the codes represent a technical component only, but certain codes represent a global service — a combination of professional and technical components. If the pathologist reviews a test result or renders an opinion of a test that is represented by a global code, the code selected should be identified with modifier -26 to indicate that only the professional component was provided.

ORGAN OR DISEASE-ORIENTED PANELS

Twelve codes (80049–80092) report panels listing definitive test components: basic metabolic; general health; electrolyte; comprehensive metabolic; obstetric; hepatic function; hepatitis; lipid; arthritis; TORCH antibody; thyroid; and thyroid with TSH. These panels neither specify clinical parameters nor do they preclude performance of other tests. Tests performed in addition to the procedures defined in a panel can be reported separately. However, panel tests should not be reported separately on the same day as single test codes listed as part of the panel. For example, a hepatic function panel code 80058 includes codes 82040, 82247, 82248, 84075, 84450, and 84460.

DRUG TESTING

The drug testing subsection lists codes (80100–80103) for qualitative screens that are usually confirmed by a second technique. Thirteen drugs or classes of drugs are listed as examples of commonly assayed qualitative screens: alcohols; amphetamines; barbiturates; opiates; benzodiazepines; cocaine and metabolites; methadones; methaqualones; phencyclidines; phenothiazines; propoxyphenes; tetrahydrocannabinoids; and tricyclic antidepressants.

Reporting Drug Screens

Qualitative screens should be reported when a provider is testing for the presence of a particular substance or substances. Coding for qualitative screening tests is based on procedure, not method or analyte. For example, if confirmation of five drugs requires three procedures, 80102 *Drug confirmation, each procedure* is identified three times. Drugs that have been confirmed through qualitative testing may also be quantitated. Quantitative testing is reported separately with codes from the chemistry section (82000–84999) or therapeutic drug assay section (80150–80299).

THERAPEUTIC DRUG ASSAYS

The therapeutic drug assays subsection (80150–80299) lists codes for quantitative assays. Several of these codes were found in the chemistry and toxicology subsection in past editions of CPT and reported as either qualitative or quantitative tests. In *CPT 1999*, the therapeutic drug assays and chemistry subsections list codes for quantitative tests only unless stated otherwise in the code description.

Coding for Drug Assays

Codes listed under therapeutic drug assays or under chemistry are used when a drug is quantitated, or measured. Screening may be used to detect a substance, but it is not a prerequisite for quantitation. For example, screening is not necessary when a known drug has been overdosed. Coding for quantitative assays is based on the substance tested. Unless the code description notes otherwise, the examination material may be from any source.

EVOCATIVE/SUPPRESSION TESTING

These procedures (80400–80440) measure the effects of administered evocative (stimulating) or suppressive agents upon the patient and represent the technical component of the service. These panels measure levels of multiple constituents or the same constituent multiple times after administering the stimulating or suppressing agent. Most of these tests are performed to evaluate specific conditions stated in the code narrative. For example, 80400 *ACTH stimulation panel* is performed for adrenal insufficiency. The physician's administration of the agent is reported separately using 90780–90784. Supplies and drugs are reported separately, (99070 or HCPCS Level II codes). To report physician attendance and monitoring during the testing, refer to the appropriate evaluation and management codes. Prolonged physician care codes may be reported separately, except when testing is performed by prolonged infusion (90780–90781).

CPT references analyte tests for information regarding the testing required for each code. For instance, following 80415 *Chorionic gonadotropin stimulation panel; estradiol response* is an instruction, indicating that an estradiol level must be performed twice on three pooled blood samples to complete the test.

CONSULTATION (CLINICAL PATHOLOGY)

Two consultation codes (80500 and 80502) are reserved for the pathologist to indicate a service, not a test. The pathology consultation is performed at the request of an attending physician and requires a written report. Code 80500 is a limited service without review of the patient's history and medical records. Code 80502 is a comprehensive service for a complex diagnostic problem, with review of the patient's history and medical records.

URINALYSIS

Codes 81000–81099 are used for specific analysis of one or more components of the urine. Select the appropriate code based on method (e.g., dip stick, tablet reagent, qualitative, semiquantitative) purpose (e.g., pregnancy test, timed-volume, bacteriuria screen) and specific constituents evaluated (e.g., bilirubin, glucose, pH). Not all urine analyses are listed in this section. For other tests, see appropriate section. For example, urine chloride can be found in the chemistry section.

CHEMISTRY

Chemistry codes (82000–84999) report only quantitative tests unless the description specifies otherwise, as is the case with the chromatography codes (82486–82489). Qualitative screens are reported by the four drug testing codes (80100–80103).

Qualitative analysis identifies the substances in a sample.

Quantitative analysis determines the concentration of a substance in the sample.

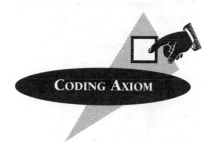

CODING AXIOM

To report physician attendance and monitoring during the evocative/suppression testing, refer to the appropriate evaluation and management codes.

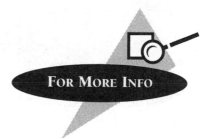

FOR MORE INFO

Urinalysis continues to be waived from the government's Clinical Laboratory Improvement Act (CLIA) regulations. See *Code It Right*'s Medicare chapter for more information about CLIA regulations.

When selecting codes for services involving multiple tests, read the code descriptions carefully. Contact the AMA or insurance payers as needed for clarification of how CPT codes and descriptions should be used.

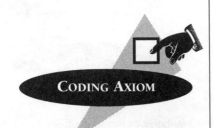

An individual code or a series of codes may be required for appropriate reporting. Glucose testing is an example:

82947	Glucose; quantitative
82948	blood, reagent strip
82950	post glucose dose (includes glucose)
82951	tolerance test (GTT), three specimens (includes glucose)
82952	tolerance test, each additional beyond three specimens

Code 82951 reports a three-specimen glucose tolerance test (GTT). This code includes obtaining the fasting blood sample, supplying and administering the oral glucose dose, and obtaining the next two samples (e.g., at one-half hour and one hour). Code 82952 reports additional samples beyond the first three. Report 82951 once and 82952 twice for a three-hour GTT in which specimens are obtained at zero, one-half, one, two, and three hours.

Multiple specimens from different sources as well as specimens obtained at different times should be reported separately. For example, total bilirubin levels (82247) obtained in the morning and afternoon would be reported twice on that date of service.

Molecular Diagnostics (83890–83912)
Molecular diagnostics (analysis of nucleic acids) are found in the chemistry section of CPT. Tests in this series are reported by procedure rather than analyte and should be coded separately for each procedure used in an analysis.

HEMATOLOGY AND COAGULATION
The hematology and coagulation subsection (85002–85999) lists those laboratory procedures specific to blood and blood-forming organs, including complete blood counts (CBC), clotting factors, clotting inhibitors, parathrombin and thrombin time, platelets, and sickling.

When 85025 *Blood count; hemogram and platelet count, automated, and automated complete differential WBC count (CBC)*, is performed on the same day as a 85007 *Blood count; manual differential WBC count (includes RBC morphology and platelet estimation)*, both codes should be reported. These two tests are sometimes performed on the same date of service because a flag (abnormal value) has been identified during the automated procedure (85025), and further testing is required. A visual microscopic examination of the blood slide (85007) for immature, atypical, or clumped cells is a component of 85007, but is not included in 85025.

Codes for bone marrow aspiration, biopsy, and smear interpretation (85095–85102) are found in this subsection. However, when reporting interpretation services read procedure descriptions carefully as cell block interpretations and bone marrow biopsy interpretations should be reported with 88305.

IMMUNOLOGY
The immunology subsection (86000–86849) identifies codes for antigen and antibody studies. Detection of antibodies to infectious agents using multiple step qualitative or semiquantitative immunoassays should be reported with codes 86602–86804.

Specific tissue typing procedures are also found in the immunology subsection, see 86805–86822.

High-volume procedures include: cardiolipin antibody; antigen complement; deoxyribonucleic acid antibody; hepatitis C antibody; delta agent hepatitis; heterophile antibodies; and streptococcus screening.

TRANSFUSION MEDICINE

Once listed in immunology, most blood bank codes are now grouped together under the transfusion medicine subsection (86850–86999). Since more blood bank procedures are likely to be performed on an outpatient basis, this subsection may expand in the future.

Be aware that the present codes do not report the supply of blood or blood products, and their cost may not be covered by insurance. Payors usually cover antibody screening, autologous blood or component collection, processing and storage, blood typing, and blood preparate. Some payors require blood to be replaced (when the unit given is replaceable) instead of paid. Some payors will not cover the cost of blood components, such as albumin, plasma, or plasmanate. There may also be restrictions on procedures involving pheresis. Check with individual payors for prior authorization and allowables and have this information available for the patients who ask about coverage of these services.

MICROBIOLOGY

These microbiology codes (87001–87999) identify services related to cultures, organism identification, and sensitivity studies. Many of the narratives are similar to those in the immunology section, so it is important to pay close attention to technique. Infectious agents identified by antigen detection, nucleic acid probe, or fluorescence microscopy are reported with codes 87260–87999 from microbiology. Infectious agents identified by antibody detection are reported with codes 86602–86804 from immunology. For example, cytomegalovirus (CMV) identified by infectious agent *antigen* detection by enzyme immunoassay technique, qualitative or semiquantitative, multiple step method is reported with 87332 from microbiology. However, CMV *antibody* detection by qualitative or semiquantitative immunoassay, multiple step method is reported with 86644.

ANATOMIC PATHOLOGY

Anatomic pathology (88000–88299) includes postmortem examinations (e.g., necropsy, autopsy), cytopathology (e.g., fluids, washing or brushing, Pap smears, fine needle aspirations, flow cytometry, etc.) and cytogenetic studies (e.g., tissue cultures for chromosome studies, etc.). Postmortem examination procedures (88000–88099) report only the physician portion of the service. To report outside laboratory services append modifier -90.

Codes for reporting cervical and vaginal screening (Pap smears) (88141–88155, 88164–88167) have undergone considerable revision and expansion in recent years. Codes 88142–88145 report cervical or vaginal specimens collected in a preservative fluid using automated twin layer preparation. These specimens may then be examined by either Bethesda or non-Bethesda reporting systems. Codes 88150–88154 report cervical or vaginal specimens (Pap smears) prepared on slides and examined using non-Bethesda reporting systems. Codes 88164–88167 report cervical or vaginal specimens (Pap smears) prepared on slides and examined using Bethesda reporting systems. All of the above codes report manual screening and rescreening using various techniques under physician supervision. Cervical or vaginal cytopathology services requiring physician interpretation are reported separately with code 88141. Definitive hormonal evaluation is also reported separately with code 88155.

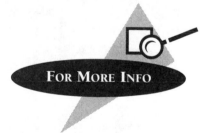

FOR MORE INFO

The Bethesda system for reporting cervical/vaginal cytologic diagnoses was developed by the National Cancer Institute. The system includes:

- Adequacy of specimen
- General categorization (optional)
- Descriptive diagnosis
- Epithelial cell abnormalities

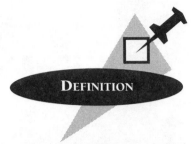

SURGICAL PATHOLOGY

The primary surgical pathology codes (88300–88309) describe gross and microscopic examination of specimens submitted for pathologic evaluation.

The specimen is the unit of service to report for surgical pathology. A specimen is defined as each tissue or tissues submitted for individual and separate evaluation. Each separate specimen requires individual examination and pathologic diagnosis. When two or more individual specimens are submitted from the same patient, each specimen is assigned an individual CPT code which should reflect the proper level of service.

Levels of service are defined by type of exam, and the type of tissue. CPT 88300 should be reported for specimens requiring only gross examination. All other surgical pathology services require both gross and microscopic examination of the tissue and are defined by the type of specimen. The type of specimen included in each level is listed in the code description. For example, tissue submitted labeled "synovium knee" is examined by the pathologist and determined to be a synovial cyst. The surgical pathology code reported is 88304 because "bursa/synovial cyst" is listed under CPT 88304.

Codes listed in 88300–88309 do not include any of the special services described by procedures 88311–88399. Procedures 88311–88399 describe additional services which should be reported separately and include the following: special stains, histochemistry, immunocytochemisty, immunofluorescent studies, electron microscopy, nerve teasing perparations, protein analysis by the western blot method, and pathology consultations during surgery.

OTHER PROCEDURES

Codes in this subsection (89050–89399) describe such procedures as crystal identification by light microscopy, duodenal intubation and aspiration, gastric intubation and aspiration, and nasal smear for eosinophils — and reproductive services such as culture and fertilization of oocytes and sperm evaluation.

Tracking Lab Work and Other Ancillary Services

Most offices do an excellent job of capturing the charges provided directly by the physician. The charges most often missed are ancillary services, such as lab, x-ray, or special studies (ECG, treadmills, cardiac rehabilitation, and sleep lab).

A moderately busy lab in an internal medicine clinic may perform an average of 50 tests per day. If overworked lab personnel fail to charge two tests per day at an average cost of $10 each, more than $5,000 may be lost each year. A simple check of the day's totals against the laboratory log sheet can prevent this revenue loss. A log sheet that tracks lab services on a daily basis should become part of the office's internal controls. This sheet can be arranged by patient name and patient number and should identify each test.

Each day, lab personnel can total the number of tests performed and transfer this information to a control sheet for the month. At the end of the month, compare these totals to the frequency reports. If the error rate is low, there is no need to be alarmed. Most busy offices, however, find at least five or six missed tests in a given category.

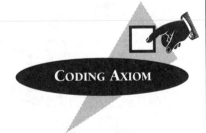

Laboratory Coding Methodology

In recent years payors have scrutinized the reporting of laboratory services for medical necessity and correct coding. Therefore, verify that all services performed have a signed physician order, are medically necessary and each is coded correctly, and supported by documentation in the medical record. Maintaining a current chargemaster or fee schedule is critical. Laboratories, (physician/clinic-based, hospital-based, or free-standing) must update their chargemasters and fee schedule annually and verify that the codes and descriptors match the services performed. Never report a service with a code that appears to be "close enough" to the actual service performed. If the descriptor does not match the service performed, review CPT to identify a more specific code. If a code cannot be identified, assign an unlisted procedure code and supply supporting documentation with the claim.

To avoid unbundling become familiar with the following subsections: Organ and Disease Oriented Panels (80049–80092), and Evocative/Suppression Testing (80400–80440). Do not report individual codes when the individual laboratory procedures are included in a panel.

DISCUSSION QUESTIONS

1. Explain the technical and professional components of pathology and laboratory procedures.

2. What is the key to appropriate coding and reimbursement for pathology and laboratory? How do you verify the information is correct?

3. How can inaccurate tracking of ancillary services negatively affect on reimbursement? What can be done to better track these services?

4. When should you report clinical pathology consultations?

5. Evocative/Suppression testing reports only the laboratory component of the services. What additional services and supplies should be reported?

6. Codes for reporting cervical and vaginal screening (Pap smears) have been significantly revised. Describe the three methods of examination.

_____

_____

_____

Specialty-Specific Scenarios

The following scenarios are designed by specialty to help you make the leap from documentation to correct code choices.

OBSTETRICS SCENARIO — OUTPATIENT

An obstetrician requests the laboratory perform an alpha-fetoprotein (AFP) triple test on a 42-year-old multigravida pregnant patient. The test results are extremely low and the physician's diagnosis is pregnancy with probable fetal Down syndrome.

Obstetrics

21. DIAGNOSIS OR NATURE OF ILLNESS OR INJURY (RELATE ITEMS 1, 2, 3 OR 4 TO ITEM 24E BY LINE)							
1	655.13				3		
2	659.63				4		

24.	A						B	C	D		E
	DATE(S) OF SERVICE						Place of Service	Type of Service	PROCEDURES, SERVICES, OR SUPPLIES (Explain Unusual Circumstances)		DIAGNOSIS CODE
	From			To					CPT / HCPCS	MODIFIER	
	MM	DD	YY	MM	DD	YY					
	6	30	98	6	30	98	11		82105	90	1,2
	6	30	98	6	30	98	11		82677	90	1,2
	6	30	98	6	30	98	11		84702	90	1,2

ICD-9-CM

655.13   Chromosomal abnormality in fetus, antepartum condition or complication

659.63   Elderly multigravida, with antepartum condition or complication

CPT

82105-90   Alpha-fetoprotein; serum — Reference laboratory

82677-90   Estriol — Reference laboratory

84702-90   Gonadotropin, chorionic (hCG); quantitative — Reference laboratory

These tests are not definitive and will be followed with a chromosomal work-up. Though probable diagnoses are not usually coded in an outpatient setting, the 655 category specifies they should be used for known or suspected fetal abnormalities affecting management of the mother. There is not a single test for an alpha-fetoprotein triple test. When this test is performed an AFP, B-hCG, and estriol should be reported. The tests on a pregnant woman's serum screen for neural tube defects such as spina bifida in the fetus (high AFP levels) and for trisomy -21 (Down syndrome, low AFP levels). The predictive value for the low AFP levels for Down syndrome improves when combined with the results of hCG and estriol on the same sample.

Modifier -90 indicates the physician is reporting laboratory tests performed outside his or her office.

OBJECTIVES

See the practical application of CPT pathology and laboratory coding

Identify the special circumstances and rules of specialties

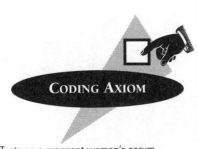

CODING AXIOM

Tests on a pregnant woman's serum screen for neural tube defects such as spina bifida and trisomy -21 (Down syndrome) in the fetus.

DERMATOLOGY SCENARIO — OUTPATIENT

A dermatologist excises two facial skin lesions on an outpatient basis in his office. The two specimens, labeled "skin lesion temple" and "skin lesion forehead," are sent to an outside lab where a pathologist performs an exam. The diagnosis is basal cell carcinoma, temple and forehead. Code the pathology services.

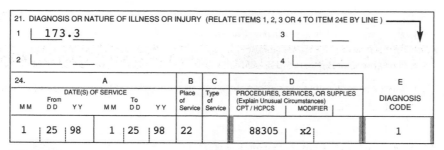

ICD-9-CM

173.3 Malignant neoplasm skin of other and unspecified parts of face

CPT

88305 Level IV — Surgical pathology, gross and microscopic examination

Code 88305 is reported twice since two separate specimens were submitted for individual and separate evaluation. The code for a Level IV exam is assigned since the tissue evaluated is a skin lesion, other than a cyst, skin tag, debrided tissue, or tissue excised during plastic repair.

ORTHOPEDIC SURGERY SCENARIO

For anaerobic bacterial culture, an orthopedic surgeon submits a screw that has been removed due to infection. Code the diagnosis and laboratory procedure.

Orthopedics

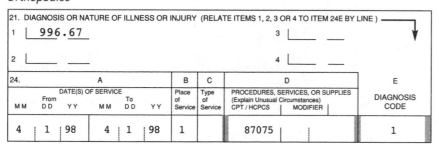

ICD-9-CM

996.67 Infection and inflammatory reaction due to other internal orthopedic device, implant or graft

CPT

87075 Culture, bacterial, any source; anaerobic (isolation)

MEDICAL SPECIALTIES CARDIOLOGY SCENARIO — OUTPATIENT

A 43-year-old man with coronary artery disease and benign essential hypertension is scheduled to have a cardiac catheterization as an outpatient at a local hospital. The cardiologist notices a low serum potassium (3.0) on the morning of the scheduled catheterization when reviewing pre-catheterization labs performed three days earlier. Review of the ECG, performed at the same time as the labs, shows a flattened T-wave. The cardiologist orders a stat serum potassium. When the results of the test are reviewed, the cardiologist reschedules the procedure. The diagnosis in the medical record is listed as hypokalemia. Code the outpatient laboratory service.

Medical Specialties

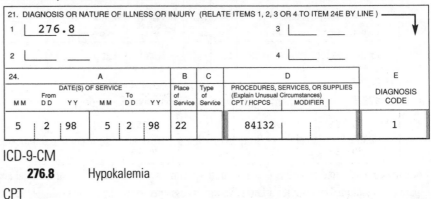

ICD-9-CM

276.8   Hypokalemia

CPT

84132   Potassium; serum

There is no mechanism in CPT for reporting stat services.

GENERAL SURGERY SCENARIO

A general surgeon orders a preoperative work-up to include: albumin, bilirubin, calcium, chloride, carbon dioxide (bicarbonate), creatinine, glucose, alkaline phosphatase, potassium, total protein, sodium, aspartate amino transferase (AST), and BUN. In addition, a complete blood count (CBC) including automated hemogram, platelet count and complete differential WBC is ordered. This is done as part of the preoperative work-up on a patient scheduled for outpatient laparoscopic cholecystectomy for chronic cholecystitis. This specimen is sent to an outpatient laboratory. Code the laboratory service.

General Surgery

21. DIAGNOSIS OR NATURE OF ILLNESS OR INJURY (RELATE ITEMS 1, 2, 3 OR 4 TO ITEM 24E BY LINE)

1. 575.11
2.
3.
4.

24. DATE(S) OF SERVICE From MM DD YY	To MM DD YY	B Place of Service	C Type of Service	D PROCEDURES, SERVICES, OR SUPPLIES (Explain Unusual Circumstances) CPT/HCPCS	MODIFIER	E DIAGNOSIS CODE
5 30 98	5 30 98	22		80054		1
5 30 98	5 30 98	22		85025		1

ICD-9-CM

575.11 Chronic cholecystitis

CPT

80054 Comprehensive metabolic panel

85025 Blood count; hemogram and platelet count, automated and automated complete differential WBC count (CBC)

The 13 laboratory tests are included in a comprehensive metabolic panel and reported with code 80054. CPT 85025 for the CBC is reported separately. It would be incorrect to report code 80050 for a general health panel even though it includes both the comprehensive metabolic panel (80054) and the CBC (85025) because the general health panel also includes a test for thyroid stimulating hormone (TSH) (84443) which was not performed. Panel codes should only be reported when all tests included in that panel are requested and performed.

INTERNAL MEDICINE — GASTROENTEROLOGY SCENARIO

A 48-year-old female presents to her internal medicine physician with complaints of upper abdominal pain, chills, and fever. In addition, she is noted to be jaundiced. Liver function tests are performed including serum albumin, total and direct bilirubin, and alkaline phosphatase. Both the bilirubin and alkaline phosphatase are elevated. The diagnosis is extrahepatic biliary duct obstruction. The patient is referred to a general surgeon. Code the laboratory services.

Internal Medicine — Gastroenterology

21. DIAGNOSIS OR NATURE OF ILLNESS OR INJURY (RELATE ITEMS 1, 2, 3 OR 4 TO ITEM 24E BY LINE)

1. 576.2
2.
3.
4.

DATE(S) OF SERVICE From MM DD YY	To MM DD YY	Place of Service	Type of Service	PROCEDURES, SERVICES, OR SUPPLIES CPT / HCPCS MODIFIER	DIAGNOSIS CODE
2 8 98	2 8 98	11		82040	1
2 8 98	2 8 98	11		82251	1
2 8 98	2 8 98	11		84075	1

ICD-9-CM

576.2 Obstruction of bile duct

CPT

82040 Albumin; serum

82251 Bilirubin; total AND direct

84075 Phosphatase, alkaline;

Tests are reported by individual codes. The hepatic function panel (80058) is not reported because not all tests included in the panel were performed.

PATHOLOGY AND LABORATORY SCENARIO

An ACTH stimulation panel for adrenal insufficiency was performed by an outpatient hospital laboratory. Three cortisol levels are obtained.

Pathology and Laboratory

21. DIAGNOSIS OR NATURE OF ILLNESS OR INJURY (RELATE ITEMS 1, 2, 3 OR 4 TO ITEM 24E BY LINE)
1. 255.4   3.
2.   4.

24. DATE(S) OF SERVICE From MM DD YY	To MM DD YY	B Place of Service	C Type of Service	D PROCEDURES, SERVICES, OR SUPPLIES (Explain Unusual Circumstances) CPT / HCPCS	MODIFIER	E DIAGNOSIS CODE
10 31 98	10 31 98	81		80400		1
10 31 98	10 31 98	81		82533		1

ICD-9-CM

255.4 Corticoadrenal insufficiency

CPT

80400 ACTH stimulation panel; for adrenal insufficiency

82533 Cortisol; total

The ACTH stimulation panel includes only two cortisols, but three cortisol levels were measured. Therefore, a cortisol code (82533) may be reported separately with the ACTH stimulation panel code (80400). Obtaining a third specimen is consistent with recommended protocols for ACTH stimulation testing.

Evocative/suppression testing reports only the laboratory component. The physician should report his or her services separately including E/M services, administration of stimulating or suppressive agents.

Because this service was performed at an outpatient hospital laboratory, the physician would not report supplies or drugs; the laboratory would.

RADIOLOGY SCENARIO

A request for a complete urinalysis on a catheter specimen is sent to a clinic laboratory by a radiologist during an IVP on a patient diagnosed with hematuria. A non-automated test is performed by tablet reagent. A microscopic examination is also done.

Radiology

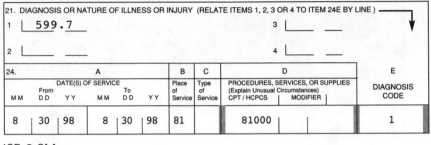

ICD-9-CM

599.7 Hematuria

CPT

81000 Urinalysis, by dip stick or tablet reagent for bilirubin, glucose, hemoglobin, ketones, leukocytes, nitrite, pH, protein, specific gravity, urobilinogen, any number of these constituents; non-automated, with microscopy

It may be necessary for the coder to request further information from the laboratory before determining the correct CPT code when more than one code is listed for similar tests.

Advanced Coding Practice

CODING PRACTICE 1

A 68-year-old male with one year status post MI and elevated serum cholesterol not controlled by diet sees his cardiologist for follow-up. Current medications include digoxin. His physician requests that the patient return in the morning for a fasting total serum cholesterol, HDL cholesterol, and triglycerides. In addition, the physician requests a digoxin level. Code the laboratory services.

24.	A				B	C	D		E
	DATE(S) OF SERVICE				Place of Service	Type of Service	PROCEDURES, SERVICES, OR SUPPLIES (Explain Unusual Circumstances) CPT / HCPCS MODIFIER		DIAGNOSIS CODE
MM DD YY		MM DD YY							

CODING PRACTICE 2

A patient with symptoms suggesting pernicious anemia is evaluated with the following laboratory tests; automated hemogram and platelet count with automated complete differential WBC, intrinsic factor antibody, serum folic acid, serum bilirubin (total and direct), cyanicobalamin, and unsaturated Vitamin B_{12} binding capacity. Tests confirm the suspected diagnosis. Code the laboratory services.

21. DIAGNOSIS OR NATURE OF ILLNESS OR INJURY (RELATE ITEMS 1, 2, 3 OR 4 TO ITEM 24E BY LINE)
1 |___ ___ ___   3 |___ ___ ___
2 |___ ___ ___   4 |___ ___ ___

24.	A		B	C	D		E
	DATE(S) OF SERVICE		Place of Service	Type of Service	PROCEDURES, SERVICES, OR SUPPLIES (Explain Unusual Circumstances)		DIAGNOSIS CODE
MM DD YY	From	MM DD YY To			CPT / HCPCS	MODIFIER	

Chapter Review

Guidelines are provided for the use of laboratory codes at the beginning of the pathology and laboratory section. Further clarification is provided in the subsections, subheadings, and in parenthetical notes. Pathology and laboratory services are provided by the physician or by technologists under the supervision of a physician. The majority of the codes represents a technical component only, but certain codes represent a global service — a combination of professional and technical components. Most offices do an excellent job of capturing the charges provided directly by the physician; however, ancillary services, including pathology and laboratory services, are sometimes missed. A system to track these services should be developed. Laboratory services are under increased scrutiny by third-party payors for both medical necessity and correct coding. Before laboratory services are performed verify that all procedures have a single physician order. Charge masters and fee schedules should be reviewed and updated annually.

KEY POINT

Pathology and laboratory services are provided by the physician or by technologists under the supervision of a physician. The majority of pathology and laboratory codes represent a technical component only, though certain codes represent a global service — a combination of technical and professional components.

8 Medicine Services

DIAGNOSTIC AND THERAPEUTIC SERVICES

CPT's medicine section (90281–99199) follows the pathology and laboratory section. The majority of services reported to Medicare and other payors are E/M and medicine codes. The diagnostic and therapeutic services include immunizations, injections, specialty-specific codes, and special services.

The medicine section has guidelines clarifying the use of codes in its section and subsections. Code categories, subcategories, and parenthetical phrases have guidelines in the same arrangement as the other sections of CPT that are unique to the category, subcategory, range of codes, or an individual code. Follow the directions in the notes and guidelines carefully to ensure accurate coding reflecting the services performed.

Subsections within the medicine section that have special instructions are:

> Immune Globulins
> Immunization Administration for Vaccines/Toxoids
> Vaccines/Toxoids
> Therapeutic or Diagnostic Infusions (Excludes Chemotherapy)
> Psychiatry
> Dialysis
> Ophthalmology
> Special Otorhinolaryngologic Services
> Echocardiography
> Cardiac Catheterization
> Non-Invasive Vascular Diagnostic Studies
> Pulmonary
> Allergy and Clinical Immunology
> Neurology and Neuromuscular Procedures
> Central Nervous System Assessments/Tests (e.g., Neuro-Cognitive, Mental Status, Speech Testing)
> Chemotherapy Administration
> Special Dermatological Procedures
> Physical Medicine and Rehabilitation
> Osteopathic Manipulative Treatment
> Chiropractic Manipulative Treatment
> Special Services and Reports
> Sedation with or without Analgesia (Conscious Sedation)

OBJECTIVES

Understand the difference between administration of vaccines/toxoids, therapeutic or diagnostic injection codes, and surgical injection codes and when each should be reported

Identify the special instructions for coding psychiatry services

Know when dialysis codes are reported and what services are included in a procedure code

Learn how to report ophthalmology codes

Determine the difference between the intermediate and comprehensive levels of services for ophthalmology

Recognize the coding rules for ENT services

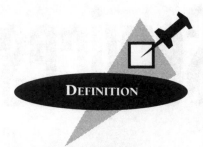

Unbundling or fragmenting is the process of coding integral services separately from a procedure or bundled service.

Coders are instructed in the medicine codes section of CPT to report each procedure separately. The word "procedure" may also describe a medical and/or E/M service.

Bundled Medicine Codes

The process of coding integral services separately from a procedure or bundled service is called unbundling or fragmenting (see Chapter 5 for further information). If the component is considered part of the package or bundled service, do not code it individually. For example, 93015 is a bundled code that includes all the components of a stress test and should be reported as such when the complete procedure is performed in the physician's office. If the components 93016 and 93018 are reported instead of the complete test (93015), the payor will probably rebundle the two codes into 93015. The reimbursement is usually greater when the codes are unbundled than when they are reported appropriately, and Medicare and private payors are becoming adept at isolating and rejecting claims in which procedures have been unbundled. However, if the procedure is performed outside the physician's office, only the services provided by the physician, e.g., interpreting the report (93018) would be reported. The facility providing the technical component would report those services.

Immunization injections

The subsection titled Immunization Injections was deleted in 1999. Services previously reported under this section have been restructured into three new subsections: Immune Globulins, Immunization Administration for Vaccines/Toxoids, and Vaccines/Toxoids. All three sections contain reporting guidelines.

IMMUNE GLOBULINS

Immune Globulin codes (90281–90399) report only the supply of the immune globulin product which includes: broad-spectrum and anti-infective immune globulins, antitoxins, and erythrocytic isoantibodies. Administration is reported separately with codes 90780–90784.

IMMUNIZATION ADMINISTRATION FOR VACCINES/TOXOIDS

Immunization administration codes (90471–90472) are reported separately in addition to the code for the vaccine or toxoid supply (90476–90749). Significant, separately identifiable E/M services should also be reported additionally.

VACCINES/TOXOIDS

Vaccines and toxoids (90476–90749) identify only the vaccine product and should be reported with an immunization administration code (90471–90472). The exact vaccine product administered must be reported. Note that code selection is also dependent on dosage, dose schedule, chemical formulation, and route of administration (e.g., intramuscular, subcutaneous, oral). Separate codes are available for reporting combination vaccines.

The following case study illustrates billing for immunizations at the time of a routine well-child exam for an established patient, age 13 months.

Immunization Injections

21. DIAGNOSIS OR NATURE OF ILLNESS OR INJURY (RELATE ITEMS 1, 2, 3 OR 4 TO ITEM 24E BY LINE)	
1 V20.2	3
2 V06.3	4

24.	A							B	C	D		E
	DATE(S) OF SERVICE							Place of Service	Type of Service	PROCEDURES, SERVICES, OR SUPPLIES (Explain Unusual Circumstances)		DIAGNOSIS CODE
	From			To						CPT / HCPCS	MODIFIER	
	MM	DD	YY	MM	DD	YY						
	2	12	98	2	12	98		11		99392		1
	2	12	98	2	12	98		11		90472		2
	2	12	98	2	12	98		11		90700		2
	2	12	98	2	12	98		11		90712		2

ICD-9-CM

V20.2 Routine infant or child health check

V06.3 Need for prophylactic vaccination with diphtheria-tetanus- pertussis with poliomyelitis (DTP + polio) vaccine

CPT

99392 Periodic preventive medicine reevaluation and management of an individual including a comprehensive history, comprehensive examination, counseling/anticipatory guidance/risk factor reduction interventions, and the ordering of appropriate laboratory/diagnostic procedures, established patient; early childhood (age 1 through 4 years)

90472 Immunization administration (includes percutaneous, intradermal, subcutaneous, intramuscular and jet injections and/or intranasal or oral administration); two or more single or combination vaccines/toxoids

90700 Diphtheria, tetanus toxoids, and acellular pertussis vaccine (DTaP), for intramuscular use

90712 Poliovirus vaccine, (any type(s)) (OPV), live, for oral use

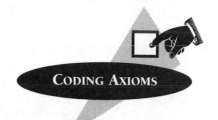

CODING AXIOMS

Therapeutic or diagnostic injection codes usually do not include the supply of materials or the office visit. These should be reported separately.

Do not use infusion therapy codes for administration of routine medications through intravenous lines. These codes also may not be used in addition to prolonged services codes.

THERAPEUTIC OR DIAGNOSTIC INFUSIONS (EXCLUDES CHEMOTHERAPY) AND INJECTIONS

Codes 90780 and 90781 identify therapeutic or diagnostic infusions. These infusions are prolonged intravenous injections requiring a physician's presence. The first code (90780) is for infusions up to one hour and the second (90781) is for each additional hour up to eight hours. When reporting 90781, indicate the number of hours in the unit column on the HCFA-1500 form or electronic bill. Remember that 90781 must be reported as a secondary code to 90780. Therapeutic or diagnostic injection codes (90782–90799) are for subcutaneous, intramuscular, intra-arterial, and intravenous injections of a therapeutic or diagnostic agent.

The materials injected are not included in the codes. When the drug is purchased and supplied by the physician, use 90281–90399 for immune globulin products, 99070 for supplies, including drugs, provided and not elsewhere listed, or the appropriate HCPCS Level II J-code for other drugs. See Chapter 10 for information regarding HCPCS coding.

Medicare bundles the administration of the medication into the E/M service. Each Medicare and Medicaid carrier has individual requirements for HCPCS Level II codes to describe the drug administered. Some carriers require the use of the CPT code for the injection and the HCPCS

Level II J-code for the drug; others use only the J code and require a modifier to designate the method of administration.

The following case study illustrates a claim to a commercial payor for a follow-up problem focused history and exam and a therapeutic injection of Depo-Provera, 150 mg, for contraception:

Therapeutic Injections

21. DIAGNOSIS OR NATURE OF ILLNESS OR INJURY (RELATE ITEMS 1, 2, 3 OR 4 TO ITEM 24E BY LINE)		
1 ⌊ V25.49	3 ⌊ __ __	
2 ⌊ __ __	4 ⌊ __ __	

24.	A						B	C	D		E
	DATE(S) OF SERVICE						Place of Service	Type of Service	PROCEDURES, SERVICES, OR SUPPLIES (Explain Unusual Circumstances)		DIAGNOSIS CODE
	From MM DD YY			To MM DD YY					CPT / HCPCS	MODIFIER	
	3 ¦ 15 ¦ 98			3 ¦ 15 ¦ 98			11		99212	¦ ¦	1
	3 ¦ 15 ¦ 98			3 ¦ 15 ¦ 98			11		90782	¦ ¦	1
	3 ¦ 15 ¦ 98			3 ¦ 15 ¦ 98			11		99070	¦ ¦	1
									—or—		
	3 ¦ 15 ¦ 98			3 ¦ 15 ¦ 98			11		J1055	¦ ¦	1

ICD-9-CM

V25.49   Encounter for contraceptive management

CPT

99212   Office or other outpatient visit for the evaluation and management of an established patient, which requires at least two of these three key components: a problem focused history; a problem focused examination; straightforward medical decision making. Counseling and/or coordination of care with other providers or agencies are provided consistent with the nature of the problem(s) and the patient's and/or family's needs. Usually, the presenting problem(s) are self limited or minor. Physicians typically spend 10 minutes face-to-face with the patient and/or family.

90782   Therapeutic or diagnostic injection (specify material injected); subcutaneous or intramuscular

99070   Supplies and materials (except spectacles), provided by the physician over and above those usually included with the office visit or other services rendered (list drugs, trays, supplies, or materials provided)

or

J1055   Depo-Provera, 150 mg, for contraception

PSYCHIATRY

While CPT codes were developed specifically for reporting physician services, codes from Psychiatry (90801–90899) are frequently used by psychologists and social workers to report their services. Payors generally reimburse nonphysician providers a percentage of the amount allowed by physicians, typically 60 percent for psychologists and 40 percent for social workers.

Psychiatry codes include psychiatric diagnostic or evaluation interview procedures (90801–90802), and psychiatric therapeutic procedures (90804–90899).

Psychiatric diagnostic interview exam (90801) includes a history, mental status, and disposition, and may include communication with family or other sources and ordering/interpretation of

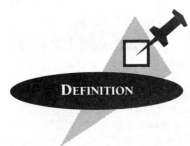

Psychiatric Therapeutic Procedures
Psychotherapy is the treatment of mental illness and behavioral disturbances in which the clinician, through definitive therapeutic communication, attempts to alleviate the emotional disturbances, reverse or change maladaptive patterns of behavior, and encourage personality growth and development.

Interactive psychotherapy involves the use of physical aids and non-verbal communication to overcome barriers to therapeutic interaction between the clinician and a patient.

Insight oriented, behavior modifying and/or supportive psychotherapy refers to the development of insight or affective understanding, the use of behavior modification techniques, the use of supportive interactions, the use of cognitive discussion of reality, or any combination of the above to provide therapeutic change.

diagnostic studies. An interactive psychiatric diagnostic interview (90802) is furnished to children or individuals who lack expressive and receptive communication skills. These procedure codes are normally reported only on the initial visit.

The most frequently reported services are therapeutic psychiatric service codes (90804–90829) for individual psychotherapy. Individual psychotherapy services are organized first by place of service (office/outpatient, inpatient/partial hospital/residential care). Within these two subcategories, they are then organized by type of psychotherapy service (insight oriented, behavior modifying, supportive, interactive), face-to-face time, and the provision of any additional medical evaluation or management services.

Other psychotherapy services (90845–90857) are used to report family and group psychotherapy services. Psychiatric services and procedures (90862–90899) are used to report medication management, electroconvulsive therapy, and hypnotherapy.

Hospital inpatient service codes (99221–99233) should be reported when the physician is involved in the medical management of an inpatient (e.g., when the attending physician reviews laboratory tests or initiates the patient's treatment plan) but does not provide psychotherapy on the same day. Do not use hospital inpatient service codes when both psychotherapy and E/M services are provided on the same day. Combined E/M and psychotherapy services should be reported with codes designated as such in the psychiatry section (90804–90822).

BIOFEEDBACK
Biofeedback codes (90901–90911) may require prior authorization. If the payor does not cover biofeedback, enlist the help of the medical director or prior authorization (or utilization) review nurses for service coverage. Documentation may be required, such as articles or printed research material about the benefits of biofeedback.

DIALYSIS
Dialysis services (90918–90999) are divided into end stage renal disease (ESRD) services, hemodialysis, peritoneal dialysis, and miscellaneous dialysis procedures. Codes for the latter three services are selected according to whether the service includes single physician evaluations or repeated evaluations. Repeated evaluations are reported despite no changes in the dialysis prescription.

The dialysis procedure (90935–90947) includes all evaluation and management services related to the patient's ESRD rendered on a day dialysis is performed, as well as all other patient care services rendered during the dialysis procedure. Office and hospital visits are reported in addition to dialysis procedures only when they are unrelated to dialysis and cannot be rendered during a dialysis session.

Codes that report ESRD related services (90918–90921) are selected according to the age of the patient and reflect services for a full month. For less than a full month, 90922–90925 are reported for each day ESRD service is provided. Procedures for other medical problems and complications unrelated to ESRD are not included in the monthly ESRD service.

GASTROENTEROLOGY
The diagnostic procedures (91000–91299) are frequently performed with consultations or other E/M services. Evaluation and management services should be reported separately. Even though

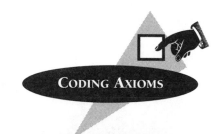

CODING AXIOMS

For a level of service to be reimbursed with dialysis treatment on the same day, a separate diagnosis supporting the level of service must be reported. For instance, 585 *Chronic renal failure* with 707.1 *Ulcer of lower limbs, except decubitus.*

gastroenterology is a medicine subspecialty, the majority of procedures performed by gastroenterologists are endoscopic and are listed in the surgery section.

OPHTHALMOLOGY

The medical services of ophthalmologists are described in codes 92002 through 92499. General ophthalmological services (92002–92014) are divided into new and established patient categories that are further subdivided by level of service.

Intermediate Level of Service

Intermediate service codes (92002 and 92012) report the evaluation of new or existing conditions that have been complicated by a new diagnostic or management problem. This new complaint may relate to the primary diagnosis. Included in the evaluation are:

- History
- General medical observation
- External examination
- Ophthalmoscopy
- Other diagnostic procedures as indicated
  - Biomicroscopy
  - Mydriasis
  - Tonometry
- Initiation of diagnostic and treatment program

Comprehensive Level of Service

Comprehensive service codes (92004 and 92014) report the evaluation of the complete visual system. This is a single service, that need not be performed at one session. Included in this evaluation are:

- History
- General medical observation
- General evaluation of the complete visual system to include:
  - External examination
  - Ophthalmoscopy
  - Gross visual field
  - Basic sensorimotor examination
- Other diagnostic procedures as indicated:
  - Biomicroscopy
  - Dilation (cycloplegia)
  - Mydriasis
  - Tonometry
- Initiation of a diagnostic treatment program

Special Ophthalmological Services

Refractions
Refractions (92015) should be reported additionally when performed at the time of a general ophthalmological service (92002–92014).

Refractions

21. DIAGNOSIS OR NATURE OF ILLNESS OR INJURY (RELATE ITEMS 1, 2, 3 OR 4 TO ITEM 24E BY LINE)			
1. 367.20		3.	
2.		4.	

24. A DATE(S) OF SERVICE						B Place of Service	C Type of Service	D PROCEDURES, SERVICES, OR SUPPLIES (Explain Unusual Circumstances) CPT / HCPCS MODIFIER	E DIAGNOSIS CODE
MM	DD	YY	MM	DD	YY				
2	18	98	2	18	98	11		92014	1
2	18	98	2	18	98	11		92015	1

ICD-9-CM

367.20   Astigmatism, unspecified

CPT

92014   Ophthalmological services: medical examination and evaluation, with initiation or continuation of diagnostic and treatment program; comprehensive, established patient, one or more visits

92015   Determination of refractive state

Medicare allows the reporting of refractions, a noncovered service, to minimize patient confusion.

Visual Field Exam
Gross visual field testing is integral to the general ophthalmic service and should not be reported separately. However, more extensive visual field examinations should be reported separately with codes, 92081–92083. CPT recognizes three coding levels for visual field exams. The three specific visual field tests (limited, intermediate, and extended) are described as unilateral or bilateral.

Lens Services and Ocular Prosthetics
Fitting and provision of contact lenses, glasses, and ocular prostheses are reported with the CPT codes 92310–92396. Use modifier -26 or 09926 with 92391 or 92396 to report the service of fitting without supply. All the codes in this section are bilateral. For prescription or fitting of one eye, append modifier -52 or 09952.

SPECIAL OTORHINOLARYNGOLOGIC SERVICES
Otorhinolaryngologic codes (92502–92599) identify the special diagnostic and treatment services not usually included in a comprehensive otorhinolaryngologic evaluation. Comprehensive ENT evaluations include basic diagnostic procedures such as otoscopy and rhinoscopy. These services are an integral part of the evaluation and management service and are not itemized separately. Special services not generally included in this total evaluation are reported separately with 92502–92599, such as audiologic function tests (92551–92598). Hearing tests using calibrated electronic equipment are reportable; use of a tuning fork is not.

Hearing test codes are inherently bilateral (binaural, both ears). If only one ear is tested, the reduced service is reported with modifier -52. Codes 92590, 92592, and 92594 are the exception, identified in CPT as monaural (one ear). If binaural, report with 92591, 92593, or 92595.

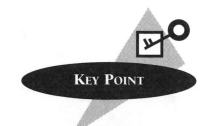

KEY POINT

Making Sense of Misunderstood Codes
Special otorhinolaryngology services codes contain procedures that are among the most misunderstood in CPT. While some codes use common terminology, such as 92507 *Speech, language or hearing therapy*, terms like 92543 *Caloric vestibular test* are less clear. Here are some tips that may help you and your payors gain a better understanding of confusing audiology codes:

- If questioned on a test or a new code, provide a definition of the test and describe the disorders for which the test is indicated. This may clarify the issue for prior authorization, and your definitions may become part of the payors protocol for the tests.

- If a screening test is performed and further testing is warranted, attach a standard definition and a statement indicating why the additional testing is necessary. Submit the documentation to the payor's prior authorization department. Documentation helps the payor determine if and when the test is appropriate.

Indications for Holter monitor include:

- Suspected dysrhythmia

- Unexplained symptoms (dizziness, syncope, or palpitations)

- Chest pain episodes

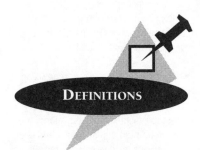

DEFINITIONS

Echocardiography records ultrasonic waves reflected from the heart and allows visualization of heart size and shape, myocardial wall thickness, motion, cardiac valve structure, and function.

Cardiac catheterizations are invasive procedures used to visualize the heart's chambers, valves, great vessels, and coronary arteries.

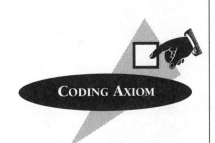

CODING AXIOM

Medicare has specific policies related to 93015–93018 when performed in a hospital. See *Code It Right*'s Medicare chapter.

CARDIOVASCULAR SERVICES

Cardiovascular services (92950–93799) include diagnostic and therapeutic services.

Therapeutic (92950–92966)

Therapeutic services are performed for treatment of a specific condition, disorder, or disease. Some of the more frequently performed services include: percutaneous placement of intracoronary stents, percutaneous transluminal coronary angioplasty (PTCA), and percutaneous transluminal coronary arthrectomy.

Percutaneous placement of coronary stents (92980–92981) include therapeutic procedures such as PTCA and arthrectomy. Therefore, procedures 92982, 92984, 92995, and 92996 should not be reported with the codes for stent placement.

PTCA (92982–92984) is used to treat coronary artery obstruction. A balloon catheter is placed in the affected artery and the balloon is inflated to flatten the plaque against the wall of the artery and open the obstruction.

Percutaneous transluminal coronary arthrectomy (92995–92996) may be used instead of the PTCA to treat coronary artery obstruction. Arthrectomy involves placing a catheter into the affected artery and using a rotary cutter to remove the plaque. When arthrectomy is performed with a PTCA, the PTCA is not reported separately as it is included in procedures 92995 and 92996.

Cardiography (93000–93278)

Cardiography services include electrocardiogram (ECG), cardiovascular stress tests, and electrocardiographic (Holter) monitoring. Cardiography codes include both a professional and a technical component. These codes have separate listings for the total component, the recording (technical component), and the review and interpretation (professional component). For example, code 93015 identifies the total service (global) for a cardiovascular stress test and includes the following components:

- The tracing (the technical component only) (93017)

- Supervision of the procedure (a portion of the professional component) (93016)

- Interpretation and report (a portion of the professional component) (93018)

The Holter monitor is a diagnostic tool that creates a continuous record of the heart's electrical activity during the patient's normal activities for a 24-hour period.

Echocardiography (93303–93350)

Echocardiography records ultrasonic waves reflected from the heart and allows visualization of heart size and shape, myocardial wall thickness, motion, cardiac valve structure, and function.

Echocardiography codes represent a global procedure. When the physician provides only supervision and interpretation, modifier -26 is added. In echocardiography, ultrasonic waves directed at the heart and great vessels provide a hard copy recording that serves as a diagnostic tool.

After an initial study, follow-up echocardiograms by the same provider or provider group are usually covered: (a) when there are new, significantly changing symptoms for the conditions listed above, or (b) at reasonable intervals when progression is expected in one of these conditions. Routine follow-up testing outside the criteria may not be covered. To code for a follow-up echocardiogram, use 93304, 93308, and 93321, if applicable.

Transesophageal echocardiography (93312–93317) involves guiding a small ultrasonic device attached to the tip of a gastroscope into the patient's esophagus, where it rests behind the heart.

Doppler echocardiography (93320–93321) provides continuous waves but also uses a sound or frequency ultrasound to record direction of blood flow through the heart chambers. Doppler echocardiography is an add-on code and should be reported in addition to two-dimension (2-D) echocardiogram (93303–93315, 93317, 93350).

Color flow mapping (93325) converts recorded flow frequencies into different colors. These color images are superimposed on M-mode or 2-D echoes, allowing more detailed evaluation of disorders. Color flow mapping is an add-on service and should be reported in addition to echocardiography (76825–76828, 93307, 93308, 93312, 93314, 93315, 93317, 93320, 93321, and 93350).

Cardiac Catheterization (93501–93572)

Cardiac catheterizations are invasive procedures used to visualize the heart's chambers, valves, great vessels, and coronary arteries. Catheter procedures produce pressure measurements and blood volumes used to evaluate cardiac function and valve patency.

The three major components of cardiac catheterization include: introduction and positioning of the catheter (93501–93536) including repositioning, injection procedures (93539–93545) and imaging supervision, interpretation, and report (93555–93556). Indicator dilution studies (93561–93562) and intravascular doppler studies (93571–93572) are other components.

Supervision and interpretation codes related to cardiac catheterization (93555 and 93556) are used with imaging performed as part of cardiac catheterization procedures. The plural presentation of the word "procedure(s)" as well as the "and/or" terminology in the descriptions of imaging services suggest the codes include imaging of one or more areas.

Aortic root aortography (93544) is the injection of a large bolus of dye into the proximal ascending aorta, just above the aortic valve. When thoracic aortography is performed without a cardiac catheterization, it should be reported using procedure 36200 and the appropriate radiologic supervision/interpretation (75600 or 75605).

Electrophysiologic Studies (EPS) (93600–93660)

Electrophysiologic studies (93600–93660) evaluate the electrical conduction system of the heart. An electrode is placed and the patient is monitored constantly with both intracardiac external ECG leads to record the cardiac response. Programmed electrical stimulation is delivered through an electrode catheter to evaluate electrical conduction pathways, formation of dysrhythmia, and automaticity and refractoriness of myocardial cells. These procedures may include induction of arrhythmia to isolate the origin of the conduction problem.

Endomyocardial Biopsy (93505)

Biopsy of the inside and middle layers of the heart is a separately reportable service. It may be performed in surgery or in the cardiac cath lab with the patient under local anesthesia. The sample is usually taken from the right or left ventricle. The patient is monitored constantly with both intracardiac and external ECG leads to record cardiac response.

KEY POINT

Cardiac catheterization includes the following services:

- Intravenous pressure
- Intracardiac pressure
- Arterial blood sample for blood gas studies
- Cardiac output (93561)
- Ergometer (to exercise patient)
- Electrode catheter (temporary pacemaker)
- Swan-Ganz insertion
- Arterial/venous cutdown
- Placement or repositioning of catheters and use of automatic power injectors

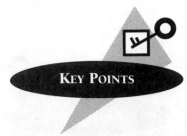

NONINVASIVE VASCULAR DIAGNOSTIC STUDIES

Noninvasive vascular studies codes (93875–93990) include the patient care required to perform the studies supervision of the studies and interpretation of results.

A duplex scan combines both two-dimensional structure of motion with time and Doppler ultrasonic signal documentation with spectral analysis and color flow velocity mapping or imaging to produce a real-time video display of organ structure and motion.

A vascular study must produce a hard copy with data analysis for the patient's record, including bidirectional vascular flow or imaging when provided. Simple hand-held (screening) devices do not meet these requirements, are part of the physical exam of the vascular system, and are not reported separately.

PULMONARY

Pulmonary codes (94010–94799) include both diagnostic and therapeutic services. All procedures include laboratory services, interpretation, and physician services. Read definitions carefully. List hospital inpatient visits, consultations, emergency department services, or office visits separately when performed on the same date as a diagnostic pulmonary service.

Specify the procedures that may be performed in requesting prior authorization for pulmonary testing. If ordering tests for a patient and unsure about which test should be performed, contact the pulmonary laboratory for clarification and CPT code numbers. Include that information in documentation for prior authorization and claim review.

Spirometry/Bronchospasm Evaluation

Spirometry (94010–94070) measures lung capacity. Code 94010 refers to the measurement of the lung's capacity and flow measurements using a spirometer. Expiratory flow rate is calculated generally in terms of liters per second. Maximal voluntary ventilation is included in this service. The graphic record produced by the spirometer goes into the patient's record.

Codes 94014–94016 were added in 1999 to report patient initiated spirometric recording per 30 day time period.

Bronchospasm evaluation (94060) includes spirometry before and after the use of a bronchodilator (either aerosol or parenteral). The final codes in this series report prolonged evaluation with multiple spirometric determinations.

ALLERGY AND CLINICAL IMMUNOLOGY

Allergy testing and immunology treatment (95004–95199) are performed according to the patient's history, physical findings, and clinical judgment of the provider. Specify the number of tests performed in the unit area of the claim or electronic billing form. Many payors require a report of the exact number of tests performed since their allowable is based on a per-test amount. Significant, separately identifiable E/M services should be reported in addition to allergen testing and immunotherapy.

NEUROLOGY AND NEUROMUSCULAR PROCEDURES

Neurologic services (95805–95999) are frequently performed with consultative or other evaluation and management services. The E/M services are reported separately.

Sleep Testing

Sleep services (95805–95811) include sleep studies and polysomnography. Both types of services include continuous and simultaneous monitoring and recording of selected physiological and pathophysiological sleep parameters for a minimum of 6 hours. For studies of less than 6 hours append modifier -52. These services are global and include tracing, interpretation, and report. For interpretation only append modifier -26. These studies are performed to diagnose a variety of sleep disorders and to evaluate a patient's response to therapies such as nasal continous positive airway pressure (NCPAP).

Polysomnography is distinguished from sleep studies by the inclusion of sleep staging, which is defined to include:

- A 1–4 lead electroencephalogram (EEG)
- An electro-oculogram (EOG)
- A submental electromyogram (EMG)

Additional parameters of sleep include:
- Electrocardiogram (ECG)
- Airflow
- Ventilation and respiratory effort
- Gas exchange by oximetry, transcutaneous monitoring, or end tidal gas analysis
- Extremity muscle activity, motor activity-movement
- Extended electroencephalogram (EEG) monitoring
- Penile tumescence
- Gastroesophageal reflux
- Continuous blood pressure monitoring
- Snoring
- Body positions, etc.

Electroencephalogram (EEG)

Electroencephalogram (EEG) codes (95812–95829, 95950–95962) include tracing, interpretation, and report. For interpretation only, append modifier -26.

Evoked Response

Evoked response (95920–95930) are global services and include tracing, interpretation and report. For interpretation only, append modifier -26. Codes 95925–95927 report bilateral studies. For unilateral studies append modifier -52.

EMG/Nerve Conduction Stuides

EMG's (95860–95875) and nerve conduction studies (95900–95904, 95934–95936) are frequently performed together. Codes for EMG studies are site specific. Nerve conduction studies should be reported for each nerve studied. F-wave studies are performed on upper extremities while H-reflex studies are performed on lower extremities. Modifier -51 should not be used when reporting nerve conduction studies (95900–95904).

Neurostimulators, Analysis — Programming

Six new codes to the Medicine section report the analysis of simple and complex implanted neurostimulators pulse generator/transmitter systems (95970–95975). These devices send small electric shocks to different sites to treat symptoms of various diseases, such as Parkinson's.

DEFINITION

Cognitive is being aware by drawing from knowledge, such as judgment, reason, perception, and memory. Several types of testing procedures, when combined, produce information about the patient's congnitive functioning.

A simple stimulator is capable of affecting three or fewer of the following conditions, while a complex neurostimular is capable of affecting more than three: pulse amplitude, pulse duration, pulse frequency, eight or more electrode contacts, cycling, stimulation train duration, train spacing, number of programs, number of channels, phase angle, alternating electrode polarities, configuration of wave form, and more than one clinical feature (e.g., rigidity, dyskinesia, and tremor.

Code 95970 reports analysis of implanted neurostimulator pulse generator system, simple or complex, without reprogramming. All other codes report analysis with intraoperative or subsequent programming. Analysis of simple devices requiring reprogramming are reported with a single code 95971. Analysis of complex devices requring reprogramming are reported based on time. Report 95972 or 95974 for the first hour and 95973 or 95975 for each additional 30 minutes.

Insertion, revision, and removal of neurostimulator pulse generators are reported using codes from the Surgery section of CPT.

CENTRAL NERVOUS SYSTEM ASSESSMENTS/TESTS

Central nervous system assessment codes (96100–96117) combine several types of testing procedures to produce information about the **cognitive** function of a patient. Tests include cognitive processes, visual motor responses, and abstractive abilities. When these tests are performed, material generated should be formulated into a report.

CHEMOTHERAPY ADMINISTRATION

Chemotherapy codes (96400-96549) are reported independent of evaluation and management services provided during the same encounter or on the same day. Most individuals receiving chemotherapy services will require a separately reportable evaluation and management service at the time of chemotherapy services.

Chemotherapy codes include preparation of the chemotherapy agent(s). However, the supply of chemotherapy agents should be reported with HCPCS Level II J-codes or with CPT code 96545.

Administration of other medications provided in conjunction with chemotherapy should be reported separately using 90780-90788. These include: antibiotics, antiemetics, narcotics, analgesics, steroidal and biological agents. Since 90780-90788 report only the administration of the medications, report the medication supplied with the appropriate HCPCS Level II J-code or with CPT code 99070.

Report special filter needles, infusion sets, and other chemotherapy supplies separately with HCPCS Level II A-codes or CPT code 99070.

Medicare and most commercial payors require HCPCS Level II codes since they are more specific than CPT codes. Indicate the exact drugs and supplies for payors who do not accept HCPCS Level II codes. Include invoices to answer questions regarding cost.

Chemotherapy codes are distiguished by several factors. First, different codes are provided for intravenous and intra-arterial injections. Regional (isolation) chemotherapy perfusion is reported with intra-arterial infusion codes. Placement of the intra-arterial catheter should be reported using the appropriate code from the cardiovascular surgery section (36620-36640). Second, separate codes are provided for infusion and push techniques. Report the code for each technique when both techniques are used. A final factor is the element of time for infusion techniques.

SPECIAL DERMATOLOGICAL PROCEDURES

When dermatology treatments are performed with a separately identifiable E/M service, both may be reported. Dermatologic services are typically consultative, so any of the five levels of consultation (99241–99263) may be appropriate. Similarly, evaluation and management levels of service appropriate to dermatologic illnesses should be coded.

PHYSICAL MEDICINE AND REHABILITATION

Evaluation Services

Codes 97001–97004 report evaluation and re-evaluation services for physical and occupational therapy. Codes 97001 and 97003 indicate the initial evaluation service. Re-evaluation services should be reported with codes 97002 and 97004.

Modalities

The modality range of codes in the physical medicine and rehabilitation subsection are organized into two groups. The first group (97010–97028) are supervised procedures that do not require direct (one-on-one) patient contact. The second group (97032–97039) requires constant attendance and direct (one-on-one) patient contact.

The description for all treatment modalities specifies application of a modality to one or more areas. In other words, when hot or cold packs are applied to the arm, leg, and neck, code 97010 should be reported once. However, when different modalities are used, such as 97010 *Application of hot or cold pack*, 97014 *Application of electrical stimulation*, and 97022 *whirlpool*, each is reported separately.

Time should be reported in 15-minute increments for treatment modalities requiring constant attendance. If more than 15 minutes are required, i.e., 30 minutes, report two units on the HCFA-1500 form. For less than 15 minutes, append the reduced service modifier -52 and adjust the usual cost of the code based on the time that was actually spent.

Therapeutic Procedures

Therapeutic procedures within the physical medicine/rehabilitation section describe the application of clinical skills or services to improve function. These procedures require direct (one-on-one) patient contact. Some therapeutic procedures have a time component and should be reported once for each 15 minutes of treatment. Others do not have a time component and should be reported only once per visit. For work hardening/conditioning (97545–97546), report 97545 for the initial two hours and 97546 for each additional hour. Procedure 97546 is considered an "add on" procedure. "Add on" procedures are never reduced in value and modifier -51 *multiple procedures* should not be appended.

Tests, Measurements, and Other Procedures

Use 97703 and 97750 to report tests and measurement. These codes are also reported in 15-minute increments, as is code 97770.

OSTEOPATHIC MANIPULATIVE TREATMENT

Codes 98925–98929 report inpatient or outpatient osteopathic manipulative treatment (OMT). Instructional notes state osteopathic manipulative treatment is a form of manual treatment applied by a physician to eliminate or alleviate somatic dysfunction and related disorders.

DEFINITION

Modality is any physical agent applied to produce therapeutic changes to biologic tissue; includes but is not limited to thermal, acoustic, light, mechanical, or electric energy.

Therapeutic procedures are a manner of effecting change through the application of clinical skills and/or services that attempt to improve function.

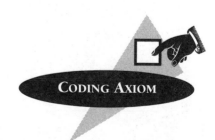

CODING AXIOM

For an E/M service to be paid separately when performed on the same day as OMT, identify the E/M service with modifier -25 *Significant, separately identifiable evaluation and management service by the same physician on the day of a procedure.*

Conditions for OMT treatment include:

- Disorders in the skeletal, arthrodial, myofascial, and visceral structures as well as related vascular, lymphatic, and neural elements

- Palpatory findings such as tenderness, asymmetry, range of motion abnormalities, and tissue texture changes

OMT may be accomplished by a variety of techniques including, but not limited to:

- Soft tissue techniques, such as stretching, gentle range of motion, and kneading

- Direct techniques, such as joint mobilization, thrust, and muscle energy

- Indirect techniques, such as myofascial release, strain/counterstrain, and cranial osteopathy

The five codes are differentiated by the number of body regions involved in the treatment. CPT guidelines refer to the following body regions: head, cervical, thoracic, lumbar, sacral, pelvic, lower extremities, upper extremities, rib cage, and abdomen and viscera.

OMT includes a component of E/M service to ascertain the effectiveness of the therapy. An E/M service may be identified separately when:

- A physician diagnoses the condition requiring manipulative therapy and provides it during the same visit.

- The condition requiring manipulative therapy fails to respond to the therapy or the condition significantly changes or intensifies and requires E/M services beyond the usual pre- and postservice work associated with the procedure.

- The physician treats a condition unrelated to the condition requiring manipulative therapy during the same visit.

CHIROPRACTIC MANIPULATIVE TREATMENT

Chiropractic manipulative treatment (CMT), reported with codes 98940–98943, is a form of manual treatment performed to influence joint and neurophysical function. CMT codes include a premanipulation patient assessment. Evaluation and management services should not be reported separately unless the patient's condition requires a separately identifiable E/M service beyond the usual pre- and postservice work normally associated with the procedure.

CMT codes are reported by region. The five spinal regions are defined as follows: cervical (includes atlanto-occipital joint); thoracic (includes costovertebral and costotransverse joints); lumbar, sacral; and pelvic (includes sacro-iliac joint). The five extraspinal regions are defined as follows: head (including temporomandibular joint); lower extremities; upper extremities; rib cage, and abdomen.

SPECIAL SERVICES AND REPORTS

Special services and reports (99000–99090) allow supplemental reporting for "services that are an adjunct to the basic services rendered." To justify use of these codes, identify the medical necessity of special circumstances. Document the information clearly and completely in the patient's medical record. Payors have individual guidelines for use of these codes.

Code 99024 reports a postoperative follow-up visit included in the global service period. It is reported mainly for record keeping purposes as providers receive no additional reimbursement for routine postoperative care. Code 99025 reports an initial (new patient) visit when a starred (*) procedure constitutes the major service at that visit. Guidelines related to starred procedures are described in Chapter 5.

Codes 99050–99058 identify emergency office calls and services provided after hours, on Sundays, or on holidays. Other codes in this category identify medical testimony, unusual travel requirements (e.g., escorting a patient on a trip of more than 10 miles), and educational services.

There are also codes for transportation of specimens (99000–99001). These codes should be reported only once per visit, regardless of the number of specimens. Not all payors reimburse additionally for transportation services.

DISCUSSION QUESTIONS

1. How do you report the supply of materials for therapeutic or diagnostic injections?

    _____

    _____

    _____

2. Are procedures for other medical problems and complications included in the monthly maintenance service for dialysis? Explain.

    _____

    _____

    _____

3. Explain the differences between the intermediate and comprehensive levels of service for ophthalmology. Are ophthalmology service codes unilateral or bilateral?

    _____

    _____

    _____

4. Cite the difference between "supervised" and "constant attendance" as related to Physical Medicine and Rehabilitation.

    _____

    _____

    _____

5. What services are an integral part of the evaluation and management for ENT?

    _____

    _____

    _____

OBJECTIVES

See the practical application of CPT medicine services coding

Identify the special circumstances and rules of specialties

Specialty-Specific Scenarios

The following surgical scenarios are designed by specialty to help you make the leap from documentation to correct code choices.

DERMATOLOGY SCENARIO

A 15-year-old male with severe acne was referred by his primary care physician to a dermatologist for consultation and possible management. The dermatologist performed a problem-focused history and examination and reviewed the records (including lab results) the patient brought with him. Treatment options were discussed with the patient and his mother who accompanied him to the visit. It was decided that the initial treatment would consist of antibiotics and actinotherapy. An actinotherapy (ultraviolet light) treatment was performed during the initial visit and the patient was to return in one month for follow-up on his response to the antibiotics that were prescribed. A written report was sent to the primary care physician with treatment recommendations. Code the ICD-9-CM and CPT codes.

Dermatology

21. DIAGNOSIS OR NATURE OF ILLNESS OR INJURY (RELATE ITEMS 1, 2, 3 OR 4 TO ITEM 24E BY LINE)
1.	706.1		3.	
2.			4.	

24.	A						B	C	D		E
	DATE(S) OF SERVICE						Place of Service	Type of Service	PROCEDURES, SERVICES, OR SUPPLIES (Explain Unusual Circumstances)		DIAGNOSIS CODE
	From			To					CPT / HCPCS	MODIFIER	
	MM	DD	YY	MM	DD	YY					
	7	6	98	7	6	98	11		99241		1
	7	6	98	7	6	98	11		96900		1

ICD-9-CM

706.1   Other acne

CPT

99241   Office consultation for a new or established patient, which requires these three key components: a problem focused history; a problem focused examination; and straightforward medical decision making. Counseling and/or coordination of care with other providers or agencies are provided consistent with the nature of the problem(s) and the patient's and/or family's needs. Usually, the presenting problem(s) are self limited or minor. Physicians typically spend 15 minutes face-to-face with the patient and/or family.

96900   Actinotherapy (ultraviolet light)

The patient required a separately identifiable consultative service prior to the actinotherapy. Both services should be reported.

NEUROLOGY SCENARIO

A 35-year-old secretary was referred to neurology by her family physician for consultation and diagnostic studies related to right hand numbness. The neurologist performed a expanded problem focused history and exam with decision making of low complexity. Nerve conduction studies included 2 sensory nerves, 2 motor nerves (one with and one without F-wave). These studies confirmed a right median nerve entrapment at the wrist (carpal tunnel). The neurologist outlined a course of therapy and requested in a written report which was sent to her family physician that the patient return in one month.

Neurology

21. DIAGNOSIS OR NATURE OF ILLNESS OR INJURY (RELATE ITEMS 1, 2, 3 OR 4 TO ITEM 24E BY LINE)

1. 354.0
2.
3.
4.

24. A DATE(S) OF SERVICE From			To			B Place of Service	C Type of Service	D PROCEDURES, SERVICES, OR SUPPLIES (Explain Unusual Circumstances) CPT / HCPCS	MODIFIER	E DIAGNOSIS CODE
MM	DD	YY	MM	DD	YY					
2	5	98	2	5	98	11		99242	–25	1
2	5	98	2	5	98	11		95900		1
2	5	98	2	5	98	11		95903		1
2	5	98	2	5	98	11		95904	x2	1

ICD-9-CM

354.0   Carpal tunnel syndrome

CPT

99242-25   Office consultation for a new or established patient, which requires these three key components: an expanded problem focused history; an expanded problem focused examination; and straightforward medical decision making. Counseling and/or coordination of care with other providers or agencies are provided consistent with the nature of the problem(s) and the patient's and/or family's needs. Usually, the presenting problem(s) are of low severity. Physicians typically spend 30 minutes face-to-face with the patient and/or family. — Significant, separately identifiable E/M service by the same physician on the same day of the procedure or other service

95900   Nerve conduction, amplitude and latency/velocity study, each nerve, any/all site(s) along the nerve; motor, without F-wave study

95903   Nerve conduction, amplitude and latency/velocity study, each nerve, any/all site(s) along the nerve; motor, with F-wave study

95904x2   Nerve conduction, amplitude and latency/velocity study, each nerve, any/all site(s) along the nerve; sensory

Neurology services are typically consultative in nature and should be reported in addition to diagnostic and/or therapeutic services.

Nerve conduction studies are reported for each nerve tested. Codes are selected based on whether the nerve is a sensory or motor nerve and whether an F-wave study is performed. Nerve conduction codes (95900–95904) are modifier -51 exempt.

MEDICAL SPECIALTY — CARDIOLOGY SCENARIO

A 32-year-old male presented to the cardiologist with a complaint of recent onset of palpitations. He was referred from his family physician for assumption of care. The cardiologist reviewed past and present social and medical history and records. After a detailed system review was performed, which failed to demonstrate any abnormality, the cardiologist prescribed a 24-hour Holter monitor. The cardiologist supplied the monitor with hook-up and recording and performed a review and interpretation of the microprocessor-based analysis. The analysis and report were supplied by another facility. The cardiologist diagnosed stress induced ectopic atrial beats and discussed a course of therapy with the patient upon follow-up visit. The follow-up visit lasted approximately 20 minutes.

Medical Specialty – Cardiology

21. DIAGNOSIS OR NATURE OF ILLNESS OR INJURY (RELATE ITEMS 1, 2, 3 OR 4 TO ITEM 24E BY LINE)

1. 785.1
2. 427.61
3.
4.

24. DATE(S) OF SERVICE From MM DD YY	To MM DD YY	B Place of Service	C Type of Service	D PROCEDURES, SERVICES, OR SUPPLIES (Explain Unusual Circumstances) CPT / HCPCS	MODIFIER	E DIAGNOSIS CODE
3 24 98	3 24 98	3		99204		1
3 24 98	3 24 98	3		93231		1
3 24 98	3 24 98	3		93233		1
3 25 98	3 25 98	3		99213		2

ICD-9-CM

785.1   Palpitations

427.61   Supraventricular premature beats

CPT

99204   Office or other outpatient visit for the evaluation and management of a new patient, which requires these three key components: a comprehensive history; a comprehensive examination; and medical decision making of moderate complexity. Counseling and/or coordination of care with other providers or agencies are provided consistent with the nature of the problem(s) and the patient's and/or family's needs. Usually, the presenting problem(s) are of moderate to high severity. Physicians typically spend 45 minutes face-to-face with the patient and/or family.

93231   Electrocardiographic monitoring for 24 hours by continuous original ECG waveform recording and storage without superimposition scanning utilizing a device capable of producing a full miniaturized printout; recording (includes hook-up, recording, and disconnection)

93233   Electrocardiographic monitoring for 24 hours by continuous original ECG waveform recording and storage without superimposition scanning utilizing a device capable of producing a full miniaturized printout; physician review and interpretation

99213   Office or other outpatient visit for the evaluation and management of an established patient, which requires at least two of these three key components: an expanded problem focused history; an expanded problem focused examination; medical decision making of low complexity. Counseling and coordination of care with other providers or agencies are provided consistent with the nature of the problem(s) and the patient's and/or family's needs. Usually, the presenting problem(s) are of low to moderate severity. Physicians typically spend 15 minutes face-to-face with the patient and/or family.

When a patient presents with symptoms and no diagnosis is made during the initial evaluation, it is appropriate to code the symptoms until a diagnosis is made.

Note that the cardiologist performed only a portion of the total 24-hour ECG monitor service — the recording and physician interpretation. The microprocessor-based analysis and report were performed by another facility. In this case, CPT provides separate codes to identify each portion of the total service as well as a single code for global service.

GENERAL SURGERY SCENARIO

A patient is seen by a general surgeon for a routine postoperative follow-up visit two weeks after discharge from the hospital, post cholecystectomy via an open laparotomy. Code the service.

General Surgery

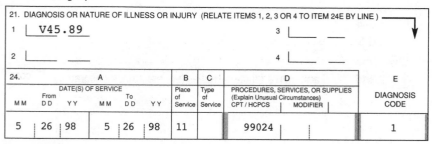

ICD-9-CM

V45.89   Other postsurgical status

CPT

99024   Postoperative follow-up visit, included in global service

For reporting purposes, it is appropriate to identify a postoperative follow-up visit when it is part of the global surgery follow-up period, although many offices do not report this to payors.

OTORHINOLARYNGOLOGY SCENARIO

An ear, nose, and throat (ENT) specialist conducts facial nerve function studies on an established patient who is being examined for facial nerve paralysis. An electroneuronography determines the patient has Bell's palsy. Code the ICD-9-CM diagnosis and CPT procedure.

Otorhinolaryngology

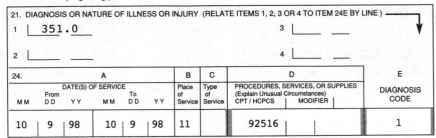

ICD-9-CM

351.0   Bell's palsy

CPT

92516   Facial nerve function studies (eg, electroneuronography)

PEDIATRIC/FAMILY PRACTICE SCENARIO

An 18-month-old established patient returns for follow-up on an acute supporative otitis media with rupture of eardrum after completing course of antibiotics. The acute infection has resolved; however, the perforation has not healed. It is noted that this child is behind on his immunization so, DTaP-HIB, MMR, and oral polio vaccines are given.

21. DIAGNOSIS OR NATURE OF ILLNESS OR INJURY (RELATE ITEMS 1, 2, 3 OR 4 TO ITEM 24E BY LINE)

| 1 | 384.20 | 3 | V06.4 |
| 2 | V06.3 | 4 | V03.81 |

24.	A					B	C	D		E
	DATE(S) OF SERVICE					Place of Service	Type of Service	PROCEDURES, SERVICES, OR SUPPLIES (Explain Unusual Circumstances)		DIAGNOSIS CODE
	From			To				CPT / HCPCS	MODIFIER	
MM	DD	YY	MM	DD	YY					
9	9	98	9	9	98			99213		1
9	9	98	9	9	98			90721		2,4
9	9	98	9	9	98			90707		3
9	9	98	9	9	98			90712		2
9	9	98	9	9	98			90472		2,3,4

ICD-9-CM

384.20   Unspecified perforation of tympanic membrane

V06.3   Need for prophylactic vaccination with diptheria-tetanus-pertussis with poliomyelitis (DTP + polio) vaccine

V06.4   Need for prophylactic vaccination with measles-mumps-rubella (MMR) vaccine

V03.81   Need for prophylatic vaccination against hemophilus influenza type B (Hib)

CPT

99213   Office or other outpatient visit for the evaluation and management of an established patient, which requires at least two of these three key components: an expanded problem focused history; an expanded problem focused examination; medical decision making of low complexity. Counseling and coordination of care with other providers or agencies are provided consistent with the nature of the problem(s) and the patient's and/or family's needs. Usually, the presenting problem(s) are of low to moderate severity. Physicians typically spend 15 minutes face-to-face with the patient and/or family.

90721   Diphtheria, tetanus toxoids, and acellular pertussis vaccine and Hemophilus influenza B vaccine (DtaP-Hib), for intramuscular use

90707   Measles, mumps and rubella virus vaccine (MMR), live, for subcutaneous or jet injection use

90712   Poliovirus vaccine, (any type(s)) (OPV), live, for oral use

90472   Immunization administration (includes percutaneous, intradermal, subcutaneous, intramuscular and jet injections and/or intranasal or oral administration); two or more single or combination vaccines/toxoids

The evaluation and management service should be reported separately.

The vaccine/toxoid products are reported with codes 90476–90749. Administration is reported separately with code 90472 since three single or combination vaccines/toxoids were administered.

RADIOLOGY SCENARIO

A patient is referred to the clinic for numbness and tingling in his arms. The tingling occurs when lying on his back or any time he brings his arms above his head. The radiologist performs a Doppler analog wave form analysis, photoplethysmography and flow velocity signals of the arteries of both arms. A duplex scan of the arteries of both arms is also performed. The impression is thoracic outlet syndrome.

Vascular

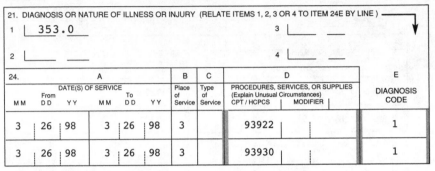

ICD-9-CM

353.0   Brachial plexus lesions

CPT

93922   Non-invasive physiologic studies of upper or lower extremity arteries, single level, bilateral (eg, ankle/brachial indices, Doppler waveform analysis, volume plethysmography, transcutaneous oxygen tension measurement)

93930   Duplex scan of upper extremity arteries or arterial bypass grafts; complete bilateral study

CPT codes for noninvasive physiologic vascular studies (i.e., Doppler) are inclusive. One study or a combination of many studies are reported with only one code that describes the vessel studied. To report unilateral studies, use modifier -52 or 09952 unless a separate code for unilateral study is available. Duplex scans are reported separately.

ONCOLOGY SCENARIO

A patient with advanced gastric cancer receives palliative chemotherapy using Adriamycin. The patient first receives IV infusion of 1000 cc of D-5-W for hydration and Kytril as an antiemetic. Adriamycin is then administered intravenously using push technique.

21. DIAGNOSIS OR NATURE OF ILLNESS OR INJURY (RELATE ITEMS 1, 2, 3 OR 4 TO ITEM 24E BY LINE)				
1 V58.1		3		
2 151.9		4		

24.						A		B	C	D		E
			DATE(S) OF SERVICE					Place of Service	Type of Service	PROCEDURES, SERVICES, OR SUPPLIES (Explain Unusual Circumstances)		DIAGNOSIS CODE
	From			To								
MM	DD	YY	MM	DD	YY					CPT / HCPCS	MODIFIER	
7	25	98	7	25	98					90780		1,2
7	25	98	7	25	98					96408		1,2
7	25	98	7	25	98					J9000		1,2
7	25	98	7	25	98					J7070		1,2
7	25	98	7	25	98					J1626		1,2
7	25	98	7	25	98					A4213		1,2
7	25	98	7	25	98					A4305		1,2
7	25	98	7	25	98					A4215		1,2

ICD-9-CM

V58.1	Encounter for chemotherapy
151.9	Malignant neoplasm stomach, unspecified

CPT

90780	IV infusion for therapy/diagnosis, administered by physician or under direct supervision of physician; up to one hour
96408	Chemotherapy administration, intravenous; push technique
J9000	Doxorubicin HCl, 10 mg (Adriamycin)
J7070	Infusion, D-5-W, 1,000 cc
J1626	Injection, granisetron hydrochloride, 100 mcg (Kytril)
A4213	Syringe, sterile, 20 cc or greater, each
A4305	Disposable drug delivery system, flow rate of 50 ml or greater per hour
A4215	Needles only, sterile, any size, each

Intravenous administration of D-5-W and Kytril (90780) is reported in addition to chemotherapy administration (90408). The code J9000 is used for Adriamycin, PFS, Adriamycin RDG, and Rubex.

Chemotherapy administration includes preparation of chemotherapy agents but does not include the supply of the chemotherapy agents. All other supplies are also reported separately.

If an E/M service is provided on the same day as chemotherapy administration, it should be reported separately.

Advanced Coding Practice

CODING PRACTICE 1

A 34-year old male status post anterior cruciate ligament (ACL) repair is referred to physical therapy for therapeutic exercises. This is the initial visit. The physical therapist does an initial evaluation and provides one-on-one supervision of 30 minutes of therapeutic exercises.

21. DIAGNOSIS OR NATURE OF ILLNESS OR INJURY (RELATE ITEMS 1, 2, 3 OR 4 TO ITEM 24E BY LINE)

1. |___ ___   3. |___ ___

2. |___ ___   4. |___ ___

24.	A						B	C	D		E
	DATE(S) OF SERVICE						Place of Service	Type of Service	PROCEDURES, SERVICES, OR SUPPLIES (Explain Unusual Circumstances)		DIAGNOSIS CODE
	From			To					CPT / HCPCS	MODIFIER	
	MM	DD	YY	MM	DD	YY					

CODING PRACTICE 2

A 57-year-old male admitted from the ER with acute myocardial ischemia without infarction is taken to the special procedure room for cardiac catheterization and possible PTCA. A combined right heart with retrograde left heart catheterization is performed with imaging supervision, interpretation, and report. A selective coronary angiography procedure is performed. There is blockage of the left anterior descending coronary artery. A PTCA is performed on this single vessel. Code the cardiologist's procedures.

21. DIAGNOSIS OR NATURE OF ILLNESS OR INJURY (RELATE ITEMS 1, 2, 3 OR 4 TO ITEM 24E BY LINE)

1 |___ ___   3 |___ ___

2 |___ ___   4 |___ ___

24.	A					B	C	D		E
	DATE(S) OF SERVICE					Place of Service	Type of Service	PROCEDURES, SERVICES, OR SUPPLIES (Explain Unusual Circumstances)		DIAGNOSIS CODE
MM	From DD	YY	MM	To DD	YY			CPT / HCPCS	MODIFIER	

Chapter Review

Among the many diagnostic and therapeutic services included under medicine are immunizations, injections, specialty specific codes, and special services. The medicine section has guidelines clarifying the use of codes in its section and subsections. The majority of codes reported to Medicare and other payors are E/M and medicine codes.

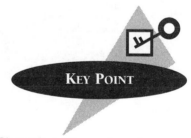

KEY POINT

Diagnostic and therapeutic services include:

• Administration of vaccines/toxoids

• Injections

• Specialty-specific codes

• Special services

9 Inpatient Coding

Introduction

As a text to medical coding, *Code It Right* prepares the student in coding conventions surrounding medical reimbursement for the office and outpatient services. A separate coding world exists for inpatient services, however, and no primer is complete without a review of the complex system underpinning today's government and third party reimbursement to hospitals.

ICD-9-CM Volumes 1 and 2 and their uses in inpatient diagnostic coding are discussed in Chapter 1 of *Code It Right*. Volumes 1 and 2 and Volume 3 — procedures — form the basis of inpatient hospital reimbursement by Medicare and some other payors. CPT codes play only a minor role in hospital reimbursement, ordinarily as a means to report the facility component of outpatient ambulatory surgical services and other outpatient procedures. In addition, some hospitals provide billing services for physician employees (ER physicians, and pathologists), specialty clinics, and centralize the coding and medical records for all of these services in one area of the hospital. In these settings, CPT codes are assigned in the usual manner for the various outpatient services.

Coding accuracy for inpatient services is an important factor in establishing medical necessity for research and statistical data, and for the financial health of the hospital. The coder's role is crucial to the success of the institution and the hospital's reimbursement for its inpatient services.

The inpatient system of reimbursement is fundamentally different from office and outpatient services because diagnoses rather than the procedures are the focus of payment.

However, in this chapter we are focusing on inpatient coding. Because inpatient diagnosis coding was covered by Chapter 1, it will not be presented here. This chapter covers inpatient procedure coding using ICD-9-CM Volume 3, inpatient reimbursement methodologies, and DRG (Diagnosis Related Groups) assignment.

DEFINITION

Inpatient reimbursement is the payment to a hospital for the hospital costs incurred to treat a patient. ICD-9-CM Volumes 1, 2, and 3 form the basis of inpatient hospital reimbursement by Medicare and other payers.

ICD-9-CM Procedure Codes

PRESENTATION
The alphabetic index to procedures is presented first. It is an alphabetical index of procedures and the corresponding codes. The tabular list of procedures is presented second, listing information from the index in numeric order along with other pertinent coding conventions. This logical placement of the alphabetic index allows for quick location of procedural terms for verification in the tabular list.

OBJECTIVES

Learn the steps of coding inpatient services

Recognize Volume 3 coding conventions

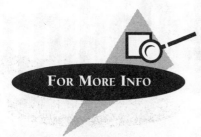

For copies of *Coding Clinic,* contact:

American Hospital Association
One North Franklin
Chicago, IL 60606
(312) 422–3000
1–800–242–2626

For copies of the *Federal Register* contact:

U.S. Government Printing Office
Superintendent of Documents
PO Box 371954
Pittsburgh, PA 15250–7954
http://www.access.gpo.gov/su_docs/

For general information about
GPO Access call:
(202) 512–1530
between 7 a.m. and 5 p.m. Eastern Time

KEY POINTS

Presentation of ICD-9-CM Vol. 3

Index To Procedures (in alphabetical order)

Tabular List of Procedures (in numerical order)

The medical record should contain a complete and thorough account of the following:

- Reason for initial hospitalization
- All diagnoses
- All procedures
- All complications
- Comorbidities (pre-existing conditions)
- Signs and symptoms
- Status upon discharge

CODING SPECIFICITY

In ICD-9-CM Volume 3, the procedures are cataloged in a series of two-digit category codes. For example, all operations on the external ear are found under category 18, and operations on valves and septa of the heart are found under category 35. Knowing the two-digit category is not enough for accurate ICD-9-CM procedure coding because all two-digit codes require further specificity, by the addition of a third-digit subcategory and frequently a fourth digit subclassification.

Third and fourth digits in Volume 3 provide coding specificity by clarifying an anatomical site or kind of procedure (e.g., plastic repair, open or closed procedure). For example, the two-digit code 45 identifies incision, excision, and anastomosis of intestine. Add a third digit 0 after the decimal point (45.0) and an enterotomy is specified. A fourth digit (45.01) identifies a specific site, an incision of the duodenum.

The index of procedures contains many diagnostic descriptors not appearing in the tabular section of Volume 3. Many terms in the index are cross-referenced to different terms that may be used to identify a procedure, such as incision of duodenum, which may be found under *Incision, duodenum* and under *Duodenotomy*. The tabular section main term is only listed under incision of duodenum. Consequently, when assigning diagnostic codes, consult the index first.

Incision	Dwyer operation
Incision — *continued*	**Drawing test** 94.08
bursa — *continued*	**Dressing**
pharynx 29.0	burn 93.57
carotid body 39.8	ulcer 93.56
cerebral (meninges) 01.39	wound 93.57
epidural or extradural space 01.24	**Drilling, bone** (*see also* Incision, bone) 77.10
subarachnoid or subdural space 01.31	**Ductogram, mammary** 87.35
cerebrum 01.39	**Duhamel operation** (abdominoperineal pull-
cervix 69.95	through) 48.65
to	**Dührssen's**
assist delivery 73.93	incisions (cervix, to assist delivery) 73.93
replace inverted uterus 75.93	operation (vaginofixation of uterus) 69.22
chalazion 08.09	**Dunn operation** (triple arthrodesis) 81.12
with removal of capsule 08.21	**Duodenectomy** 45.62
cheek 86.09	with
chest wall (for extrapleural drainage) (for	gastrectomy — *see* Gastrectomy
removal of foreign body) 34.01	pancreatectomy — *see* Pancreatectomy
as operative approach — *omit code*	**Duodenocholedochotomy** 51.51
common bile duct (for exploration) 51.51	**Duodenoduodenostomy** 45.91
for	proximal to distal segment 45.62
relief of obstruction 51.42	**Duodenoileostomy** 45.91
removal of calculus 51.41	**Duodenojejunostomy** 45.91
common wall between posterior left atrium	**Duodenorrhaphy** 46.71
and coronary sinus (with roofing of	**Duodenoscopy** 45.13
resultant defect with patch graft) 35.82	through stoma (artificial) 45.12
conjunctiva 10.1	transabdominal (operative) 45.11
cornea 11.1	**Duodenostomy** 46.39
radial (refractive) 11.75	**Duodenotomy** 45.01
cranial sinus 01.21	**Dupuytren operation**
craniobuccal pouch 07.72	fasciectomy 82.35
cul-de-sac 70.12	fasciotomy 82.12
cyst	with excision 82.35
dentigerous 24.0	shoulder disarticulation 84.08
radicular (apical) (periapical) 24.0	**Duraplasty** 02.12
Dührssen's (cervix, to assist delivery) 73.93	
duodenum 45.01	
ear	

TABULAR LISTINGS

Volume 3's tabular listing classifies groups of procedures by body system and then by miscellaneous diagnostic and therapeutic procedures like x-rays, tests, or monitoring:

Chapter 1	**Operations on the Nervous System (01–05)**
Chapter 2	**Operations on the Endocrine System (06–07)**
Chapter 3	**Operations on the Eye (08–16)**
Chapter 4	**Operations on the Ear (18–20)**
Chapter 5	**Operations on the Nose, Mouth, and Pharynx (21–29)**
Chapter 6	**Operations on the Respiratory System (30–34)**
Chapter 7	**Operations on the Cardiovascular System (35–39)**
Chapter 8	**Operations on the Hemic and Lymphatic System (40–41)**
Chapter 9	**Operations on the Digestive System (42–54)**
Chapter 10	**Operations on the Urinary System (55–59)**

Conventions

Each space, typeface, indention, and punctuation mark determines how to interpret ICD-9-CM Volume 3 codes. These conventions were developed to help match correct codes to the procedures encountered. Many of the coding conventions in Volume 3 are the same as those for diagnosis coding in Volumes 1 and 2. The major difference are the types of notes. These additional types of notes are described here along with a review of the conventions detailed in Chapter 1.

Format

ICD-9-CM has an indented format. Subterms are indented two spaces to the right of the term to which they are linked. Continuations of lines that are too long to fit the column are indented four spaces.

37.74   Insertion or replacement of epicardial lead [electrode] into epicardium

> Insertion or replacement of epicardial lead by:
> sternotomy
> thoracotomy

Type Face

Bold type identifies all codes and main terms in the Tabular List of Volume 3, separating it from subordinate information or notes.

43.9   Total gastrectomy

Punctuation

[ ]   Brackets enclose synonyms, alternative wordings, or explanatory phrases. The brackets may be regular [ ] or italicized *[ ]*.

52.14   Closed [endoscopic] biopsy of pancreatic duct

( )   Parentheses enclose supplementary (nonessential) modifiers that do not affect the code number (even if they are absent). Parentheses also enclose many *see also* references.

71.21   Percutaneous aspiration of Bartholin's gland (cyst)

}   A brace encloses a series of terms modified by the statement appearing to the right of the brace.

04.07   Other excision or avulsion of cranial and peripheral nerves

> Curettage
> Debridement } of peripheral nerve
> Resection

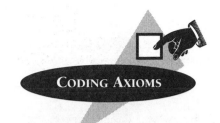

CODING AXIOMS

A two-digit ICD-9-CM procedure code is not acceptable. The coder must code to the third and fourth digits for procedures.

Because the index offers a more diverse list of terms, consult it first when seeking an ICD-9-CM procedure code. Then verify the code in the Volume 3 tabular section.

KEY POINT

HCFA maintains the Volume 3 codes, which include operative, diagnostic, and therapeutic procedures. Annual code revisions reflect the goal of a procedure coding system that can be used with equal efficiency both in hospitals and primary care settings.

Notes

To assign procedure codes at the highest level of specificity, you must follow instructional notes. These include:

Category Notes provide instructions specific to all codes in the category.

The following fourth-digit subclassification is for use with appropriate categories in section 77 to identify the site. Valid fourth digits are in [brackets] under each code:

0	unspecified site
1	scapula, clavicle, and thorax [ribs and sternum]
2	humerus
3	radius and ulna
4	carpals and metacarpals
5	femur
6	patella
7	tibia and fibula
8	tarsals and metatarsals
9	other

These fourth-digit subclassifications are followed by the three-digit codes for category 77.

Includes appears immediately under a three-digit code title to provide further definition or to give an example of the category contents. The word is indented 10 spaces, in plain typeface, and is followed by a colon. The Medicode edition shows includes as: `INCLUDES`

14.2   **Destruction of lesion of retina and choroid**

      `INCLUDES`   destruction of chorioretinopathy or isolated chorioretinal lesion

Excludes indicates terms that are not to be coded under the referenced term. The "Excludes" is surrounded by a box for easy identification and the corresponding note appears in italics. This note does not prevent you from using the excluded code in addition to the code from which it was excluded when both conditions are present. The Medicode hospital edition shows:
`EXCLUDES`

31.42   **Laryngoscopy and other tracheoscopy**

      `EXCLUDES`   *that with biopsy (31.43–31.44)*

Omit code is found only in the Alphabetic index of Volume 3 and is an instruction to omit codes which are considered to be the surgical approach.

    Incision (and drainage)
      abdominal wall 54.0
        as operative approach — *omit code*

Synchronous procedure notes indicate that components of the procedure must be coded separately.

02.02	**Elevation of skull fracture fragments**
	Code also any synchronous debridement of brain (01.59)

Symbols

Medicode's edition of ICD-9-CM Volume 3 is color-coded to indicate the need for additional digits. A red stop sign indicates a code is not as specific as possible and requires a third or fourth digit.

● 77	**Incision, excision, and division of other bones**

ASSIGNING PROCEDURE CODES

The five-step process for assigning procedure codes can be summarized as follows:

Step 1: Determine the Main Terms

Analyze the operative report and procedure statements for those words or main terms that identify the procedure. Think of the main term as a common denominator – a total procedure classification. Once you've located this general term, follow the alphabetical list to the specific condition. Examples of main terms include:

Excision	**Manipulation**
Fixation	**Reduction**
Lysis	**Repair**

Step 2: Look up the Main Term In the Index

Main terms in the index of procedures appear in bold type. Some procedures have more than one listing. If the term describing a condition can be expressed in more than one form, all forms appear in the main entry.

> **Pneumogram, pneumography**

Step 3: Follow Cross-references

Follow cross-references to the alternate term when the procedure is not located under the first term you find. There are three types of cross-references:

See indicates that you should see the procedure listed instead of the term found. You must follow the instruction to assign the correct term.

> **Ankylosis, production of** — *see* **Arthrodesis**

See also indicates that additional information is available. This cross-reference provides an additional procedure and code when the main term or subterm is insufficient, or when there is an alternate term. The additional information helps select the correct code.

> **Closure** — *see also* **repair**

When a single code does not fully describe a given procedure, use multiple codes to identify all components of the procedure. However, the procedure statement must mention the presence of all the elements for each code to be used.

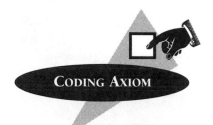

CODING AXIOM

Use multiple codes to identify all components of the procedure when a single code does not fully describe a given procedure.

KEY POINT

Medicode's Volume 3 Icons

● Additional digits required

↗ OR Procedure

▼ Non-OR Procedure

⊘ Noncovered

▢ Nonspecific OR procedure

The five-step process for assigning procedure codes can be summarized as follows.

1. Determine the main terms that describe the procedure performed.

2. Look up the main term in the index of procedures.

3. Follow cross-references, such as see, and see also.

4. Review subterms or modifiers.

5. Verify the code listed in the index to procedures by looking it up in the tabular section of Volume 3 checking all code also, excludes, and other notes.

See category directs you to a category, not just a single code. Again, do not assign an appropriate code unless you follow this instruction.

Apheresis, therapeutic — *see* **category 99.7**

Step 4: Review Subterms or Modifiers

A main term may be followed by one or more subterms that further describe the patient's condition. These supplemental words, called modifiers, may describe the method, type of closure, or synonyms. There are two types of modifiers:

Nonessential Modifiers

These subterms are listed immediately to the right of the main term and are enclosed in parentheses. They serve as examples to help translate written terminology into numeric codes and do not affect the selection of the procedure code.

Amputation (cineplastic) (closed flap) (guillotine)

Essential Modifiers

These subterms are listed below the main terms and are indented two spaces. They are generally presented in alphabetical order, with the exceptions of with and without, which appear before the alphabetized modifiers. Each additional essential modifier clarifies the previous one and is indented two additional spaces to the right. These descriptive terms affect code selection and describe essential differences in site, method, or type of procedure.

Lysis
  adhesions
    bladder (neck) (intraluminal) 57.12
      external 59.11
Ligation
  fallopian tube (bilateral) (remaining) (solitary) 66.39
    by endoscopy (culdoscopy) (hysteroscopy) (laparoscopy) (peritoneoscopy) 66.29
    with
      crushing 66.31
        by endoscopy (laparoscopy) 66.21
      division 66.32
        by endoscopy (culdoscopy) (laparoscopy) (peritoneoscopy) 66.22
      Falope ring 66.39
        by endoscopy (laparoscopy) 66.29

When a main term in the index has only one essential modifier, it appears on the same line as the main term separated by a comma.

Litholapaxy, bladder 57.0

Step 5: Cross-Reference the Index to Procedures in the Tabular Section of Volume 3

The tabular section is the authoritative ICD-9-CM Volume 3 coding reference. It contains procedure codes, full descriptions, additional instructional notes, and examples of terms assigned to each code. These are intended to enhance the verification process and ensure proper code selection. There are times, however, when a descriptive term listed in the index is not found in the tabular section. In these instances, trust the index as the most often updated and use the number listed there.

DISCUSSION QUESTIONS

1. What is the first step to inpatient coding?

   _____

   _____

   _____

2. What should you consult first when assigning a procedure code?

   _____

   _____

   _____

3. What should be listed when a single code does not fully describe a given procedure?

   _____

   _____

   _____

Clinical Applications of Coding Rules

The rules for procedure coding must be applied to a broad variety of procedures. Just as the medical record tells a written story of procedures that occurred during the hospitalization of the patient, the numerical codes assigned by the medical coder must tell the same story in code. The most important factor in ICD-9-CM procedure coding is understanding the rules. Knowing how to correctly sequence and report procedures must be the goal for all coders. The entire record of the current admission must be reviewed before selecting a principal procedure.

Volume 3 procedures have a hierarchical order. The hierarchy is dependent on a classification assigned to a procedure and is demonstrated in the surgical partitioning of a MDC. They are:

- Surgery
- Procedural risk
- Anesthesia risk
- Non-significant procedures

PRINCIPAL PROCEDURE

The principal procedure is the procedure that is performed for definitive treatment, not for diagnostic or exploratory purposes or necessary in treating a complication. If two procedures may be the principal procedure, then the one most closely related to the principal diagnosis should be designated as the principal procedure.

When a definitive procedure and a diagnostic procedure, both related to the principal diagnosis, are performed, the definitive procedure is sequenced as the principal procedure regardless of the order in which the procedures were performed or listed in the medical record.

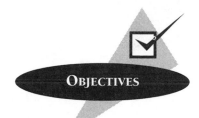

OBJECTIVES

Define the term principal procedure

Master the order of coding for DRGs

Distinguish the differences in using hard copy or software products for DRG assignment

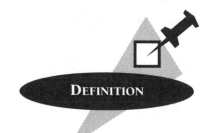

DEFINITION

Principal procedure is the procedure performed for definitive treatment rather than one performed for diagnostic or exploratory purposes, or necessary to take care of a complication. If there appear to be two procedures that are principal procedures, then the one most related to the principal diagnosis should be considered the principal procedure.

When a definitive, or therapeutic procedure was not performed for the principal diagnosis but was performed for a complication code, the principal procedure is the one performed for the complication.

Principal procedures are usually performed in an operating room.

When a definitive operating room procedure is not performed, but a therapeutic procedure is, the therapeutic procedure is listed as the principal procedure.

Diagnostic procedures are sequenced as the principal procedure only when no definitive or therapeutic procedure has been performed.

Secondary procedures that are performed after the assignment of the principal procedure should be sequenced as follows:

- Other definitive procedures, related or unrelated to the principal diagnosis, matching complications and secondary diagnoses codes when applicable
- Therapeutic procedures
- Diagnostic procedures
- Other procedures, such as tests, measurements, or procedures that may be part of another procedure are usually not coded for hospital inpatients (However, the facility may require coding of additional services for statistics, research, grants, or studies. Request a list from the facility for any other procedures that must be coded and reported.)

All significant procedures should be coded. Significant procedures are those that carry an operative or anesthetic risk or require specially trained personnel or equipment.

DEFINITIONS

There are three types of inpatient reimbursement methodologies:

Fee-for-Service is when the payor reimburses the full charge for medical services.

Per Diem refers to reimbursement based on a set rate per day rather than on a charge-by-charge basis.

Prospective Payment System depends on historical data of case mix and regional differences, such as diagnosis related groups (DRGs).

Inpatient Reimbursement Methodologies

There are three basic inpatient reimbursement methodologies, although many variations exist within these three broad categories. One method is to reimburse based on cost or billed charges. The second is to reimburse a fixed amount per day, also called a per diem reimbursement. The third method is the prospective payment system (PPS).

Fee-For-Service/Cost/Billed Charge Reimbursement
Fee-for-service, also referred to as cost or billed charge, reimbursement is based on the actual expenses a hospital incurs for a specific patient during a single admission plus an added amount to cover administrative costs and provide a profit. Under this method of reimbursement, all costs for documented services are covered including: room, meals, nursing care, procedures, pharmaceuticals, supplies, etc. However, given that all billed charges are allowed or covered, hospitals have little incentive to contain costs.

Per Diem Reimbursement
A per diem reimbursement is a fixed amount paid per day for hospital care. Usually payors allow varying per diem amounts based on type of service. For example, an intensive care bed day would be paid at a higher rate than a medical/surgical bed day or a newborn bed day. This method of reimbursement does not provide for a fixed rate for each admission. It does provide hospitals with an incentive to provide cost effective care by limiting the amount paid for each day of service.

Prospective Payment System (PPS)

Under a prospective payment system (PPS), the amount paid for services is set in advance. Prospective payment was not a new concept for payors when it was introduced as a method for reimbursing inpatient services. Payors had applied this methodology to reimbursement of physician services for some time by setting maximum allowables for various services, including: office visits, surgical procedures and maternity care. In other words, the insurance companies set in advance the amount they would pay for a given physician service.

In order to develop a prospective payment system for inpatient services, a method of categorizing inpatient services needed to be developed. This was accomplished by the system of diagnosis related groups (DRGs) as described in the next section. DRGs categorize the patient by type of case (a case being defined as a single admission for a single patient). Cases with similar characteristics were grouped together and a fixed reimbursement amount was calculated for each type of case.

The goal behind developing a prospective payment system was to contain the ever-increasing cost of healthcare. By setting a fixed predetermined payment rate for each type of case, payors felt they would be better able to control healthcare costs.

DRGs

The prospective payment system for inpatient services used today by the federal government (Medicare) and many other third-party payors is called the DRG system.

Diagnosis related groups (DRGs) provide the basis for payment to hospitals for Medicare, Medicaid, and an increasing number of commercially insured patients. The federal government adopted DRGs more than a decade ago to curb rising hospital costs associated with reasonable cost and line-item reimbursement methods. Through DRGs, hospitals are reimbursed a flat-rate based on a patient's diagnosis and treatment. Assuming patients with similar illnesses undergoing similar procedures will require similar care, each category of illness/treatment is assigned a DRG that is the main factor in determining reimbursement.

Before DRGs, hospitals were paid based upon itemized services following treatment and release. The payor and provider tallied the costs in retrospect — after the care was provided. Because DRG payments are standardized by diagnosis and treatment, DRGs allow payors and providers to predict reimbursement prospectively — before the care is provided. This type of reimbursement is called a prospective payment system (PPS). Hospitals still itemize bills for their patients, but today, reimbursement now falls largely under the umbrella of the DRG assignment.

Personnel in medical records departments now influence the financial health of hospitals, as DRGs are based upon the ICD-9-CM codes assigned to diagnoses and procedures. Documentation is crucial. Hospital executives closely evaluate case mix — the clientele the hospital serves — since the nature and severity of overall patient illnesses play heavily in budget projections.

EVOLUTION OF DRGs

The implementation of a DRG-based payment system was prompted by Medicare administrators, who in the 1960s identified significant differences among hospitals in the costs incurred to care for patients. Intuitively, administrators knew that the more complex a hospital's patient mix, the higher its cost of doing business. For example, tertiary care facilities and teaching hospitals tend

OBJECTIVE

Understand the evolution of DRGs and MDCs

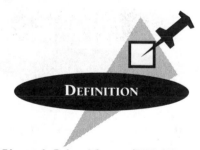

DEFINITION

Diagnosis Related Groups (DRGs) The basis of inpatient reimbursement is DRGs, a complex scheme of over 500 patient mix classifications. The philosophy behind DRGs is that payment to inpatient facilities should accurately correlate the patient case mix to the resources the patients consume. See *Code It Right*'s appendix for a list of DRGs.

Clinical Data Abstraction Centers (CDACs) perform DRG validation of the correct use of ICD-9-CM codes. CDACs collect data from a nationwide random sampling of 30,000 claims. They evaluate the data and send their findings to each state's **Professional Review Organization (PRO)**. The PRO evaluates the data and identifies those hospitals and other parties in their state that may have areas of coding problems. The PRO works with the hospital on a local program or cooperative project to make improvements in the area(s) identified. The projects can be made up of multiple parties working together as an opportunity for improvement. This program can be hospital-initiated as well – the hospital can go to the PRO and ask for help.

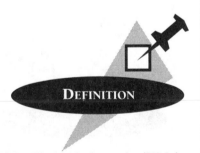

Major Diagnostic Categories (MDCs)
The original DRGs developed at Yale were begun by dividing all possible principal diagnoses into mutually exclusive categories, referred to as Major Diagnostic Categories (MDCs). These broad classifications of diagnoses are typically grouped by body system. (See *Code It Right's* appendix for a list of MDCs).

to admit patients referred from other facilities. Although these "sicker" patients clearly contributed to higher costs, there was no established method to define the case mix and its exact association with the higher costs. For this reason, a means to closely define and measure hospital's patient case mix was undertaken.

Case Mix Complexity
Researchers at Yale University developed the early application of the ICD-9-CM version of DRGs on the concept of patient case mix complexity. The researchers identified patient attributes that contributed most to resource demands. Key among them were the following:

- Severity of illness
- Prognosis
- Treatment difficulty
- Need for intervention
- Resource intensity

Patient Classifications
The next step was to classify patients based on information routinely collected in hospital medical records to identify a manageable number of patient groups that shared demographic, diagnostic, and therapeutic attributes. In short, the goal was to identify classes of clinically similar patients who consume hospital resources in a similar fashion.

Major Diagnostic Categories (MDCs)
The original DRGs developed at Yale divided all possible principal diagnoses into mutually exclusive categories, referred to as major diagnostic categories (MDCs). These broad classifications of diagnoses are typically grouped by body system. See *Code It Right's* appendix for a list of MDCs.

Surgical and Nonsurgical
Once the MDCs were defined, each category was further evaluated to identify additional patient characteristics that might affect consumption of hospital resources. The principal deciding factor was whether the patient was treated in an operating room (OR). The performance of OR procedures requires a host of inpatient resources such as anesthesia services, the recovery room, and the operating suite itself. A distinction was then made which allowed the MDCs to be further separated into categories of medical or surgical cases.

The picture that began to emerge for the Yale researchers was a decision-making tree for DRG assignment. Once a surgical category had been established for a patient, further specification was based on the type of procedure performed — the surgical hierarchy. Medical patients were further defined according to principal diagnosis when admitted to the hospital. Both the medical and surgical classes within an MDC are organized by principles of anatomy, surgical approach, diagnostic approach, pathology, etiology, or treatment process.(See *Code It Right's* appendix for an example of Major Diagnostic Category 6 Diseases and Disorders of The Digestive System, Surgical and Medical partitioning.)

Complications and Comorbidities (CCs)
The medical and surgical classes were further tested to determine whether complications or comorbidities (CCs) would affect consumption of hospital resources. For example, patients admitted for congestive heart failure may exhibit numerous CCs, such as kidney failure or urinary retention, which affect their length of stay in the hospital as well as their use of other services. A

comprehensive list of diagnoses generally considered a CC was generated. It soon became apparent, however, that the validity of CCs is dependent upon the principal diagnosis. Over time, government and private parties developed a list of CC exclusions for inappropriate associations with the principal diagnoses.

Other Variables
A patient's age was determined to be a defining factor in DRG assignment. Pediatric patients and patients over 70 were often assigned a DRG that evaluated age. The patient's status upon discharge from the hospital was also considered a variable in the definition of a DRG. Burn patients transferred to another facility, for example, were designated a separate DRG. Similarly, separate DRGs were designated for patients who leave the hospital against medical advice.

Following extensive testing, the DRG system was launched nationwide in 1983 with implementation of the Medicare prospective payment system. HCFA became the lead agency for the maintenance and modification of DRGs, as it is for maintenance and modification of ICD-9-CM, Volume 3.

ALL PATIENT DRGs
Senior populations covered by Medicare were the focus of the original DRG design. In response to interest from a healthcare industry serving a broader clientele, revisions were made to the system, now referred to as All-Patient DRGs (AP-DRGs). Early features of AP-DRGs included MDC 24, specifically devoted to the human immunodeficiency virus (HIV), as well as the restructuring of the MDC governing newborns. The CCs exclusion methodology was further refined. There are currently 25 MDCS and four pre-MDCs.

DRGs continue to evolve to better reflect patient profiles and to accommodate annual code changes in ICD-9-CM. DRG updates become effective in January of each year and publication of proposed and final changes appear regularly in the AHA's *Coding Clinic* as well as in the *Federal Register*.

Refinements that would further divide DRGs by degrees of severity are being considered by HCFA. In one system being considered, the current 511 AP-DRGs would be expanded to 652 All Patient Refined (APR)-DRGs. Under this restructuring, some DRGS would be shifted to other MDCs. New MDCs would be added. CCs would be divided into levels of severity: CC and MCC, for major complication or comorbidity. These changes, which represent a hybrid of several methodologies developed nationally, are still being evaluated.

ICD-10
While plans are made to launch a new system of expanded DRGs, other changes in current coding systems could require a complete overhaul of the DRG system within a few years. HCFA intends to implement ICD-10-CM, a new alphanumeric coding system for diseases and procedures in October 2001. ICD-10 is being clinically modified by the National Center for Healthcare Statistics (NCHS), and the procedural part of ICD-10, administered by HCFA, is currently being tested at sites across the United States.

Since DRGs are all based on ICD-9-CM codes, the change to ICD-10-CM would greatly affect DRG decision trees and assignments. The same issues of mapping will be at work when ICD-10-CM is adopted. Once HCFA formally presents the proposed DRG and ICD-10 changes, the hospital industry can begin to analyze the effects these changes will have on their businesses.

AP-DRGs: All Patient Diagnosis Related Groups were developed in response to interest from the healthcare industry serving a broader clientele than the senior populations covered by Medicare. The federal program was the focus of the original DRG design.

Under Medicare PPS, any revision of the DRG system must redistribute reimbursement among hospitals according to the case mix, but may not increase or decrease aggregate Medicare payments to hospitals. Individual hospitals, however, could see significant changes in reimbursement under the new DRGs depending on their case mix.

Additionally, private payors may lag behind Medicare in any adoption of a new DRG system. Since these new designations would likely be assigned three-digit numbers, hospital information systems will be challenged to differentiate between new and old DRGs if both systems are used concurrently. The ability to map from the old system to the new one would also be critical for utilization, finances, quality assurance, and case-mix study.

DISCUSSION QUESTIONS

1. Explain the basis of inpatient hospital reimbursement by Medicare and some other payors.

    _____

    _____

    _____

2. What are DRGs and MDCs and how are they used?

    _____

    _____

    _____

3. How do other variables such as surgical or nonsurgical, complications and comorbidities, or age, affect DRG assignment?

    _____

    _____

    _____

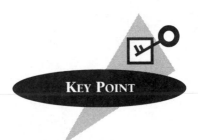

KEY POINT

Hospital Payment
When inpatient claims are paid by DRG reimbursement method, reimbursement is based upon an average for all cases that are alike in most respects. This means that for one case the hospital may lose money, but for another that is similar the hospital may make money. This payment method also means that no matter how many resources are used, only one dollar amount will be paid. Even if the case is over the length of stay or is a cost outlier, the hospital receives very little additional reimbursement. In any case the hospital never receives what would be considered a fee-for-service reimbursement under a DRG reimbursement scheme.

Coding for DRGs

Using a Hard Copy to Assign a DRG
In practice, most inpatient coders rarely consult hard copy references, relying instead on centralized computer systems and coding software. Both approaches are similar, however. Lookups are approached either by diagnosis or procedure and are cross-checked. Code all diagnoses sequencing them by:

STEP 1
Principal diagnosis, and all secondary diagnoses, complications, or comorbidities sequenced after the principal diagnosis.

STEP 2
Code all significant procedures following sequencing rules. The coding reference, whether hard copy or electronic, will probably feature some level of support material to steer the user toward the most specific code selection. Medicode's edition of Volume 1 (tabular) references features an indicator for codes that affect DRG assignment, acceptable or non-acceptable principal diagnosis, and CCs.

STEP 3

Determine whether a valid OR procedure was performed. Volume 3 tabular references usually feature an indicator for codes that affect DRG assignments by identifying OR or non-OR procedures.

STEP 4

Looking at the principal diagnosis code, the coder assigns the correct MDC. Reference sources list the MDC to which a principal diagnosis is assigned. One reference is *Medicode's DRG Guide*.

STEP 5

The coder determines, based on procedures performed or not performed, whether to follow the medical or surgical partitioning of the MDCs. Reference sources list procedures that will affect a DRG in a given MDC. These are printed copies of MDCs with the decision trees for ultimate assignment of a DRG. See *Code It Right's* appendix for an example of an MDC with partitioning for a DRG assignment.

1. Medical Partition

   If no procedures were performed and the medical partitioning is followed, the coder will follow the logic through the tree, taking age, secondary codes for any comorbidities and complications, and discharge status into consideration and apply them to the medical MDC. Some medical trees are straightforward and do not consider age, CCs, or other factors in the assignment of a DRG. After the logic has been followed, the tree will end in the DRG applicable to the case coded.

2. Surgical Partition

   If an invalid OR procedure was performed that will affect the DRG, then the surgical partitioning of the MDC is followed.

   a. The coder will follow the logic through the surgical partitioning of the tree, taking age, secondary codes that apply to any comorbidities and complications, procedures, and classification of procedures, and discharge status into consideration, if applicable to the particular surgical MDC.

   b. After the logic has been followed, the tree will end in the DRG that applies to the case that has been coded.

Using Software to Assign a DRG

Software products called encoders are available to help assign a DRG. Encoders lead coders through a series of questions to ultimately assign diagnoses and procedures codes. However, the coder still must go through the medical record and determine the principal diagnosis and the secondary diagnoses. The coder must take into account complications and comorbidities, the principal procedure, and any applicable secondary procedures.

The encoder then uses the information the coder provides and translates it into codes and corresponding code descriptions. The encoder then (unseen by the coder) assigns an MDC, the medical or surgical partitioning, and follows the tree through the decision-making process based on information the coder entered into the product, (e.g., age) and assigns a DRG. The encoder is faster at following the same steps as the coder would if performing a hard copy assignment of the DRG.

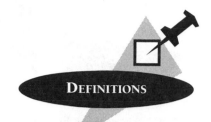

DEFINITIONS

An **encoder** is a software product that helps assign a DRG. Encoders lead coders through a series of questions to ultimately assign diagnoses and procedure codes. However, the coder still must go through the medical record and determine the principal and secondary diagnosis.

GMLOS: geometric mean length of stay

AMLOS: arithmetic mean length of stay

OT: outlier threshold

RW: a comparative assigned weight to indicate relative resource consumption associated with a given DRG

DRG: diagnosis related group

MDC: major diagnostic category

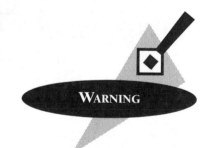

WARNING

Software products are more accurate in assigning DRGs than manual assignments of a DRG. However, if the software product is flawed or an update to the software is incorrect, the coder is still responsible for assigning the correct DRG. This means the coder must know whether the software has produced the correct DRG.

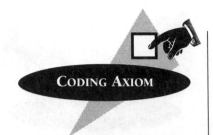

There are two hospital units that are exempt from DRGs: rehabilitation and psychiatric units.

The encoder provides the DRG assignment, MDC, principal diagnosis, and secondary diagnosis. Any CCs and principal and secondary procedures are listed in sequence with their corresponding code descriptions.

The encoder allows the coder to switch the diagnoses and procedures. This feature shows the coder how a change made to the code sequencing would affect the DRG assignment. This may be necessary if the coder entered the incorrect principals, for example. However, the code sequence should not be changed to optimize the DRG value. The code sequence may be changed when two diagnoses or procedures of equal weight have been performed, in which case it is legitimate to use the code which will produce the greatest revenue to the facility.

Typically, the DRG is presented along with its geometric mean length of stay (GMLOS), arithmetic mean length of stay (AMLOS), relative weight (RW) and its outlier threshold (OT). These components figure in the reimbursement calculation for that particular DRG. The length of stay is averaged for the given DRG and the GMLOS and is weighted to allow for outliers and other factors that skew data. The RW is a comparative assigned weight to indicate relative resource consumption associated with the given DRG. The higher the relative weight, the greater the reimbursement. The relative weight multiplied by a regional conversion factor produces the dollar amount that will be paid to the facility. Factors that can influence the DRG are length of stay, cost outliers, and transfer of the patient. There are also two hospital units that are exempt from DRGs: the rehabilitation and psychiatric units. Teaching facilities receive a payment above those paid to other facilities; however, the amount of payment is not dependent on the DRG weight. These factors, and proposed adjustments to them, are published in the *Federal Register* and in the AHA *Coding Clinic*.

DISCUSSION QUESTIONS

1. Explain how to sequence diagnoses correctly.

   _____

   _____

   _____

2. MDCs were developed prior to DRGs. What is the major distinguishing point between the two classifications?

   _____

   _____

   _____

3. Describe the three basic methodologies of inpatient reimbursement.

   _____

   _____

   _____

4. Highlight the differences in using hard copy or software for DRG assignment.

   _____

   _____

   _____

5. What sources should your office have on hand to determine appropriate DRG assignment?

_____

_____

_____

OBJECTIVES

See the application of ICD-9-CM procedural coding logic

Identify the special circumstances and rules of specialties

Specialty-Specific Scenarios

The following scenarios are designed by specialty to help you make the leap from documentation to correct code choices.

UROLOGY SPECIALTY SCENARIO — INPATIENT

A 68-year-old Medicare patient is admitted to the hospital for surgery for urinary stress incontinence. Her physician performs the admission history and physical and lists the diagnoses:

> **Urinary stress incontinence**
> **Benign essential hypertension**

The patient is taken to surgery the day after admission. A Marshall-Marchetti-Krantz is performed. No complications are noted in the operative report. The patient is discharged on post-op day three. Code the ICD-9-CM diagnoses and procedures.

ICD-9-CM diagnosis
625.6	**Stress incontinence, female**
401.1	**Benign essential hypertension**

ICD-9-CM procedure
59.5	**Retropubic urethral suspension**

In ICD-9-CM Volume 3, a Marshall-Marchetti-Krantz procedure may be found under:

> **Marshall-Marchetti (-Krantz)** operation 59.5
> **Operation**
>   Marshall-Marchetti (-Krantz) (retropubic urethral suspension) 59.5
> **Repair**
>   stress incontinence (urinary) NEC
>   by
>   retropubic urethral suspension 59.5
> **Suspension**
>   urethrovesical
>   Marshall-Marchetti (-Krantz) 59.5

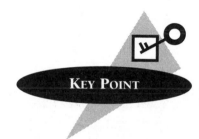

KEY POINT

The move from documentation to correct code choices involves researching the ways a procedure may be defined, the type of procedure, how it is performed, and the anatomy involved.

Not all procedures are as easily accessed in ICD-9-CM Volume 3. The key is researching the ways a procedure may be defined, the type of procedure, how it is performed, and the anatomy involved. The above example has more than one listing in the index. The procedure is listed as an eponym (originator's name), operation, repair, and suspension. The procedure is also a retropubic urethral or urethrovesical suspension. Always look under related terms.

This case would be followed through the surgical partitioning of the applicable MDC.

RECONSTRUCTIVE SURGERY SCENARIO

A 27-year-old male incurs serious injuries while operating machinery at his farm. A reconstructive surgeon admits the patient to the hospital and reimplants his right foot after the traumatic complete amputation. He repairs a complicated open wound of the right thigh requiring extensive debridement and fat, fascia, and skin grafting. The patient is discharged on hospital day seven. Code the ICD-9-CM diagnoses and procedures.

ICD-9-CM diagnoses

896.1	**Unilateral, complicated traumatic amputation of foot (complete) (partial)**
890.1	**Open wound of hip and thigh, complicated**
E919.0	**Agricultural machines**
E849.1	**Farm**

ICD-9-CM procedure

84.26	**Foot reattachment**
86.22	**Excisional debridement of wound, infection, or burn**
83.82	**Graft of muscle or fascia**
86.63	**Full-thickness skin graft to other sites**

Procedures in the index and tabular sections of Volume 3 may be general or specific. Repairs are coded by type. Although specific codes exist for plastic operation on hand with graft of muscle or fascia (82.72) and full-thickness skin graft to hand (86.61), there is only a general listing for grafts to the leg or thigh.

The index lists:

Graft
    fat pad (NEC)
        with skin graft — *see* Graft, skin, full-thickness

This information verifies that a fat pad is included when coding a full-thickness skin graft. The information is not repeated in the tabular section under the code number and description.

Be sure to check code exclusions to make sure the procedures may be reported or are reported with separate codes.

This case would be followed through the surgical partitioning of the applicable MDC.

ORTHOPEDIC SURGERY SCENARIO

A 70-year-old patient is admitted to the hospital three weeks status post total hip arthroplasty for removal of an infected right total hip prosthesis. The surgery is performed and a culture of the femoral and acetabular components of the hip prosthesis shows an infection by staphylococcus aureus. The patient is treated for the infection in the hospital with IV antibiotics. He is discharged on postoperative day seven to a skilled nursing facility for further care and antibiotic therapy. Code the ICD-9-CM diagnoses and procedure code.

ICD-9-CM diagnoses

996.66	**Infection and inflammatory reaction due to internal joint prosthesis**
041.11	**Staphylococcus aureus**

ICD-9-CM procedure
    80.05   **Arthrotomy for removal of prosthesis, hip**

Note that the procedural fourth digit specifies the prosthesis was removed from the hip. Always code to the highest level of specificity.

A complication code is used as the principal diagnosis since the complication was the reason for the admission (i.e., the infection was due to the hip prosthesis). Information regarding the type of infection is important for tracking nosocomial infections (an infection acquired in the hospital) for quality assurance.

The discharge status of the patient is reported for each hospital stay. Patients discharged to another facility, especially another acute care facility, may prompt a split in DRG payment.

The case would be followed through the surgical partitioning of the applicable MDC.

MEDICAL SPECIALTIES CARDIOLOGY SCENARIO

A 65-year-old male with a history of angina asks to be worked into the office schedule of his cardiologist, due to tightness in his chest and night sweats. The physician reviews past medical history which is significant for a myocardial infarction (MI) four years ago. An extended examination of head, heart, lungs, and abdomen is obtained. As a part of the exam in the office, the physician provides a 12-lead ECG and pulsed wave Doppler echocardiography with color flow mapping. The patient is diagnosed as having acute unstable angina with an impending MI, coronary atherosclerosis, benign essential hypertension, and a personal history of an MI. The patient is immediately admitted to the cardiac care unit of the local hospital at 6 p.m. On the day after his admission he is scheduled to go to the heart catheter lab for percutaneous transluminal coronary angioplasty (PTCA), but he has a massive myocardial infarct of the anterior wall. Although the patient is initially stabilized within an hour of the infarction, he goes into ventricular fibrillation. The patient is defibrillated but a cardiac arrest ensues. Cardiopulmonary resuscitation is attempted for 30 minutes by the physician and the resuscitation team, but cardiac death occurs at 7 a.m. Code the ICD-9-CM diagnosis and procedure codes.

ICD-9-CM diagnosis
411.1	**Intermediate coronary syndrome**
410.11	**Acute myocardial infarction of other anterior wall, initial care episode**
427.41	**Ventricular fibrillation**
427.5	**Cardiac arrest**
414.01	**Coronary atherosclerosis of native coronary artery**
412	**Old myocardial infarction**
401.1	**Benign essential hypertension**

ICD-9-CM procedure
99.60	**Cardiopulmonary resuscitation**
99.62	**Other electric countershock of heart**

DEFINITIONS

Principal diagnosis: main reason the patient was admitted to the hospital, after study.

Principal procedure: the procedure that is performed for definitive treatment not for diagnostic or exploratory purposes, or was necessary in treating a complication; the one that is most closely related to the principal diagnosis.

Complication: a condition that arose during hospitalization that will prolong the length of the hospital stay by at least one day in 75 percent of the cases.

Cardiac death is not separately reported since it codes to the heart disease (e.g., coronary atherosclerosis). The Volume 2 index specifies:

Death
cardiac — *see* Disease, heart

Disease
heart
artery — *see* Arteriosclerosis, coronary

Arteriosclerosis, arteriosclerotic (artery)
coronary (artery) 414.00
native (artery) 414.01

The facility determines which nonoperating room procedures are coded.

This case would be followed through the medical partitioning of the applicable MDC.

GENERAL SURGERY SCENARIO

An 80-year-old woman with an acute bowel obstruction is taken to the OR where her surgeon resects two feet of necrotic proximal jejunum. Before the physician can reconnect the bowel, the patient becomes hemodynamically unstable due to heart failure and the case is terminated. The duodenum is closed with bowel clips and the patient is taken to the ICU. After 24 hours of aggressive medical management, she is stable and taken back to the OR for completion of the procedure. Code the ICD-9-CM diagnoses and procedure codes for the two separate dates.

ICD-9-CM diagnoses
1st surgery

560.2	**Intestinal obstruction without mention of hernia, volvulus**
997.1	**Cardiac complications, during or resulting from a procedure**
V64.1	**Surgical or other procedure not carried out because of contraindication**

2nd surgery

863.39	**Other injury to small intestine with open wound into cavity**
428.0	**Congestive heart failure**

Code sequence

560.2	**Intestinal obstruction without mention of hernia, volvulus**
997.1	**Cardiac complications, during or resulting from a procedure**
428.0	**Congestive heart failure**
863.39	**Other injury to small intestine with open wound into cavity**
V64.1	**Surgical or other procedure not carried out because of contraindication**

ICD-9-CM procedure
1st surgery

45.62	**Other partial resection of small intestine**

2nd surgery

45.91	**Small-to-small intestinal anastomosis**

The principal diagnosis is an intestinal obstruction, which is sequenced first. The cardiac complication is sequenced second. The congestive heart failure is sequenced third because it is also a complication. The open wound code is sequenced fourth because hospital resources were used for treatment. The V code indicating the surgery or procedure was not carried out due to contraindication is sequenced last.

The principal procedure is the resection of the small intestine and is the first procedure sequenced. The anastomosis is coded as the second procedure. Guidelines under intestinal anastomosis specify to code also any synchronous resection (45.31–45.8, 48.41–48.69). However, in this case, the resection was performed during the previous surgical session and therefore would not be reported a second time. In addition, end-to-end anastomosis is excluded. In this case, the anastomosis is reported additionally because it was performed during a separate surgical session. The diagnosis codes indicate the circumstances of the second procedure consuming additional hospital operating room resources.

The diagnosis and procedure codes in this scenario lead the coder to:

MDC 6
Diseases and Disorders of the Digestive System (DRGs 146–167, 170–184, 188–190)

Surgical DRG 148
Major Small and Large Bowel Procedures with CC

HEAD AND NECK SURGERY SCENARIO
A patient with a biopsy-proven primary malignant neoplasm (intrinsic) of the larynx is admitted to the hospital. Her medical record states she uses tobacco; smoking one and a half packs of cigarettes per day for 30 years, and has chronic obstructive bronchitis. The day after the admission she is taken to the operating room where a laryngotomy (laryngofissure) is performed. It is mentioned in the operative report that the patient had an intraoperative hemorrhage with a blood loss of 1200 cc and two units of packed red blood cells were given. Code the ICD-9-CM diagnosis and procedure codes.

ICD-9-CM diagnoses
- **161.0** **Malignant neoplasm of glottis**
- **998.1** **Hemorrhage or hematoma complicating a procedure**
- **491.20** **Obstructive chronic bronchitis, without mention of acute exacerbation**
- **305.1** **Tobacco use disorder**

ICD-9-CM procedure
- **30.29** **Other partial laryngectomy**

Sequencing of codes are as listed above. The proper code for a partial laryngotomy (laryngofissure) is not listed under partial or laryngotomy. It can be found under:

Laryngofissure 30.29
Laryngectomy

partial (frontolateral) (glottosupraglottic) (lateral) (submucous) (supraglottic) (vertical) 30.29

The patient's smoking history should be coded as listed in the medical record.

This case would be followed through the surgical partitioning of the applicable MDC.

PATHOLOGY SPECIALTY SCENARIO

A specimen is submitted to the hospital pathology department from the operating room for gross and microscopic examination. The specimen is labeled larynx, partial. The pathologist examines the specimen and the final diagnosis is secondary malignant neoplasm of the larynx, primary site not identified. Code the ICD-9-CM diagnoses and procedure code(s).

ICD-9-CM diagnoses
197.3	**Other respiratory organs, secondary malignant neoplasm**
199.1	**Other, malignant neoplasm without specification of site**

ICD-9-CM procedure
90.39	**Microscopic examination of specimen from ear, nose, throat, and larynx, other microscopic examination**

Occasionally, a primary malignancy site cannot be identified, and the pathologist can find only a secondary malignancy site. The primary malignancy code is in the neoplasm table listed under unknown.

The secondary malignant neoplasm is sequenced first since it is the reason the patient was admitted to the hospital, (e.g., for excision of the malignant neoplasm of the larynx).

Frequently, procedures that are not performed in the operating room are not coded for inpatient stays. The facility decides which non-operating room procedures will be coded as determined by ongoing studies and statistical gathering information needed by the hospital. The pathology report is an important part of the total inpatient hospitalization and should be used as the definitive document for coding the nature of tumor (e.g., malignant, benign), and whether it is primary, secondary, etc.

Gross examination is not listed in Volume 3 of ICD-9-CM.

This case would be recorded using all the information in the medical record and would be followed through the surgical partitioning of the applicable MDC.

RADIOLOGY SPECIALTY SCENARIO

A physician requests an anterior, posterior, and lateral chest x-ray as part of an admission workup on a patient. The patient is admitted to the hospital through the ED for congestive heart failure. The radiologist's interpretation of the x-ray states congestive heart failure (CHF), right lower lobe pneumonia, r/o bacterial cause. Code the ICD-9-CM diagnoses and procedure code(s).

ICD-9-CM diagnoses
428.0	**Congestive heart failure**
482.9	**Bacterial pneumonia unspecified**

ICD-9-CM procedure
87.49	**Other chest x-ray**

The chest x-ray is a diagnostic tool used in an inpatient hospital setting. A chest x-ray may not be coded for inpatients, but the information in the interpretation and report clarifies the story of the patient's hospitalization. Diagnoses found on x-rays are coded when identified by the attending physician as a diagnosis, especially if the condition was treated. If the attending physician does not mention a diagnosis that appears on an x-ray or other report and the coder feels it may be a significant finding, it is appropriate to ask the physician whether it should be included. If the physician agrees, the coder should write an addendum in the medical record. The coder should use all of the doucumentation for a hospital stay to make the correct coding decisions.

This case would be recorded using all the information in the medical record. If an operating procedure was not ultimately performed, the coding would be followed through the medical partitioning of the applicable MDC.

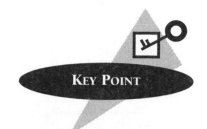

Advanced Coding Practice

CODING PRACTICE 1

A 42-year-old woman with a long history of back pain treated conservatively is admitted to the hospital for surgery of herniated lumbar disks because of progressive radiculopathy of the right leg. An MRI obtained one week prior to admission had demonstrated herniation at the L4-5 and L5-S1 interspaces. A hemilaminectomy with decompression of nerve root(s), including excision of herniated disks is performed at each level. A posterior interbody arthrodesis is performed at each level. Morselized bone obtained from the iliac crest is grafted into the surgical site. Code ICD-9-CM diagnosis and procedure codes for this inpatient hospitalization.

21. DIAGNOSIS OR NATURE OF ILLNESS OR INJURY (RELATE ITEMS 1, 2, 3 OR 4 TO ITEM 24E BY LINE)
1
2
3
4

24.	A DATE(S) OF SERVICE						B Place of Service	C Type of Service	D PROCEDURES, SERVICES, OR SUPPLIES (Explain Unusual Circumstances) CPT / HCPCS | MODIFIER	E DIAGNOSIS CODE
	From MM | DD | YY			To MM | DD | YY						

CODING PRACTICE 2

A 77 year old male was admitted for evaluation of a syncopal episode. On admission he was noted to have a bradycardia with a heart rate of 46-54. An ECG showed a Wenckenbach atrioventricular block. A dual chamber permanent pacemaker system was placed. Code the ICD-9-CM diagnosis and procedure codes.

21. DIAGNOSIS OR NATURE OF ILLNESS OR INJURY (RELATE ITEMS 1, 2, 3 OR 4 TO ITEM 24E BY LINE)
1 |___ .___   3 |___ .___
2 |___ .___   4 |___ .___

24.	A						B	C	D		E
	DATE(S) OF SERVICE						Place of Service	Type of Service	PROCEDURES, SERVICES, OR SUPPLIES (Explain Unusual Circumstances)		DIAGNOSIS CODE
	From			To					CPT / HCPCS	MODIFIER	
MM	DD	YY	MM	DD	YY						

Chapter Review

The inpatient system of reimbursement is different from office and outpatient services since the facility costs rather than the professional services of physicians are the focus of payment. The basis of inpatient reimbursement is diagnosis related groups (DRGs), a complex scheme of more than 500 patient mix classifications. Sound ICD-9-CM diagnostic coding is critical to the success of any inpatient coding program, largely because much of the decision making methodology hinges on the patient's medical condition during hospitalization. Knowing how to correctly sequence and report procedures must be the goal for all coders.

10 HCPCS

What Is HCPCS?

The term HCPCS can be confusing. HCPCS (pronounced "hick-picks") is most accurately used as the acronym for the entire three-level HCFA Common Procedure Coding System. HCPCS is also most commonly used to identify HCPCS Level II national codes, the topic of this chapter.

PURPOSE OF HCFA COMMON PROCEDURE CODING SYSTEM

HCPCS is a uniform method for healthcare providers and medical suppliers to report professional services, procedures, and supplies. HCFA developed this system in 1983 to:

- Meet the operational needs of Medicare/Medicaid
- Coordinate government programs by uniform application of HCFA's policies
- Allow providers and suppliers to communicate their services in a consistent manner
- Ensure the validity of profiles and fee schedules through standardized coding
- Enhance medical education and research by providing a vehicle for local, regional, and national utilization comparisons

OVERVIEW OF HCFA COMMON PROCEDURE CODING SYSTEM

To see how HCPCS fits within the entire HCFA coding system, we provide the following overview of each of the three levels, their official names and their popular, commonly used names.

HCPCS Level I /CPT

Level I is the American Medical Association's (AMA) CPT (*Physicians' Current Procedural Terminology*), which was developed and is maintained and copyrighted by the AMA. CPT provides five-digit codes with descriptive terms for reporting services performed by healthcare providers and is the country's most widely accepted procedure coding reference. CPT was first published in 1966 and is updated annually. (Further information about CPT can be found in Chapter 2.)

In CPT, procedures are grouped within six major sections: evaluation and management (E/M), anesthesia, surgery, radiology, pathology and laboratory, and medicine. They are then broken into subsections according to body part, service, or condition (e.g., mouth, amputation, or septal defect).

OBJECTIVES

Understand the three levels of the Health Care Financing Administration (HCFA) Common Procedure Coding System

Know how HCPCS fits within the entire HCFA system

Learn how HCPCS will be beneficial in obtaining accurate reimbursement

DEFINITIONS

HCFA: Health Care Financing Administration

HCPCS (pronounced "hick-picks") is the acronym for the three-level HCFA Common Procedure Coding System. It is also the most commonly used name for the HCPCS/Level II/National Codes — just one part of the larger, three-level HCFA coding system.

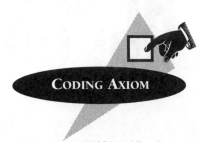

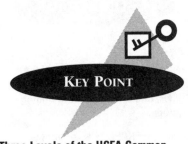

KEY POINT

Three Levels of the HCFA Common Procedural Coding System

Level I   CPT codes

Level II   National codes

Level III   Local codes

HCPCS Level II/National Codes

CPT does not contain all the codes needed to report medical services and supplies, so HCFA developed the second level of codes. The HCPCS Level II national codes found in *HCPCS 1998*, total over 2,800. If an appropriate HCPCS Level II code exists, it takes precedence over a CPT code in Medicare billing.

HCPCS codes begin with a single letter (A through V) followed by four numbers. They are grouped by the type of service or supply they represent and are updated annually by HCFA. HCPCS codes are now required for reporting most medical services and supplies provided in an outpatient setting to Medicare and Medicaid patients. An increasing number of private insurance carriers are also encouraging or requiring the use of HCPCS codes.

HCPCS Level III/Local Codes

Under physician payment reform, HCFA has eliminated most of the locally assigned Level III codes. Carriers are now required to report to and receive approval from HCFA before assigning local codes. When they are used, Level III codes are assigned and maintained by individual state Medicare carriers and supercede Level I or Level II codes. Like Level II, these codes begin with a letter (W through Z for local codes) followed by four digits.

Individual carriers assign these codes to describe new procedures that are not yet available in Level I or II. These codes can be introduced on an as-needed basis throughout the year. Carriers must send written notification to the physicians and suppliers in their area when these local codes are required.

MORE ABOUT HCPCS

Each section of codes is designated by a letter code except for the last section, the Table of Drugs.

HCPCS Codes

A codes include ambulance and transportation services, chiropractic services, medical and surgical supplies, administrative, and miscellaneous and investigational services and supplies.

B codes include enteral and parenteral therapy.

D codes include diagnostic, preventive, restorative, endodontic, periodontic, prosthodontic, prosthetic, orthodontic, and surgical dental procedures. These codes are supplied to HCFA and copyrighted by the American Dental Association.

E codes include durable medical equipment such as canes, crutches, walkers, commodes, decubitus care, bath and toilet aids, hospital beds, oxygen and related respiratory equipment, monitoring equipment, pacemakers, patient lifts, safety equipment, restraints, traction equipment, fracture frames, wheelchairs, and artificial kidney machines.

G codes include temporary procedures and professional services which are being reviewed prior to inclusion in CPT.

J codes include drugs that cannot be self-administered, chemotherapy drugs, immunosuppressive drugs, inhalation solutions, and other miscellaneous drugs and solutions.

K codes are temporary codes for durable medical equipment and drugs. Once these codes are approved for permanent inclusion in HCPCS, they typically become A, E, or J codes.

L codes include orthotic and prosthetic procedures and devices, as well as scoliosis equipment, orthopedic shoes, and prosthetic implants.

M codes include office services and cardiovascular and other medical services.

P codes include certain pathology and laboratory services.

Q codes are miscellaneous temporary codes.

R codes are diagnostic radiology services codes.

V codes include vision, hearing, and speech-language pathology services.

The Table of Drugs lists all drugs found in HCPCS by their generic name, with amount, route of administration, and code number. Brand name drugs are also listed in the table with a reference to the appropriate generic drug.

WHY SHOULD OUR PRACTICE USE HCPCS?

The following points summarize why your practice should be using HCPCS:

- The use of HCPCS is mandated by HCFA for use on Medicare claims and is also required by most state Medicaid offices.

- HCPCS codes improve a provider's ability to communicate services or supplies correctly without resorting to narrative descriptions.

- Their use reduces resubmission of claims for correction or review. If an inaccurate code is submitted, the claim's adjudicator must assign a code. That code, or its description, may be incorrect.

- Up-to-date and accurate HCPCS codes on office routing slips allow office staff to assign fees quickly and efficiently to services and supplies, saving both time and money.

- Consistent submission of "clean claims" (claims having all correct information necessary for processing) helps avoid an audit by a carrier due to frequent lack of specificity of claims.

- Use of HCPCS is essential for accurate and complete reimbursement from Medicare. For example, an injection billed to Medicare with only a CPT code will not be reimbursed correctly. The drug administered must be identified with the correct Level II/HCPCS code.

- Supplies billed to Medicare as "other than incidental to an office visit" (CPT code 99070) are not reimbursed unless identified with Level II/HCPCS or Level III/Local codes.

DISCUSSION QUESTIONS

1. What is HCPCS an acronym for?

   _____

   _____

2. Explain how HCPCS Level II fits in the national coding system.

   _____

   _____

3. Level III supercedes which levels of codes? Why?

   _____

   _____

   _____

OBJECTIVES

Learn what information is given with a HCPCS code

Understand how to use HCPCS modifiers

Recognize the concept of a facility-based procedure

How to Use HCPCS

HCPCS ICONS

The Medicode version of HCPCS uses CPT conventions to indicate new, revised, and deleted codes. A black circle (●) precedes a new code to be used only for services or supplies provided on or after January 1, of the given year; a black triangle (▲) precedes a code with revised terminology; codes deleted from last year's active list appear in parentheses with a cross-reference to an active code if HCFA has determined one.

Other pertinent information is given with each HCPCS code. Codes that are not covered by or valid for Medicare are so noted. When "Carrier Discretion" is noted, contact the carrier for specific coverage information on those codes. "Special Coverage Instructions" means that special coverage instructions apply to that code. These special instructions are typically given in the form of *Coverage Issues Manual* (CIM) and *Medicare Carriers Manual* (MCM) reference numbers. Some codes are cross-referenced to other Level II/HCPCS codes, specific CPT codes, or to CPT in general. These are indicated with "Cross-reference" plus the CPT or HCPCS code.

Color-coded Coverage Instructions

Medicode's HCPCS provide colored symbols for each coverage and reimbursement instruction. A legend to these symbols is provided on the bottom of each two-page spread.

⊘ Codes that are not covered by or valid for Medicare are now preceded by this symbol. The pertinent CIM and MCM reference numbers are also given explaining why a particular code is not covered. These numbers refer to appendixes A and B, where we have listed the complete CIM and MCM references, whenever possible.

➥ Issues that are left to "Carrier Discretion" are noted with this symbol. Contact the carrier for specific coverage information on those codes.

? This is the symbol for "Special Coverage Instructions" and means that special coverage instructions apply to that code. These special instructions are also typically given in the form of CIM and MCM reference numbers. Again, appendixes A and B list the complete CIM and MCM references.

☑ Many codes in HCPCS report quantities that may not coincide with quantities available in the marketplace. For instance, a HCPCS code for a disposable syringe reports one syringe, but the syringe is generally sold in a box of 100, and "100" must be indicated in the quantity box on the HCFA claim form to ensure proper reimbursement. This symbol indicates that care should be taken to verify quantities in this code.

MODIFIERS

Modifiers should, or in some cases must, be used to identify circumstances that alter or enhance the description of a service or supply. There are also three levels of HCFA coding system modifiers — one for each level of codes.

Level I/CPT modifiers are two numeric digits (e.g., -22 *Unusual Procedural Services*) and are described in detail in CPT. They are also maintained and updated on an annual basis by the AMA.

Level II/HCPCS modifiers are two alphabetic or alphanumeric digits (AA–VP). There are also several one digit modifiers. They are recognized by carriers nationally and are updated annually by HCFA.

Level III /Local modifiers are assigned by individual Medicare carriers and are distributed to physicians and suppliers through carrier newsletters. The carrier may change, add, or delete these local modifiers as needed.

-AA Anesthesia services performed personally by anesthesiologist
-AB Medical direction of own employee(s) by anesthesiologist (not more than four employees)
-AC Medical direction of other than own employees by anesthesiologist (not more than four individuals)
-AD Medical supervision by a physician: more than four concurrent anesthesia procedures
-AE Direction of residents in furnishing not more than two concurrent anesthesia services - attending physician relationship met
-AF Anesthesia complicated by total body hypothermia
-AG Anesthesia for emergency surgery on a patient who is moribund or who has an incapacitating systemic disease that is a constant threat to life (may warrant additional charge)
-AH Clinical psychologist
-AJ Clinical social worker
    (-AK. This modifier was deleted in 1999)
    (-AL. This modifier was deleted in 1999)
-AM Physician, team member service
    (-AN. This modifier was deleted in 1999)
-AP Determination of refractive state was not performed in the course of diagnostic ophthalmological examination
▲ -AS Physician assistant, nurse practitioner, or clinical nurse specialist services for assistant at surgery
-AT Acute treatment (this modifier should be used when reporting service 98940, 98941, 98942)
    (-AU. This modifier was deleted in 1999)
    (-AV. This modifier was deleted in 1999)

DEFINITIONS

Coverage Issues Manual (CIM) and *Medicare Carriers Manual* (MCM) list special coverage instructions for codes. The CIM is a HCFA publication containing national coverage decisions which sets forth whether specific medical items, services, treatment procedures, or technologies can be paid for by Medicare program. The CIM is used by Part A Intermediaries and Part B Carriers. The MCM is the manual HCFA provides to Medicare carriers. It contains instructions for processing and payment of Medicare claims, preparing reimbursement forms, billing procedures, and Medicare regulations. As processes and regulations change, HCFA issues revisions to the manual. The most reliable sources for revisions to Medicare information are carrier bulletins and newsletters. These publications are usually issued on a monthly or quarterly basis and contain pertinent changes to Medicare payment policies, other local Medicare policies, drug reimbursement updates, and compliance issues. Most carriers also compile Medicare policy and/or billing manuals that can be obtained upon request.

(-AW. This modifier was deleted in 1999)

(-AY. This modifier was deleted in 1999)

-BP The beneficiary has been informed of the purchase and rental options and has elected to purchase the item

-BR The beneficiary has been informed of the purchase and rental options and has elected to rent the item

-BU The beneficiary has been informed of the purchase and rental options and after 30 days has not informed the supplier of his/her decision

-CC Procedure code change (use 'CC' when the procedure code submitted was changed either for administrative reasons or because an incorrect code was filed)

-E1 Upper left, eyelid

-E2 Lower left, eyelid

-E3 Upper right, eyelid

-E4 Lower right, eyelid

-EJ Subsequent claim (for epoetin alfa-epo-injection claim only)

-EM Emergency reserve supply (for ESRD benefit only)

-EP Service provided as part of Medicaid early periodic screening diagnosis and treatment (EPSDT) program

-ET Emergency treatment (dental procedures performed in emergency situations should show the modifier 'ET')

-F1 Left hand, second digit

-F2 Left hand, third digit

-F3 Left hand, fourth digit

-F4 Left hand, fifth digit

-F5 Right hand, thumb

-F6 Right hand, second digit

-F7 Right hand, third digit

-F8 Right hand, fourth digit

-F9 Right hand, fifth digit

-FA Left hand, thumb

-FP Service provided as part of Medicaid family planning program

-G1 Most recent URR reading of less than 60

-G2 Most recent URR reading of 60 to 64.9

-G3 Most recent URR reading of 65 to 69.9

-G4 Most recent URR reading of 70 to 74.9

-G5 Most recent URR reading of 75 or greater

● -G6 ESRD patient for whom less than six dialysis sessions have been provided in a month

-GA Waiver of liability statement on file

-GC This service has been performed in part by a resident under the direction of a teaching physician

-GE This service has been performed by a resident without the presence of a teaching physician under the primary care exception

● -GH Diagnostic mammogram converted from screening mammogram on same day

● -GJ "OPT OUT" physician or practitioner emergency or urgent service

● -GN Service delivered personally by a speech-language pathologist or under an outpatient speech-language pathology plan of care

● -GO Service delivered personally by an occupational therapist or under an outpatient occupational therapy plan of care

● -GP Service delivered personally by a physical therapist or under an outpatient physical therapy plan of care

● -GT Via interactive audio and video telecommunication systems

● -GX Service not covered by Medicare

-K0 Lower extremity prosthesis functional level 0 - does not have the ability or potential to ambulate or transfer safely with or without assistance and a prosthesis does not enhance their quality of lefe or mobility

-K1 Lower extremity prosthesis functional level 1 - has the ability or potential to use a prosthesis for transfers or ambulation on level surfaces at fixed cadence. Typical of the limited and unlimited household ambulator

-K2   Lower extremity prosthesis functional level 2 - has the ability or potential for ambulation with the ability to traverse low level environmental barriers such as curbs, stairs or uneven surfaces. Typical of the limited community ambulator

-K3   Lower extremity prosthesis functional level 3 - has the ability or potential for ambulation with variable cadence. Typical of the community ambulator who has the ability to transverse most environmental barriers and may have vocational, therapeutic, or exercise activity that demands prosthetic utilization beyond simple locomotion

-K4   Lower extremity prosthesis functional level 4 - has the ability or potential for prosthetic ambulation that exceeds the basic ambulation skills, exhibiting high impact, stress, or energy levels, typical of the prosthetic demands of the child, active adult, or athlete

-KA   Add on option/accessory for wheelchair

-KH   DMEPOS item, initial claim, purchase or first month rental

-KI   DMEPOS item, second or third month rental

-KJ   DMEPOS item, parenteral enteral nutrition (PEN) pump or capped rental, months four to fifteen

-KK   Inhalation solution compounded from an FDA approved formulation

-KL   Product characteristics defined in medical policy are met

-KM   Replacement of facial prosthesis including new impression/moulage

-KN   Replacement of facial prosthesis using previous master model

-KO   Single drug unit dose formulation

-KP   First drug of a multiple drug unit dose formulation

-KQ   Second or subsequent drug of a multiple drug unit dose formulation

● -KS   Glucose monitor supply for diabetic beneficiary not treated with insulin

-LC   Left circumflex coronary artery

-LD   Left anterior descending coronary artery

-LL   Lease/rental (use the 'LL' modifier when DME equipment rental is to be applied against the purchase price)

-LR   Laboratory round trip

-LS   FDA-monitored intraocular lens implant

-LT   Left side (used to identify procedures performed on the left side of the body)

-MS   Six month maintenance and servicing fee for reasonable and necessary parts and labor which are not covered under any manufacturer or supplier warranty

-NR   New when rented (use the 'NR' modifier when DME which was new at the time of rental is subsequently purchased)

-NU   New equipment

-PL   Progressive addition lenses

-Q2   HCFA/ORD demonstration project procedure/service

-Q3   Live kidney donor: services associated with postoperative medical complications directly related to the donation

-Q4   Service for ordering/referring physician qualifies as a service exemption

-Q5   Service furnished by a substitute physician under a reciprocal billing arrangement

-Q6   Service furnished by a locum tenens physician

-Q7   One class a finding

-Q8   Two class b findings

-Q9   One class b and two class c findings

-QA   FDA investigational device exemption

-QB   Physician providing service in a rural HPSA

-QC   Single channel monitoring

-QD   Recording and storage in solid state memory by a digital recorder

-QE   Prescribed amount of oxygen is less than 1 liter per minute (LPM)

-QF   Prescribed amount of oxygen exceeds 4 liters per minute (LPM) and portable oxygen is prescribed

-QG   Prescribed amount of oxygen is greater than 4 liters per minute (LPM)

-QH   Oxygen conserving device is being used with an oxygen delivery system

-QK   Medical direction of two, three, or four concurrent anesthesia procedures involving qualified individuals

● -QL   Patient pronounced dead after ambulance called

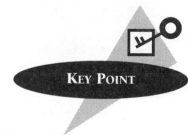

KEY POINT

PET Scan Modifiers

Use the following single digit alpha characters, in combination as two-character modifiers to indicate the results of a current PET scan and a previous test.

-N   Negative

-E   Equivocal

-P   Positive, but not suggestive of extensive ischemia

-S   Positive and suggestive of extensive ischemia (>20% of the left ventricle)

Ambulance Origin and Destination Modifiers

Single-digit modifiers for ambulance transport are used in combination in boxes 12 and 13 of HCFA form 1491. The first digit indicates the transport's place of origin, and the destination is indicated by the second digit.

-D   Diagnostic or therapeutic site other than 'P' or 'H' when these codes are used as origin codes

-E   Residential, domiciliary, custodial facility (other than an 1819 facility)

-G   Hospital-based dialysis facility (hospital or hospital-related)

-H   Hospital

-I   Site of transfer (e.g., airport or helicopter pad) between types of ambulance vehicles

-J   Non hospital-based dialysis facility

-N   Skilled nursing facility (SNF) (1819 facility)

-P   Physician's office (includes HMO non-hospital facility, clinic, etc.)

-R   Residence

-S   Scene of accident or acute event

-X   (Destination code only) intermediate stop at physician's office on way to the hospital (includes HMO nonhospital facility, clinic, etc.)

-QM   Ambulance service provided under arrangement by a provider of services
-QN   Ambulance service furnished directly by a provider of services
-QP   Documentation is on file showing that the laboratory test(s) was ordered individually or ordered as a CPT-recognized panel other than automated profile codes 80002-80019, G0058, G0059, and G0060.
-QR   Repeat clinical diagnostic laboratory test performed on the same day to obtain subsequent reportable test value(s) (separate specimens taken in separate encounters)
-QS   Monitored anesthesia care service
-QT   Recording and storage on tape by an analog tape recorder
-QU   Physician providing service in an urban HPSA
-QW   CLIA waived test
-QX   CRNA service: with medical direction by a physician
-QY   Anesthesiologist medically directs one CRNA
-QZ   CRNA service: without medical direction by a physician
-RC   Right coronary artery
-RP   Replacement and repair -RP may be used to indicate replacement of DME, orthotic and prosthetic devices which have been in use for sometime. The claim shows the code for the part, followed by the 'RP' modifier and the charge for the part.
-RR   Rental (use the 'RR' modifier when DME is to be rented)
-RT   Right side (used to identify procedures performed on the right side of the body)
-SF   Second opinion ordered by a professional review organization (PRO) per section 9401, p.l. 99-272 (100% reimbursement - no medicare deductible or coinsurance)
-SG   Ambulatory surgical center (ASC) facility service
-T1   Left foot, second digit
-T2   Left foot, third digit
-T3   Left foot, fourth digit
-T4   Left foot, fifth digit
-T5   Right foot, great toe
-T6   Right foot, second digit
-T7   Right foot, third digit
-T8   Right foot, fourth digit
-T9   Right foot, fifth digit
-TA   Left foot, great toe
-TC   Technical component. Under certain circumstances, a charge may be made for the technical component alone. Under those circumstances the technical component charge is identified by adding modifier 'TC' to the usual procedure number. Technical component charges are institutional charges and not billed separately by physicians. However, portable x-ray suppliers only bill for technical component and should utilize modifier TC. The charge data from portable x-ray suppliers will then be used to build customary and prevailing profiles.
-UE   Used durable medical equipment
-VP   Aphakic patient

FACILITY-BASED PROCEDURES

HCFA has released a national listing of procedures that are considered to be "facility-based." When a physician elects to perform one of these procedures in the office, a supply tray is allowed for payment. The supplies are considered to be mostly disposable and not routinely used in an office. There are about 70 CPT codes for which a surgical tray can be reported to Medicare for payment. Among the procedures for which a supply tray may be provided are: incisional biopsy of breast, muscle, bone, or superficial lymph node, select endoscopic procedures, hallux valgus correction, and chemotherapy administration. Get a copy of the list from your Medicare carrier.

DISCUSSION QUESTIONS

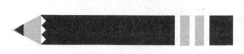

1. Which conventions do HCPCS codes use to indicate new, revised, and deleted codes?

_____

_____

_____

2. Why is it important to know which procedures are facility-based?

_____

_____

_____

3. What type of information does the *Coverage Issues Manual* (CIM) and *Medicare Carriers Manual* (MCM) contain? Why is the information important?

_____

_____

_____

Specialty-Specific Scenarios

INSTRUCTIONS

The following pages test your ability to code services and supplies correctly with the appropriate levels of HCPCS and ICD-9-CM diagnosis coding. A properly completed HCFA-1500 claim form and a written explanation of correct coding accompanies each answer. Be aware, however, that while we have tried to make these examples applicable to each geographic area, they are subject to current, individual carrier guidelines and should be regarded only as generic examples.

GYNECOLOGY SCENARIO

A disabled, 46-year-old, established Medicare patient with menopausal syndrome is seen by the clinic's nurse for a 5 mg intramuscular injection of depo-estradiol cypionate. Code the ICD-9-CM diagnosis and HCPCS Levels I CPT and II codes for this service.

Gynecology

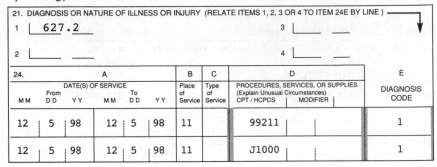

21. DIAGNOSIS OR NATURE OF ILLNESS OR INJURY (RELATE ITEMS 1, 2, 3 OR 4 TO ITEM 24E BY LINE)				
1.	627.2		3.	
2.			4.	

24.	A						B	C	D		E
	DATE(S) OF SERVICE						Place of Service	Type of Service	PROCEDURES, SERVICES, OR SUPPLIES (Explain Unusual Circumstances)		DIAGNOSIS CODE
	From			To					CPT / HCPCS	MODIFIER	
	MM	DD	YY	MM	DD	YY					
	12	5	98	12	5	98	11		99211		1
	12	5	98	12	5	98	11		J1000		1

ICD-9-CM

627.2 Menopausal or female climacteric states

HCPCS Levels I (CPT) and II

99211 Office or other outpatient visit for the evaluation and management of an established patient, that may not require the presence of a physician. Usually, the presenting problem(s) are minimal. Typically, 5 minutes are spent performing or supervising these services.

J1000 Injection, depo-estradiol cypionate, up to 5 mg

or

99211 Office or other outpatient visit for the evaluation and management of an established patient, that may not require the presence of a physician. Usually, the presenting problem(s) are minimal. Typically, 5 minutes are spent performing or supervising these services.

90782 Therapeutic or diagnostic injection (specify material injected); subcutaneous or intramuscular

J1000 Injection, depo-estradiol cypionate, up to 5 mg

Medicare bundles the administration of the medication into the E/M service provided, but allows separate payment for the drug administered. Each Medicare carrier has individual requirements for the use of HCPCS Level II codes to describe the drug administered. Some carriers require the use of the CPT code for the administration and the HCPCS Level II J code; others use only the J code and require a Level II HCPCS modifier to designate the method of administration.

PLASTIC/RECONSTRUCTIVE SCENARIO

An 8-year-old male fell off his bike onto the street and sustained a 4.5 cm complicated laceration to the cheek on the right side of his face. He is examined in the emergency room by the emergency physician who calls a reconstructive physician to repair the laceration. The physician performs a complex repair of the laceration. Code the ICD-9-CM diagnosis and HCPCS codes for the reconstructive physician.

HCPCS Level I (CPT)

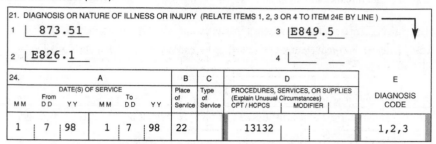

or

HCPCS Level II

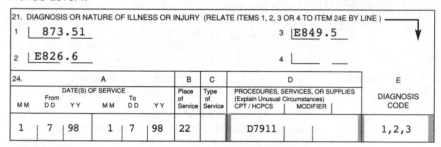

ICD-9-CM

873.51	Open wound of face, cheek, complicated
E826.1	Pedal cycle accident injuring pedal cyclist
E849.5	Place of occurrence, street and highway

HCPCS Level I (CPT)

13132	Repair, complex, forehead, cheeks, chin, mouth, neck, axillae, genitalia, hands and/or feet; 2.6 cm to 7.5 cm

or

HCPCS Level II

D7911	Complicated suture – up to five cm

OBJECTIVES

Code medical encounter scenarios accurately

Understand which coding system level to use for each scenario

ORTHOPEDIC SCENARIO

A 72-year-old established patient was seen in her orthopedist's office on an emergency basis for a minimally displaced closed fracture of the radius and ulna of the right forearm. The fracture was diagnosed after anteroposterior and lateral x-rays of the forearm were obtained by the physician's staff. The patient also had a puncture wound of the right, upper arm that occurred when a branch stabbed her as she fell six feet out of a tree she was pruning at home. From the patient's verbal history, it had been over 20 years since her last tetanus immunization. She couldn't remember when her last diphtheria immunization was given, but it was more than 20 years ago.

The patient's arm was prepped, the fracture site was injected with lidocaine, and the fracture easily reduced. Post-reduction x-rays (taken by the physician's staff) demonstrated good alignment of the bones.

A long arm fiberglass splint was then applied. The patient was given a diphtheria and tetanus toxoid immunization, and instructions to return in one week. Code the ICD-9-CM diagnosis, CPT, and HCPCS Level II codes.

Orthopedics

21. DIAGNOSIS OR NATURE OF ILLNESS OR INJURY (RELATE ITEMS 1, 2, 3,4 OR 5 TO ITEM 24E BY LINE)			
1	813.23	3	E884.9
2	880.03	4	E849.0

24.	A						B	C	D		E
	DATE(S) OF SERVICE						Place of Service	Type of Service	PROCEDURES, SERVICES, OR SUPPLIES (Explain Unusual Circumstances)		DIAGNOSIS CODE
	From			To					CPT / HCPCS	MODIFIER	
MM	DD	YY	MM	DD	YY						
9	14	98	9	14	98		11		25565		1,2,3,4
9	14	98	9	14	98		11		99058		1,2,3,4
9	14	98	9	14	98		11		73090	x2	1,2,3,4
9	14	98	9	14	98		11		90718		1,2,3,4
9	14	98	9	14	98		11		A4590		1,2,3,4
9	14	98	9	14	98		11		90471		1,2,3,4

ICD-9-CM

813.23   Fracture, radius with ulna, closed, shaft

880.03   Open wound of upper arm, without mention of complication

E884.9   Other fall from one level to another (tree)

E849.0   Place of occurrence, home

HCPCS Level I (CPT)

25565   Closed treatment of radial and ulnar shaft fractures; with manipulation

99058   Office services provided on an emergency basis

73090   Radiologic examination; forearm, anteroposterior and lateral views (x 2 units)

90718   Tetanus and diphtheria toxoids (Td) adsorbed for adult use, for intramuscular or jet injection

90471   Immunization administration (includes percutaneous, intradermal, subcutaneous, intramuscular and jet injections and/or intranasal or oral administration); single or combination vaccine/toxoid

HCPCS Level II

A4590   Special casting material (e.g., fiberglass)

Four ICD-9-CM diagnosis codes apply to this scenario. The codes and sequence should reflect the primary diagnosis and the most resource-intensive codes: the fracture and its repair. Secondary codes should reflect other conditions for which treatment is provided, in the order of their importance to the clinical picture. In this case, E codes should first report the fall. Reported second is the place of occurrence, the patient's home. This lets the payer (in this case, Medicare) know where the accident occurred so they can determine whether they are the primary insurer for this accident. Generally, homeowners insurance does not cover accidents or injuries to the homeowner.

CPT code 99058 reports office services provided on an emergency basis, but does not include the actual medical or surgical service performed. The musculoskeletal codes for fracture management include medical examination, open or closed treatment of the fracture, application of the first cast or traction device, and normal uncomplicated follow-up care.

There are many variables in managing fractures. Closed management (or reduction) means no surgical incision is necessary and that treatment is in the form of a manipulation, cast, splint, or traction application. Open management (or reduction) requires a surgical reduction with or without internal skeletal fixation. When the initial medical evaluation and/or management of the fracture is provided on the same day, the medical service is included in the surgical package.

When cast application is performed as an initial service, it is not coded. Removal of the first cast and/or traction device is included in the surgical package. X-ray services and expensive casting materials (e.g., fiberglass) may be reported when provided by the physician.

Note that there is not a HCPCS Level II code that describes a diphtheria and tetanus immunization.

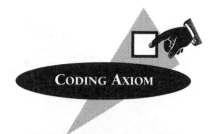

CODING AXIOM

Services should always be fully coded and entered on the superbill so that if there is a question from a payer, it can be answered by anyone. Encounters should never be partially coded.

MEDICAL SPECIALTIES/INTERNAL MEDICINE SCENARIO

An elderly established patient presented to his physician with a sore throat. A strep infection was diagnosed using a quick strep test in the office. The physician administered an injection of 1,200,000 units of penicillin G benzathine to treat the infection. Report the appropriate ICD-9-CM diagnosis, CPT and HCPCS Level II codes for the office visit, test, and injection.

Internal Medicine

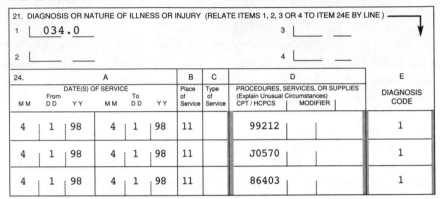

ICD-9-CM

034.0   Streptococcal sore throat

HCPCS Level I (CPT)

99212   Office or other outpatient visit for the evaluation and management of an established patient, which requires at least two of these three key components: a problem focused history; a problem focused examination; straightforward medical decision making. Counseling and/or coordination of care with other providers or agencies are provided consistent with the nature of the problem(s) and the patient's and/or family's needs. Usually, the presenting problem(s) are self limited or minor. Physicians typically spend 10 minutes face-to-face with the patient and/or family.

86403   Particle agglutination; screen, each antibody

HCPCS Level II

J0570   Injection, penicillin G benzathine, up to 1,200,000 units

MEDICAL SPECIALTIES/FAMILY PRACTICE SCENARIO

A Medicare patient noted a small lump in her right breast and scheduled an appointment with her local rural physician. After examining the patient, the physician opted to do an incisional biopsy of the lesion during the same appointment. Code the ICD-9-CM diagnosis and HCPCS codes.

Family Practice

21. DIAGNOSIS OR NATURE OF ILLNESS OR INJURY (RELATE ITEMS 1, 2, 3 OR 4 TO ITEM 24E BY LINE)

1 | 611.72   3 |

2 | 4 |

24.		A				B	C	D			E
	DATE(S) OF SERVICE					Place	Type	PROCEDURES, SERVICES, OR SUPPLIES (Explain Unusual Circumstances)			DIAGNOSIS
	From			To		of	of				CODE
MM	DD	YY	MM	DD	YY	Service	Service	CPT / HCPCS	MODIFIER		
4	1	98	4	1	98	11		19101	QB	RT	1
4	1	98	4	1	98	11		A4550			1
4	1	98	4	1	98	11		99000			1

ICD-9-CM

611.72   Lump or mass in breast

HCPCS Levels I (CPT) and Level II

19101-QB-RT   Biopsy of breast; incisional — Physician providing service in a rural health professional shortage area — Right side

A4550   Surgical tray

99000   Handling and/or conveyance of specimen for transfer from the physician's office to a laboratory

The physician correctly reported the biopsy with 19101 and added HCPCS Level II modifier -QB, identifying a physician providing service in a rural health professional shortage area. Modifier -RT indicates the procedure was performed on the right side of the body. Generally, the modifier that will affect reimbursement is listed first when two or more modifiers are used. The physician also reported A4550 for the surgical tray used in this minor surgical procedure since CPT 19101 is on the Medicare facility-based list of codes that qualify nationally for surgical tray reimbursement. (This list is available through your carrier). If the physician had made the common mistake of using 99070 *Supplies and materials (except spectacles)*, this charge would likely have been denied. Because the HCFA bonus payment applies only to medical services, the physician did not apply modifier -QB to A4550. The tissue sample was to be transported to a laboratory for analysis; consequently, the physician also reported 99000 for handling and conveyance of the specimen.

GENERAL SURGERY

A week following a suture repair of a perforated ulcer, a patient is discharged from the hospital. Three days later, she presents at her physician's office as an emergency walk-in patient, having experienced severe vomiting and diarrhea during the past 24 hours. The patient informs the physician during his detailed history and examination that her entire family recently had a bout of severe vomiting and diarrhea, but recovered within a 24-hour period. The physician orders a "stat" automated CBC with a manual differential WBC count and complete (non-automated) urinalysis. When the results return from the clinic laboratory, the physician concludes the patient suffers from viral gastroenteritis and dehydration, status post suture repair of perforated gastric ulcer. He places her in an observation room in the minor surgery suite of the clinic, and starts an IV with 1000 ccs of Ringer's lactate, into which he injects 25 mg of IV promethazine hydrochloride for the nausea. The patient remains in observation. The physician and clinic nurses checked on her frequently. After six hours, the physician discontinues the IV and examines the patient, who states she felt much better. He gives instructions for her care, makes final notes, writes a prescription, and discharges the patient to home. How should these services be coded?

21. DIAGNOSIS OR NATURE OF ILLNESS OR INJURY (RELATE ITEMS 1, 2, 3 OR 4 TO ITEM 24E BY LINE)

1. `008.8`   3. `V45.89`

2. `276.5`   4. _____

24.	A DATE(S) OF SERVICE						B Place of Service	C Type of Service	D PROCEDURES, SERVICES, OR SUPPLIES (Explain Unusual Circumstances)		E DIAGNOSIS CODE
	From MM	DD	YY	To MM	DD	YY			CPT / HCPCS	MODIFIER	
	3	4	98	3	4	98	11		99214	–24	1,2,3
	3	4	98	3	4	98	11		90780	–79	1,2,3
	3	4	98	3	4	98	11		90781	–79	1,2,3
	3	4	98	3	4	98	11		90784	–79	1,2,3
	3	4	98	3	4	98	11		85022		1,2,3
	3	4	98	3	4	98	11		81000		1,2,3
	3	4	98	3	4	98	11		A4305		1,2,3
	3	4	98	3	4	98	11		A4215		1,2,3
	3	4	98	3	4	98	11		J7120		1,2,3
	3	4	98	3	4	98	11		J2550		1,2,3

ICD-9-CM

008.8   Intestinal infections due to other organism, not elsewhere classified

276.5   Volume depletion

V45.89   Other postsurgical status

HCPCS Level I (CPT)

99214-24   Office or other outpatient visit for the evaluation and management of an established patient, which requires at least two of these three key components: a detailed history; a detailed examination; medical decision making of moderate complexity. Counseling and/or coordination of care with other providers or agencies are provided consistent with the nature of the problem(s) and the patient's and/or family's needs. Usually, the presenting problem(s) are of moderate to high severity. Physicians typically spend 25 minutes face-to-face with the patient and/or family. — Unrelated E/M service by the same physician during a postoperative period

90780-79 IV infusion for therapy/diagnosis, administered by physician or under direct supervision of physician; up to one hour — Unrelated procedure or service by the same physician during the postoperative period

90781-79 IV infusion for therapy/diagnosis, administered by physician or under direct supervision of physician; each additional hour, up to eight (8) hours (List separately in addition to code for primary procedure) — Unrelated procedure or service by the same physician during the postoperative period

90784-79 Therapeutic or diagnostic injection (specify material injected); intravenous — Unrelated procedure or service by the same physician during the postoperative period

85022 Blood count; hemogram, automated, and manual differential WBC count (CBC)

81000 Urinalysis, by dip stick or tablet reagent for bilirubin, glucose, hemoglobin, ketones, leukocytes, nitrite, pH, protein, specific gravity, urobilinogen, any number of these constituents; non-automated with microscopy

HCPCS Level II

A4305 Disposable drug delivery system, flow rate of 50 ml or greater per hour

A4215 Needles only, sterile, any size, each

J7120 Ringer's lactate infusion, up to 1,000 cc (x 2 units)

J2550 Injection, promethazine HCl, up to 50 mg

Code 99214 should be used to report the E/M services even though the patient remained in the clinic for IV therapy. Codes for observation care (99218–99220) should not be used because these codes are specific for Hospital Observation Services. Coding guidelines for Hospital Observation Services specify: When observation status is initiated in the course of an encounter in another site of service (e.g., emergency department, physician's office, nursing facility) all E/M services provided by the supervising physician in conjunction with initiating observation status are considered part of the initial observation care when performed on the same date. The key word in this instruction is "initiating" which means that care is begun outside the hospital observation unit, but the patient is eventually transferred to the hospital for observation care. In this case, all E/M care provided on the same date of service would be reported with a single E/M code from Hospital Observation Services (99218–99220). However, in the above example, the patient was treated in the minor surgery room at the clinic and not transferred to the hospital. Therefore, outpatient E/M services (99201–99215) should be reported, not hospital observation services.

Codes 90780 and 90781 should be reported for the IV therapy. Administration and physician supervision is included in this code. CPT states that prolonged detention codes may not be reported with 90780 and 90781.

Note: Modifiers -24 and -79 have been added to the E/M and medicine codes to indicate that the procedure or service by the same physician was unrelated to the prior surgery during the postoperative period.

OTORHINOLARYNGOLOGY SCENARIO

A patient who has difficulty swallowing has a scheduled flexible esophagoscopy with brushing. The procedure is performed by an ENT physician in his office after the patient is injected with 5 mg of diazepam. Code the ICD-9-CM diagnosis and HCPCS codes.

Otorhinolaryngology

21. DIAGNOSIS OR NATURE OF ILLNESS OR INJURY (RELATE ITEMS 1, 2, 3 OR 4 TO ITEM 24E BY LINE)

1	787.2		3	
2			4	

24.	A								B	C	D		E
	DATE(S) OF SERVICE								Place of Service	Type of Service	PROCEDURES, SERVICES, OR SUPPLIES (Explain Unusual Circumstances)		DIAGNOSIS CODE
	From			To							CPT / HCPCS	MODIFIER	
	MM	DD	YY	MM	DD	YY							
	6	5	98	6	5	98			11		43200		1
	6	5	98	6	5	98			11		90782		1
	6	5	98	6	5	98			11		A4550		1
	6	5	98	6	5	98			11		J3360		1

ICD-9-CM

787.2 Dysphagia

HCPCS Level I (CPT)

43200 Esophagoscopy, rigid or flexible; diagnostic, with or without collection of specimen(s) by brushing or washing (separate procedure)

90782 Therapeutic or diagnostic injection (specify material injected); subcutaneous or intramuscular

HCPCS Level II

A4550 Surgical tray

J3360 Injection, diazepam, up to 5 mg (Valium, Zetran)

If this is a Medicare patient, 43200 could be reported with A4550 because 43200 is on Medicare's facility-based national list.

PATHOLOGY AND LABORATORY SCENARIO

A 66-year-old Medicare patient had a Pap smear submitted to a laboratory for testing. Information on the lab request slip indicates the patient has had abnormal Pap smears in the past, with the last one performed six months prior to the current smear. Code the ICD-9-CM diagnoses, CPT and HCPCS Level II codes for the laboratory.

Pathology and Laboratory

21. DIAGNOSIS OR NATURE OF ILLNESS OR INJURY (RELATE ITEMS 1, 2, 3 OR 4 TO ITEM 24E BY LINE)

1. V72.6
2. V15.89
3.
4.

24.	A DATE(S) OF SERVICE						B Place of Service	C Type of Service	D PROCEDURES, SERVICES, OR SUPPLIES (Explain Unusual Circumstances) CPT / HCPCS MODIFIER	E DIAGNOSIS CODE
	MM	From DD	YY	MM	To DD	YY				
	8	21	98	8	21	98	11		88150	1,2
	8	21	98	8	21	98	11		88141	1,2

ICD-9-CM

V72.6 Laboratory examination

V15.89 Other specified personal history presenting hazards to health

HCPCS Level I (CPT)

88150 Cytopathology, slides, cervical or vaginal; manual screening under physician supervision

88141 Cytopathology, cervical or vaginal (any reporting system); requiring interpretation by physician (List separately in addition to code for technical service)

or

HCPCS Level II

P3001 Screening Papanicolaou smear, cervical or vaginal, up to three smears, requiring interpretation by physician

This scenario does not specify whether Medicare is the primary or secondary insurer. If Medicare is primary, the following applies:

A screening Pap smear (use P3000 *Screening Papanicolaou smear, cervical or vaginal, up to three smears; by technician under physician supervision* or P3001 *Screening Papanicolaou smear, cervical or vaginal, up to three smears requiring interpretation by physician*) and related medically necessary services provided to a woman for the early detection of cervical cancer (including collection of the sample of cells and a physician's interpretation of the test results) are covered under Medicare Part B when ordered by a physician under one of the following conditions:

- She has not had such a test during the preceding three years. Use ICD-9-CM diagnosis codes: V72.6 *Laboratory examination* and V76.2 *Special screening for malignant neoplasms, cervix*; or

- There is evidence, on the basis of her medical history or other findings, that she is at high risk of developing cervical cancer and her physician recommends that she have the test performed more frequently than every three years (use ICD-9-CM codes; V72.6 *Laboratory examination* and V15.89 *Other specified personal history presenting hazards to health*).

If the patient has Medicare as secondary insurance, report the same ICD-9-CM codes, but use 88150 with 88141 to report the procedure.

RADIOLOGY SCENARIO

Portable x-ray equipment was taken to a nursing home from a radiology freestanding clinic. A Medicare patient had a three view x-ray of the left hip performed. Her diagnosis on the radiology request form was continued pain in the left hip, three weeks status post total hip arthroplasty. Code the ICD-9-CM diagnosis, CPT and HCPCS Level II codes for the radiologist.

Radiology

21. DIAGNOSIS OR NATURE OF ILLNESS OR INJURY (RELATE ITEMS 1, 2, 3 OR 4 TO ITEM 24E BY LINE)							
1 719.45					3		
2 V43.64					4		

24.	A						B	C	D		E
	DATE(S) OF SERVICE						Place of Service	Type of Service	PROCEDURES, SERVICES, OR SUPPLIES (Explain Unusual Circumstances)		DIAGNOSIS CODE
	From			To							
	MM	DD	YY	MM	DD	YY			CPT / HCPCS	MODIFIER	
	11	6	98	11	6	98	32		73510	–LT	1,2
	11	6	98	11	6	98	32		R0070		1,2

ICD-9-CM

719.45   Pain in joint, pelvic region and thigh

V43.64   Organ or tissue replaced by other means, hip

HCPCS CPT Level I (CPT)

73510-LT   Radiologic examination, hip, unilateral; complete, minimum of two views — Left side

HCPCS Level II

R0070   Transportation of portable x-ray equipment and personnel to home or nursing home, per trip to facility or location, one patient seen

HCPCS modifier -LT was used with the radiology code to specify the procedure was performed on the left side of the body. Note that although the patient had a three view x-ray of the hip performed, the code nomenclature specifies a minimum of two views must be taken in order to report the code. Additional views beyond two are therefore included in this code. This is the case with multiple x-ray codes; read codes carefully before making your coding selection.

CPT does not have a code that specifies the use of portable x-ray equipment. If the service is submitted to a payer who does not accept HCPCS Level II codes, use 76499 *Unlisted diagnostic radiologic procedure*, and submit a cover letter and documentation.

The following HCFA guidelines should be used when reporting portable x-ray equipment:

The three diagnostic radiology services codes are used to report the transportation and setting-up of portable x-ray equipment (in the HCPCS book). Only a single, reasonable transportation charge is allowed for each trip the portable x-ray supplier makes to a particular location.

When more than one patient has x-rays at the same location (e.g., nursing home), prorate the single allowable transportation charge among all patients. For example, if two patients received x-rays at the same location, allow one-half of the reasonable transportation charge for each patient. Use any information regarding the number of patients receiving x-rays in each location that the supplier visits during each trip, or that the supplier of the x-ray may volunteer on the bill, or claim for reimbursement. If such information is not indicated, assume that at least four

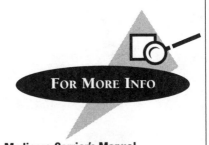

FOR MORE INFO

Medicare Carrier's Manual
2070.4
Coverage of Portable X-Ray Services Not Under the Direct Supervision of a Physician

5244.
Reasonable Charges for Portable X-Ray Services

patients had x-rays at the same location, and allow only one-fourth of the reasonable transportation charge for any one patient.

No transportation charge can be allowed unless the portable x-ray equipment used was actually transported to the location where the x-ray was taken. For example, do not report a transportation charge when the x-ray equipment is stored in a nursing home for use as needed.

Advanced Coding Practice

CODING PRACTICE 1
A 28-year-old female is seen by her OB/GYN for implantation of intradermal contraceptives. A Norplant system is used. Code the implantation and supplies.

21. DIAGNOSIS OR NATURE OF ILLNESS OR INJURY (RELATE ITEMS 1, 2, 3 OR 4 TO ITEM 24E BY LINE)

1 ⌊___ ___

2 ⌊___ ___

3 ⌊___ ___

4 ⌊___ ___

24. A DATE(S) OF SERVICE							B Place of Service	C Type of Service	D PROCEDURES, SERVICES, OR SUPPLIES (Explain Unusual Circumstances)		E DIAGNOSIS CODE
From MM	DD	YY	To MM	DD	YY				CPT / HCPCS	MODIFIER	

CODING PRACTICE 2

A patient requiring temporary home oxygen services requires an oxygen concentrator with a flow rate not to exceed 4 liters per minute with 50 feet of oxygen tubing and a nasal cannula. The patient is recovering from adverse effects of methotrexate which caused an interstitial fibrosing alveolitis but is responding well to steroids. It is expected he will require oxygen for no more than a month.

In addition, the patient temporarily requires a portable liquid oxygen system with four liquid oxygen units.

21. DIAGNOSIS OR NATURE OF ILLNESS OR INJURY (RELATE ITEMS 1, 2, 3 OR 4 TO ITEM 24E BY LINE)					
1		3			
2		4			

24. A DATE(S) OF SERVICE From MM DD YY To MM DD YY	B Place of Service	C Type of Service	D PROCEDURES, SERVICES, OR SUPPLIES (Explain Unusual Circumstances) CPT/HCPCS MODIFIER	E DIAGNOSIS CODE

Chapter Review

HCPCS (pronounced "hick-picks") is the acronym for the three-level HCFA Common Procedure Coding System. It is also the most commonly used name for the HCPCS/Level II/National Codes — just one part of the larger, three-level HCFA coding system. This system is a uniform method for healthcare providers and medical suppliers to report professional services, procedures, and supplies. The Health Care Financing Administration (HCFA) developed this system in 1983 for several reasons: to meet the operational needs of Medicare/Medicaid, coordinate government programs by uniform application of HCFA's policies, allow providers and suppliers to communicate their services in a consistent manner, ensure the validity of profiles and fee schedules through standardized coding, and enhance medical education and research by providing a vehicle for local, regional, and national utilization comparisons. The *Medicare Carrier's Manual* and *Coverage Issues Manual* list special coverage instructions on codes. HCPCS modifiers identify circumstances that alter or enhance the description of a service or supply.

11 Medicare Coding

ICD-9-CM and HCPCS coding must be understood before attempting to code for Medicare. Outpatient coding is based on ICD-9-CM diagnosis codes and the *Health Care Financing Administration* (HCFA) *Common Procedure Coding System* (HCPCS). HCPCS encompasses all of CPT in Level I in addition to Level II national codes and Level III local codes. Coding for inpatient Medicare services is based on ICD-9-CM diagnosis and procedure codes which combine to make up one of 511 diagnosis related groups (DRGs) that is Medicare's basis for payment of inpatient claims.

ICD-9-CM, CPT, and HCPCS codes have been discussed in previous chapters. An understanding of these types of codes helps distinguish any differences when coding for reimbursement by private payors and for Medicare inpatient and outpatient services.

General Medicare Information

The laws of the Medicare program are found in Title XVIII of the Social Security Act. HCFA administers Medicare, which provides health coverage to people age 65 and over and those who have permanent kidney failure and certain people with disabilities. The Medicare program is the largest public payer for healthcare. Despite the growing numbers depending on Medicare, annual health care spending has slowed markedly from 12.2 percent in 1994 to 7.2 percent in 1997 due to programs that fight fraud and abuse and also, provisions in the Balanced Budget Acts of 1996 and 1997.

Fraud and abuse costs Medicare millions each year. HCFA is stepping up its campaign to fight the misuse of program funds highlighted by two recent audits. The first audit found a 14 percent error rate in claims payment, which, if applied to all payments, would mean that $23 billion was spent inappropriately in 1996. A second study the same year, revealed that 40 percent of the services provided by home health agencies (in an audited four states) didn't meet the requirements for Medicare payment. The services were medically unnecessary in many cases or were provided to beneficiaries who were not homebound. Provisions in the BBA establish new guidelines to prevent the abuses.

MEDICARE PART A AND PART B

Medicare Part A coverage includes inpatient hospital, skilled nursing facilities, hospice, and home health. Part B coverage provides payment for physician and outpatient hospital services and medical equipment. Generally, participants covered by Part A are automatically enrolled in Part B. A monthly premium is charged for those enrolled in Part B, which is an amount subject to annual change. Regional offices provide HCFA with a decentralized administration of Medicare programs. Each regional office manages private insurance companies that contract with the government to

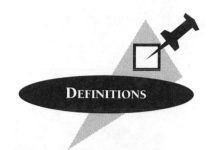

DEFINITIONS

Medicare Part A: coverage includes inpatient hospital, skilled nursing facilities, hospice, and home health.

Medicare Part B: coverage provides payment for physician, outpatient hospital services, and medical supplies and equipment.

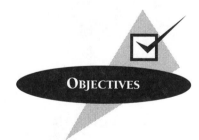

OBJECTIVES

Understand the difference between Medicare Part A Intermediaries and Part B Carriers

Learn to determine if Medicare is the secondary insurer

Distinguish between participating and non-participating

Know the reasons for the Medicare Fee Schedule and RBRVS

Watch for change with UPINs and PINs

process and make payment for Medicare services. Physicians submit their claims to carriers for Part B reimbursement, and hospitals submit their claims to intermediaries for reimbursement of Part A. In some cases, healthcare plans have risk contracts with Medicare to make payment on Part B claims.

MEDICARE REIMBURSEMENT ISSUES

Each November, Medicare notifies physicians by letter of significant changes in Medicare reimbursement practices for the upcoming year. The same information is available from the *Federal Register*. Throughout the year, physicians are notified of policy changes, coding guidelines, and other changes by their individual Medicare carrier's newsletter. These newsletters may be the only formal notification of change and should be kept in a binder for reference. Because physicians who provide services for Medicare patients are liable to abide by all rules and regulations of HCFA, it is imperative that reimbursement personnel read these documents.

Medicare claims and payments are handled by insurance organizations under contract to the Federal government. HCFA has established separate systems for paying claims for covered services and supplies in Parts A and B. The organizations that handle Part A are called "intermediaries". The organizations that handle Part B are called "carriers." The names and addresses of carriers are available from any Social Security Office.

Medicare's system for paying physicians is based on a fee schedule that is updated annually. The fee schedule assigns a dollar value to each physician service based on work, the cost of running a practice, and the cost of malpractice insurance. The fees that appear on the schedule are the Medicare approved amounts for services covered by Part B.

Under the Part B payment system, the patient is responsible for paying the first $100 each calendar year for services and supplies covered by Medicare. After the $100 deductible is met, Medicare starts paying a share of the patient's medical expenses. Part B generally pays 80 percent of the Medicare approved amount for all covered services received during the rest of the year. The patient is responsible for the other 20 percent, which is called the co-insurance. The patient is also responsible for all permitted charges in excess of the Medicare-approved amount (as shown on the fee schedule), and for all charges for services and supplies not covered by Medicare.

MANAGED CARE

Medicare beneficiaries may receive physician and other healthcare services through managed care plans that have contracts with Medicare, such as health maintenance organizations (HMOs) and competitive medical plans (CMPs).

In a managed care plan, a network of healthcare providers (physicians, hospitals, skilled nursing facilities) offer medical services to plan members on a prepaid basis. Services usually must be obtained from the professionals and facilities that are part of the plan. Medicare pays the plan a fixed monthly amount and the plan provides for all covered services. Additionally, manage care plans generally charge enrollees a monthly premium and nominal copayments for services, rather than collecting the annual deductible from the patient and the coinsurance under the fee-for-service care.

Most plans serving Medicare beneficiaries are required to offer all Medicare hospital and medical benefits available in the plan's service area. Some plans also provide benefits beyond what Medicare reimburses, such as dental care, hearing aids, and eyeglasses.

MEDICARE+CHOICE PROGRAM

The Medicare+Choice (M+C) program expands the healthcare options available to Medicare beneficiaries. Under this program, eligible individuals may elect to receive Medicare benefits through enrollment in one of many private health plans affecting choices beyond the original Medicare programs or plans available through managed care organizations. Among these alternatives: Medicare Saving Account plans which combine a high deductible M+C health insurance plan and a contribution to an M+C MSA, and M+C private fee-for-service plans.

THE BALANCED BUDGET ACT AND REIMBURSEMENT

Section 4523 of the Balanced Budget Act of 1997 (BBA) provides authority for HCFA to implement a prospective payment system (PPS) under Medicare for hospital outpatient services, certain Part B services furnished to hospital inpatients who have no Part A coverage, and partial hospitalization services furnished by community mental health centers.

All services paid under the new PPS are classified into groups called Ambulatory Payment Classes or APCs. Services in each APC are similar clinically and in terms of the resources they require. A payment rate is established for each APC. Depending on the services provided, hospitals may be paid for more than one APC for an encounter.

Section 4523 of the BBA also changed the way beneficiary coinsurance is determined for the services included under the PPS. Under the plan, a coinsurance amount will initially be calculated for each APC based on 20 percent of the national median charge for services in the APC. The coinsurance amount for an APC will not change until such time as the amount becomes 20 percent of the total APC payment. HCFA plans to implement the PPS in January 2000.

Section 4432(a) of the Balanced Budget Act (BBA) of 1997 modified how payment will be made for Medicare skilled nursing facility (SNF) services. SNFs are no longer be paid on a reasonable cost basis or through low volume prospectively determined rates, but rather on the basis of the PPS.

DETERMINING IF MEDICARE IS THE SECONDARY INSURER

Some people who have Medicare also have group health or other types of coverage that may make Medicare a secondary payor on their healthcare claims. Medicare may be the secondary payor for individuals, as follows:

- Age 65 or older, with employment status, (or whose spouse has employment status) with coverage under a group health plan
- Under age 65, disabled but with employment status, (or whose family member has employment status) with coverage under a large group health plan
- Have permanent kidney failure, and are covered under a group health plan through current or former employment or through the current or former employment of a parent or spouse

It is difficult to identify which payor is primary and which is secondary without asking the appropriate questions. Add these questions to the back of your Medicare patient information sheet for patients to answer and sign.

- Is the patient a veteran? Has the VA authorized the services to be rendered?
- Is this accident/illness/condition related to work or covered by the Black Lung program?

DEFINITIONS

Medicare Secondary Payer (MSP) Program
Medicare becomes secondary when patients are 65 or older and have group health benefits through their own employer or their spouse's.

Medigap policy is a health insurance policy, or other health benefit plan, offered by a private company to those entitled to Medicare benefits. The policy provides payment for Medicare deductibles, coinsurance amounts, or noncovered Medicare services.

KEY POINT

Medicare is also secondary when:

- A patient's treatment is covered by automobile no-fault or liability insurance.
- The patient receives VA (Veterans Administration) benefits.
- The patient receives or is entitled to workers' compensation or Black Lung medical benefits.
- Disabled beneficiaries younger than age 65 receive health insurance coverage under a "large group health plan" (LGHP).

- Is this accident/illness/condition related to an auto accident or other kind of accident?

- Is the patient over 65 and working, or is the patient's spouse working? If so, are there group benefits?

- Is the patient eligible for benefits through the ESRD program, or undergoing kidney dialysis?

- Is the patient disabled?

If the patient answers "yes" to any of these questions, then Medicare is probably not the primary insurer. But, you should call your local Medicare carrier to verify primary or secondary insurer status.

MEDIGAP AND SUPPLEMENTAL INSURANCE

A Medigap policy, as defined by HCFA, is a health insurance policy, or other health benefit plan, offered by a private company to those entitled to Medicare benefits. The policy provides payment for Medicare charges not payable due to deductibles, coinsurance amounts, or other Medicare imposed limitations.

Under the Omnibus Budget Reconciliation Act of 1987 (OBRA '87), Medicare specifically excludes two types of coinsurance or supplemental policies or plans from qualifying as a "Medigap" policy:

- Those offered by an employer to current or former employees.

- Those offered by trade or union organizations to current or former employees.

The manner in which secondary payments are obtained is affected by participation or nonparticipation with the Medicare program.

Medicare Assignment

Each time a patient uses the services of a physician, the physician submits the Medicare claim to the carrier either on "assigned" or "unassigned" basis. When a claim is assigned, it means the physician has agreed to accept the Medicare-approved amount as payment in full. The physician bills the patient for the 20 percent of the approved amount plus any unmet portion of the Part B deductible. On assigned claims, Medicare pays its share directly to the physician.

An unassigned claim means the physician has not agreed to accept the Medicare approved amount as full payment and can charge more than the Medicare-approved amount, but not more than the limiting charges. The physician bills the patient for the full amount and files the claim with the carrier. Medicare reimburses the patient its share of the charges.

PARTICIPATION

While some physicians and medical suppliers accept assignment on a case-by-case basis or not at all, others sign Medicare participation agreements that require the physician to accept assignment on all Medicare claims. These physicians and suppliers are called participating physicians and suppliers and their names and addresses are listed in the Medicare Participating Physician/Supplier Directory.

There are exceptions in choosing whether to accept assignment. For example, all physicians and qualified laboratories must accept assignment from clinical diagnostic laboratory tests covered by Medicare. Physicians and certain other practitioners and suppliers must take assignment on all claims for services furnished to Medicare beneficiaries who are eligible for medical assistance

Providers mandated by Medicare to accept assignment for services provided to Medicare patients:

- Hospitals — inpatient and outpatient facility services

- Ambulatory surgical centers — facility services

- Clinical laboratories — all tests, regardless of provider type (physician or laboratory)

- Limited license practitioners — physician assistant, nurse practitioner, certified registered nurse anesthetist, etc.

through the state Medicaid program including beneficiaries enrolled in the Qualified Medicare Beneficiary program.

A participation contract is binding for one calendar year. Physicians can change their status only during a designated period of time each year. The physician must notify the carrier in writing to discontinue participation, or the contract will continue indefinitely.

Physicians who participate in the Medicare program are rewarded by the government in several ways. Among the benefits are:

- Receiving payments directly from Medicare, Medigap, and most secondary insurers
- Claims processing time is shorter
- Receiving Explanation of Medicare benefits/payment voucher (aids in verification of coding accuracy)
- Payment allowable is 5 percent higher than for a nonparticipating physician
- Free electronic media claims submission telephone lines
- Medicare carrier works directly with physician's office
- Physician can appeal unsatisfactory claims without patient approval

Limiting Charges

While physicians who do not accept assignment of a Medicare claim can charge more than physicians who do, there is a limit to the amount they can charge for services covered by Medicare. They are permitted to charge only 15 percent more than the Medicare-approved amount, and the patient must pay that extra amount. This is called the "limiting charge" and the patient does not have to pay more than this amount.

Limiting charge information also appears on the Explanation of Medicare Part B Benefits (EOMB) form generally sent to the patient by the carrier after the patient receives the Medicare-covered service.

Medicare carriers are required to screen physician bills for overcharges and notify the physician and the patient within 30 days of the overcharge. The physician is required to refund the overcharge within 30 days or credit the patient's account. Physicians who knowingly, willfully and repeatedly charge more than the legal limit are subject to sanctions.

NONPARTICIPATION

Several states have laws requiring mandatory assignment or limiting the amount physicians can bill the patient to the Medicare allowable. Currently, Connecticut, Massachusetts, Minnesota, New York, Ohio, Pennsylvania, Rhode Island and Vermont have charge limit laws. Medicare further requires physicians who do not take assignment for elective surgery to give the patient a written estimate of cost prior to surgery if the total charge will be $500 or more. If a patient does not receive a written estimate, the patient is entitled to a refund of any amount paid in excess of the Medicare-approved amount for surgery.

Advantages to nonparticipation include:

- Charging patient up to the limiting charge amount (greater than the participating allowed amount)

- Accepting assignment on individual claims (not locked in to all claims)
- Collecting entire amount from the patient at the time of service (no need to wait for Medicare processing)

Disadvantages to nonparticipation include:

- If limiting charge is exceeded, physician can be sanctioned or fined
- Allowed amount is 95 percent of a participating physician's amount
- Must collect payment from the patient
- Explanation of Medicare Benefits is sent to the patient (last source to verify coding accuracy and payment amount)
- Limited carrier cooperation on claim status
- Patient permission to appeal required
- Explanation of Medicare Benefits tells patients how much money they would have saved if they had gone to a participating physician
- The patient may not understand the payment is for physician reimbursement

MEDICAL NECESSITY

Medicare does not pay for services that are "medically unnecessary," according to Medicare standards. Patients are not liable to pay for such services if the service is performed without prior written notification from the physician. The patient must sign the notification to indicate that the patient fully understands Medicare's decision and the patient's subsequent financial responsibility.

MEDICARE PAYMENT NOTICE

Physicians are required by law to submit the claim within a year after providing a service. The claim is submitted to the carrier that services the area where the covered service or supply was provided, not necessarily the carrier for the patient's area. If for some reason, the claim is not filed as required, the patient can still send it to the carrier as long as it is sent prior to the close of the calendar year following the year in which the service was provided. If the service was furnished in the last quarter of the year, the patient has until the close of the second year following the year in which the service was furnished to submit the claim. The patients and physicians under assignment receive an Explanation of Medicare Part B benefits. This details the action taken on the claim. The notice also shows what services were covered, what charges were approved, how much was credited toward the annual deductible, and the amount Medicare paid.

HCFA is also developing new statements called the Medicare Summary Notice (MSN). The MSN will list all claims filed during each month for each beneficiary. One notice will cover inpatient and outpatient facility services, another will include all Part B physician and other services, and a third will cover durable medical equipment (DME). The MSN will replace the Part A Medicare Benefits Notice, the EOMB and benefit denial letters. The new notices are being phased in over the next several years, though some Medicare contractors are already sending them to beneficiaries.

LOCAL VS. NATIONAL MEDICARE POLICY

Medicare carriers use both national and local policies to make medical coverage decisions. Early in 1995, HCFA updated the guidelines that carriers use to develop local medical review policy. A national coverage policy outlines Medicare coverage decisions that apply to all states and regions.

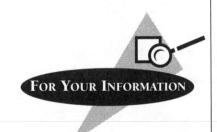

For Your Information

Medicare Summary Notice (MSN)
HCFA is developing this new statement which will list all claims filed during each month for each beneficiary.

National coverage policy indicates whether and under what circumstances items/services are covered. These policies are published in HCFA regulations in the *Federal Register*, contained in HCFA rulings, or issued as program memorandums, manual issuances to the *Coverage Issues Manual*, or the *Medicare Carriers Manual*.

A local medical review policy is used in the absence of a national coverage policy to identify local Medicare medical coverage decisions when needed. Developing local Medicare policy includes: creating a draft policy based upon review of medical literature, understanding local practice, soliciting comments from the medical community and Carrier Advisory Committee, responding to and incorporating comments into final local policy, and notifying providers of the policy effective date. It is the responsibility of the Carrier Medical Director, with assistance from carrier staff, to determine when a local policy is needed.

Here are the Medicare guidelines for the development of national and local medical review policy, as listed in the *Medicare Carriers Manual*, Section 7501.1 and part of 7501.2:

7501.1 NATIONAL COVERAGE POLICY

A. Definition National Coverage Policy — The primary authority for all coverage provisions is the statute. A national coverage policy is a statement of national policy regarding Medicare coverage which is:

- Published in HCFA regulations and the *Federal Register* as a final notice
- Contained in a HCFA ruling
- Issued as a program instruction, such as manual issuances in the *Coverage Issues Manual* or *Medicare Carriers Manual*

National coverage policy indicates whether and under what circumstances items/services are covered. Apply all pertinent statutory provisions, regulations, and national coverage policy when adjudicating claims.

When a national coverage policy indicates that a given item/service is covered under specific circumstances, cover the item/service under those circumstances. The authority and responsibility to interpret national coverage policy and apply them to individual cases are retained by the carrier. However, when making individual case determinations, no discretion is given to deviate from national policy if absolute words such as "never" or "only if" are used in the policy.

Requirements for prerequisite therapies listed in national coverage policy (e.g., "conservative treatment has been tried, but failed") must be adhered to when making decisions to cover an item/service.

When new national coverage policy is published, notify as soon as possible the provider community of the effective date. Do not solicit comments or in any way alter or revise the national coverage policy.

B. Statutory Exclusions From Coverage — The statutory authority for the majority of Medical Review is Section 1862(a)(1)(A) of the Act, which excludes coverage for "items or services that are not reasonable and necessary for the diagnosis or treatment of illness or injury or to improve the functioning of a malformed body member."

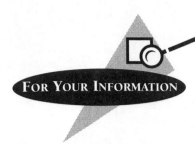

Medicare covers preventive services according to these limits:

- Pap smear — once every 3 years — once per year for high risk for cancer of the cervix — or an abnormal pap smear in preceeding 3 years

- Colorectal cancer screening — Fecal occult blood test (once per year) — Flexible sigmoidoscopy (once every 4 years), Coloposcopy (once every 2 years for high risk)

- Diabetes — glucose monitors, self-management training

- Medicare covers screening mammograms for the early detection of breast cancer. No doctor's order required. For 65 and over, Medicare covers one screening mammogram every two years. Age and risk determine frequency of mammogram for women under 65 covered by Medicare. Medicare does not cover screenings for women under 65. Medicare covers diagnostic mammograms when you show any signs of breast cancer

- Bone mass measures – varies with health status

- Hepatitis B for high risk

- Flu shots (once per year)

- Pneumococcal (one may cover life)

These are statutory exceptions to this exclusion which are specified in the full test of section 1862(a) for the following services:

- Hospice care, which is not reasonable and necessary for the palliation or management of terminal illness

- Screening mammography, which is performed more frequently than is covered

- Screening pap smear and screening pelvic exam, which is performed more frequently than is provided

- Prostate cancer screening tests which are performed more frequently than is covered

- Colorectal cancer screening tests, which are performed more frequently than is covered

- Frequency and duration of home health services which are in excess of normative guidelines

C. Least Costly Alternative — This national policy provision must be applied when determining payment for all durable medical equipment (DME). (See Section 2100.2.) The carrier has the discretion to apply this principle to payment for non-DME items and services as well.

7501.2 Local MR Policy (LMRP) — LMRPs are those policies which are used to make local medical coverage decisions. When needed and in the absence of a national coverage policy for a particular item/service, develop a LMRP to indicate whether the item/service is covered and under what clinical circumstances it is considered to be reasonable, necessary, and appropriate. The process for developing LMRP includes the development of draft policy based on review of medical literature and an understanding of local practice, soliciting comments from the medical community, including the Carrier Advisory Committee (CAC), responding to and incorporating comments into final policy, and notifying providers of the policy effective date. (See Section 7503.)

The carrier's LMRP must be clear, concise, and not restrict or conflict with national policy. If a national policy states that a given time is "covered for diagnoses/conditions A, B and C," this may not be used as a basis to develop LMRP to cover only "diagnoses/conditions A, B and C." When a national policy does not exclude coverage for other diagnoses/conditions, allow for individual consideration unless the LMRP supports automatic denial for some or all of those other diagnoses/conditions.

A. Identify Items/Services For Which a LMRP is Needed — It is the responsibility of the Carrier Medical Director (CMD), with assistance from staff, to determine when a LMRP is needed.

MEDICARE FEE SCHEDULE FOR PHYSICIANS

The reasonable charge payment method was based on historical charging patterns of physicians. In 1992, this payment method was replaced with the Medicare Fee Schedule (MFS). Under the MFS, payment allowables are determined through the application of relative value units (RVUs).

The MFS slows the rise in cost for services and standardizes payment to physicians regardless of specialty or location. Payments vary through geographic adjustments. Different payment for the same service performed by physicians of different specialties is eliminated.

Resource Based Relative Value Scale

The MFS is based on the Resource Based Relative Value Scale (RBRVS). A national total RVU is given for each procedure (HCPCS Level I (CPT), Level II national codes) provided by a physician.

Each total RVU has three components: physician work, practice expense, and malpractice insurance.

The physician work RVUs were produced from Harvard University studies under a cooperative agreement with HCFA. The practice expense and malpractice RVUs were developed by applying historical practice cost percentages to a base allowed charge for each service taken from historical Medicare charges.

HCFA has supplied Medicare final rules for the practice expense RVU in the November 2, 1998 Federal Register. Under the new Medicare payment rule, physician fees will increase an average of 2.9 percent in 1999. The January 1, 1999 implementation date is the first year in a four-year transition to resource-based practice expense payments. The 1999 practice expense relative value unit will be 75 percent of 1998 charge-based relative value units and 25 percent of resource-based units. The percentages will shift to 50/50 in the year 2000, and to 25/75 in 2001. Practice-expense payments will be fully resource-based in 2002. Practice expense payments amount to about $20 billion and account for more than 40 percent of payments each year under the fee schedule.

Geographic Adjustment Factor

HCFA's Geographic Adjustment Factors consist of an index called the Geographic Practice Cost Index (GPCI). The 89 Medicare localities have three specific GPCIs – one each for physician work, practice expense, and malpractice.

GPCIs measure the differences in physician costs for practice expenses and malpractice insurance in geographic localities compared to a national average. The GPCI for physician work measures one-fourth of the difference between the relative value of a physician's work effort in each of the different areas and the national average. The locality GPCI is used to adjust the national RVU.

Conversion Factor

The conversion factor is the national multiplier that converts the geographically adjusted relative value units into MFS dollar amounts and applies to all services paid under the MFS. Once the national RVU is GPCI-adjusted for the location, the total RVU is multiplied by the national conversion factor.

The conversion factor is used to make national adjustments and yearly updates to Medicare payment. The conversion factor for 1999 is $34.73.

SITE-OF-SERVICE DIFFERENTIAL

In 1996, HCFA extended the site-of-service differential to office-based services on the Ambulatory Surgical Center (ASC) list if those services are performed in an ASC or hospital setting. The practice expense RVU for a procedure that is furnished outside the office is reduced by 50 percent. In 1997, HCFA is providing two types of practice expense: one for "non-facility" (physician's office) and one for "facility" (hospital outpatient department) eliminating carrier calculation of the reduction.

PROVIDER-BASED AND TEACHING PHYSICIANS

Medicare does not cover a service provided by a resident without the presence of the attending physician. If an attending physician is physically present when a resident performs a service, however, payment may be made for the physician's fees. Medicare payment is the same whether the physician performs the service or the resident performs the service in the presence of an

Medicare Fee Schedule (MFS) slows the rise in cost for services and standardizes payment to physicians regardless of specialty or location.

Resource Based Relative Value Scale (RBRVS) The MFS is based on the Resource Based Relative Value Scale (RBRVS). A national total relative value unit (RVU) is given for each procedure provided by a physician. Each total RVU has three components: physician work, practice expense, and malpractice insurance.

attending physician. Services performed by provider-based and teaching physicians are reimbursed under the same regulations as other physicians under the MFS.

These are Medicare's definitions:

- Resident — an individual who participates in an approved graduate medical education program or a physician who is not in an approved GME program but who is authorized to practice only in a hospital setting.

- Teaching hospital — hospital engaged in an approved GME residency program in medicine, osteopathy, dentistry, or podiatry.

- Teaching physician — physician — other than the resident — who involves residents in the care of his or her patients.

MEDICARE INPATIENT PAYMENT

Payment for Medicare recipients receiving inpatient care is based on a prospective payment system. Reimbursement depends on ICD-9-CM diagnosis and procedure codes that make up 511 Diagnosis Related Groups (DRGs). See chapters 1 and 9 of *Code It Right* for information on coding inpatient services based on DRG payment.

OTHER RBRVS CONTRACTS

Two types of contracts are especially popular with payors today — RBRVS and capitation. The following discussion provides a better understanding of some of the advantages and disadvantages of non-Medicare RBRVS contracts.

RBRVS

RBRVS, adopted by HCFA for computation of the MFS, is used by payors to establish their own fee schedules for contracting with providers. Up to 75 percent of non-Medicare payors are currently or will soon be using RBRVS. While many payors establish their own conversion factors for RBRVS (often higher than Medicare's), others use the Medicare conversion factors. How this new wave of payor contracting might affect your practice depends on how prepared you are when RBRVS comes knocking at your door.

The use of RBRVS by non-Medicare payors has been in two forms. Each has its own set of rewards or drawbacks for the provider or payor side. The advantages and disadvantages can be seen in the following discussion.

The RBRVS Fee Schedule — Payor or Medicare's Conversion Factor
Advantages
Payor
- RBRVS methodology is resource based and used to compute the Medicare Fee Schedule.
- Published and updated in the *Federal Register*, the fee schedule can be accessed through the GPO website.
- Comparison with existing fee schedules is relatively simple, although comparison is time consuming it is well worth the effort, especially for large payors.
- It adapts easily to a spreadsheet format so that different conversion factors can be inserted and changed as necessary, depending upon specialty and other factors.

- More contracts using the same fee schedule allow easier access when trying to locate specialty-specific conversion factors in databases. A significant amount of time is saved over dealing with several different fee schedules and conversion factors.

- It can be used as a national fee schedule (instead of just in a local area).

Provider

- A fee schedule that is familiar to providers and is currently used by Medicare for compensation.

- Published and updated in the *Federal Register*, the fee schedule is easy to access for a reasonable fee.

- Comparison with a provider's current fee schedule is relatively simple if the provider has the personnel to do the work (or, an RBRVS conversion can be purchased). However, some conversion will be necessary with any product.

- The fee schedule can be updated by the provider quickly, especially if entered into a spreadsheet format.

- It is advantageous to a provider when most contracts are based on the same fee schedule by making it easier to compare reimbursement from various payors and to assign an equitable conversion factor.

Disadvantages

Payor

- Providers may be suspicious of the fee schedule if they do not have the time and resources available to do fee schedule comparisons.

- Questions from providers about the compensation and coding rules associated with the Medicare RBRVS fee schedule may slow down the processing of claims.

- It is difficult to get providers to accept RBRVS if the Medicare conversion factor is used because of the low reimbursement rate.

- Providers who do accept the fee schedule may believe they are being inadequately reimbursed and have bad feelings about the payor when asked to accept Medicare rates, especially if they are in an area where an HMO has a large member base. Providers may believe they are forced to accept the Medicare rate, or wind up without enough patients to keep their practice viable.

Provider

- Providers may not have personnel available for the time required to do the fee schedule comparison.

- The negotiated contract may only be updated yearly and, depending upon the payor, may be late in being updated (even though Medicare publishes quarterly updates).

- Providers seldom have the resources (e.g., information) that large payors have, such as the average conversion factor for a given specialty in a community. Thus, providers do not know where they stand in relationship to other providers in the same specialty and are often left with taking the payor's word that the proposed reimbursement rate is fair.

- Providers believe that if payors base fee schedules on the MFS they should also adopt Medicare's payment guidelines. Otherwise, providers may believe that payors are not only reimbursing at a low rate, but that they are also taking advantage of old global surgery and other rules which further discount the services providers perform. They do not necessarily understand that RBRVS is a relative value study and was adopted by Medicare; the fee

KEY POINT

Initially, payors may have set up RBRVS fee schedules to compare prices with Medicare; the price comparison was often used to detect possible cost-shifting by providers as Medicare started using RBRVS methodology. But it didn't take long for payors to realize that RBRVS spelled the opportunity for a low cost, easily accessed and converted relative value study legislated for use by one of the country's largest payors — Medicare.

schedule did not have Medicare's coding guidelines with it. They were added after for their own use.

- Primary care and other providers with RBRVS contracts based totally on Medicare, including the Medicare conversion factor, may believe that they should also be able to utilize Medicare's payment guidelines, especially those that deal with modifiers and the global surgery rule.

How To Convert A Fee Schedule To RBRVS

Chances are good that many contracts offered in the future will be based on RBRVS. Healthcare providers are advised to assure they are adequately compensated by having a RBRVS "crosswalk" in place.

RBRVS Crosswalk

A crosswalk is one method to determine how a practice might be affected by an RBRVS contract. It allows providers to compare fees between the type of fee schedule they are using now and one based on RBRVS. The best way to make the comparison is to enter the current fee schedule in a software spreadsheet program, then add other columns with RBRVS data and compare them. Current contracted fee rates can be added to allow an overall comparison to RBRVS. Use column A to represent the code, column B the code description, and column C the MFS relative value units (read carefully to include all of the factors built into the relative value units (e.g., work, etc.). Leave column D blank to insert a conversion factor. In column E, insert the present fee for service rate (rounded to the nearest dollar). To arrive at the conversion factor, divide the fee in column E by the MFS/RVUs.

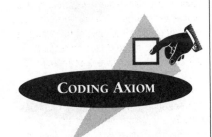

Example

A	B	C	D	E
Code	Code Desc.	MFS/RVUs	Conv. Factor	Your Fee
99201	OFF/OUTPT EXAM	.86	72.15	$62
99202	OFF/OUTPT EXAM	1.38	72.80	$100
99203	OFF/OUTPT EXAM	1.92	72.68	$140
99211	OFF/OUTPT EXAM	.38	73.69	$28
99212	OFF/OUTPT EXAM	.75	72.06	$54
99213	OFF/OUTPT EXAM	1.08	72.92	$79

At this point, unused columns to the right of your fee can be used to list other contracts. Leave a blank column (column F) to figure the conversion factor; be sure to enter the same code for the contract you are checking. In column G list the payor contract fee, then divide the fee by the MFS/RVUs to fill in column F. To find the percentage being paid at the contract rate divide your fee by the payor contract fee. In the example listed below, payment would be at 75 percent of your fee for service charge.

To find the percentage you are paid per contract over what you charge:

A	F	G	H
Code	Conv. Factor	Payor Contract Fee	% Contract Payment
99201	54.43	$43	75%

MEDICARE PAYMENT ADVISORY COMMISSION

The Medicare Payment Advisory Commission (MEDPAC) was established under the Balanced Budget Act of 1997 to assume advisory and other functions of the Prospective Payment Assessment Commission (ProPAC) and the Physician Payment Review Commission (PPRC). MEDPAC was set up to study fee-for-service and hospital prospective payment issues and review and make recommendations on Medicare+Choice capitated care plans.

CODING MEDICARE CLAIMS

All claims submitted to Medicare require diagnostic (ICD-9-CM) codes. Claims for certain services, especially when local policy has been established, may be denied based on diagnosis, so correct code selection is important. In the next several years, the current system will be replaced by the clinically modified ICD-10. Information about the new system is available from the National Center of Health Statistics (NCHS), which is a department under the Centers for Disease Control (CDC). You may also want to refer to Medicode's new publication, "*ICD•10 Made Easy.*"

Inpatient Claims

Inpatient claims for Medicare recipients are coded according to coding rules listed in the *Code It Right* chapters on ICD-9-CM coding. The claims are grouped into of the 511 DRGs and submitted for reimbursement.

Outpatient Physician Claims

Outpatient physician procedures are coding using HCPCS Level I (CPT) codes and Level II national codes (A through V). Local codes (W through Z) should be used when individual carriers have assigned them. Follow CPT coding rules and append Medicare and CPT modifiers to codes as appropriate.

Outpatient Hospital Claims

Use the annotated version of CPT for Hospital Outpatient Services to code outpatient hospital services. Check the new 1999 modifiers as they apply to payment for approved "Ambulatory Surgical Center (ASC).

Know the Rules for Filing Claims

Use caution when applying CPT codes to Medicare claims. HCFA's correct coding initiative (CCI) provides edits that determine the appropriateness of CPT code combinations for Medicare claims. Many of these edits are designed to detect "fragmentation" or separate coding of the component parts of a procedure, instead of reporting single codes that include the entire procedure.

Also, pay attention to the rules for completing the proper claims forms. The HCFA-1500 is the standard claims form for filing Part B claims. HCFA is currently working with the National Claim Committee to revise the HCFA-1500, due to the requirements of a changing century. HCFA now requires 8-digit birth dates on the form (the patient's birth date, other insured's date of birth, and the insured's date of birth). Carriers must convert the other dates to the 8-digit requirement. Claims without the 8-digit dates will be returned. The reasoning is simple. Date-related transactions occur millions of times a day as HCFA processes nearly a billion claims for its 38 million Medicare beneficiaries in a year. Many computers use just two digits to record the year. If not fixed, these computers will recognize "00" as 1900. Those who depend on HCFA for healthcare coverage and hundreds of thousands of healthcare providers could have cash flow problems because of delayed Medicare payments.

KEY POINT

HCFA's Correct Coding Initiative
Implemented January 1, 1996, the goal of HCFA's Correct Coding Initiative is to identify and eliminate the incorrect coding of medical services. The initiative installs a new set of edits into each of the Medicare carriers' automated claims processing systems. Due to copyright issues, carriers cannot publish the tables of codes. Carriers can only publish corrections to the Correct Coding Initiative tables. Code specific chapters only include correct coding edits. The mutually exclusive code combinations are listed in the General Coding Policies section.

NATIONAL PROVIDER IDENTIFIER

Health plans assign identification numbers to healthcare providers — individuals, groups, or organizations that provide medical or other health services or supplies. The result is that providers who do business with multiple health plans have multiple identification numbers. To simplify the system, HCFA has established a new system — National Provider Identification (NPI) — for healthcare providers that will be used by all health plans. The NPI is an 8-position alphanumeric identifier. The eighth position is a check digit that can help detect keying errors. It contains no embedded intelligence; that is, it contains no information about the healthcare provider such as the type of healthcare provider or State where the healthcare provider is located.

Healthcare providers and all health plans and healthcare clearinghouses will use the NPIs in the administrative and financial transactions specified by the Health Insurance Portability and Accountability Act. HIPAA mandates standards for the electronic transmission of healthcare information, which includes the national identifier.

According to HCFA, the use of a standard, unique provider identifier would enhance the campaign against fraud and abuse in healthcare programs. HCFA identifies the following benefits:

- Payments for excessive or fraudulent claims can be reduced by standardizing enumeration, which would facilitate sharing information across programs or across different parts of the same program.
- A healthcare provider's identifier would not change with moves or changes in specialty. This facilitates tracking of fraudulent healthcare providers over time and across geographic areas.
- A healthcare provider would receive only one identifier and would not be able to receive duplicate payments from a program by submitting claims under multiple provider identifiers.

The NPI program would affect health plans according to their size and the date the final rule is published in the *Federal Register*:

- Small health plan must comply with the requirements of 36 months after the effective date of the final rule
- Larger health plans must comply with the requirements 24 months after the effective date of the final rule
- Healthcare clearinghouse and healthcare provider must begin using the standard 24 months after the effective date of the final rule

COMMON WORKING FILE

While most providers will never come into direct contact with Medicare's Common Working File (CWF), it is important to understand what HCFA expects to accomplish with this system.

HCFA has traditionally maintained centralized files on each Medicare beneficiary. Medicare carriers and intermediaries query this file before making claims payments. The CWF divides this centralized file into nine regional hosts who contract with the government to maintain and operate the system much like Medicare carriers and intermediaries.

Once Medicare claims pass through carrier and intermediary processing and are ready to be finalized, the claims are transmitted to CWF, which edits for validity, entitlement, remaining

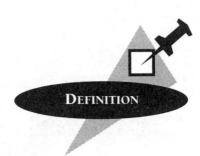

benefits, and deductible status. Approval or rejection is transmitted back to the processor within 24 hours. This shortened response time means claims are paid more quickly.

Objectives of Common Working File
With CWF, HCFA can study effects of Medicare program changes more readily. Objectives include:

- Complete beneficiary entitlement, utilization, and specific claims history
- Information quickly to Medicare carriers and intermediaries
- Part A and Part B claim comparisons to prevent overpayments, duplicate payments, and payment for noncovered services
- Curbing of payment for unnecessary services through prepayment claims edit screens
- Detection of Medicare Secondary Payor claims
- Volume tracking to gauge the Medicare Volume Performance Standard
- Future Medicare information tracking and evaluation of program changes
- A centrally managed database for research and policy development

DISCUSSION QUESTIONS

1. Explain the difference between Medicare Part A intermediaries and Part B carriers.

_____

_____

_____

2. Explain the criteria for establishing Medicare as the secondary payor.

_____

_____

_____

3. What is the difference between a claim that is "assigned" versus a claim that is "unassigned"?

_____

_____

_____

4. The HCFA-1500 form must be revised for the change in century. What has HCFA done to accommodate claims submission in the year 2000?

_____

_____

_____

5. What is the NPI and who does it affect?

_____

_____

_____

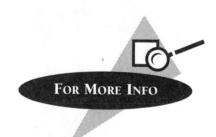

For information on *CPT For Hospital Outpatient Services*, contact:

The Department of Coding & Nomenclature
American Medical Association
515 North State Street
Chicago, Illinois 60610
1-800-621-8335

Medicare claims may be submitted electronically. For more information, contact your local carrier.

Medicare Special Coding Information

Medicare guidelines affect specific areas of CPT and ICD-9-CM coding. The following is an explanation of some of Medicare's special coding circumstances. ICD-9-CM is listed first. The information is then listed in the same order as CPT: evaluation and management, anesthesia, surgery, radiology, pathology and laboratory, and medicine. Information on Medicare-specific rules applying to modifiers is listed after the CPT sections; consult CPT section guidelines to determine if a modifier is applicable to a particular section. To compare CPT and Medicare modifier guidelines consult Chapter 2 *CPT Introduction and Modifiers* and Chapter 10 *HCPCS*.

ICD-9-CM

All physician specialties and all nonphysician practitioners must provide diagnostic codes for physician services. Payment for Medicare recipients receiving inpatient care is based on the PPS. Reimbursement depends on ICD-9-CM diagnosis and procedure codes that make up 511 Diagnosis Related Groups (DRGs). See chapters 1 and 9 of *Code It Right* for information on coding inpatient services based on DRG payment methodology.

EVALUATION AND MANAGEMENT

In 1997, E/M documentation guidelines were revised by the American Medical Association (AMA), which holds the copyright to CPT, and HCFA, the federal agency that controls Medicare and Medicaid spending. Their attempt to simplify E/M coding, however, did not come to fruition by the anticipated effective date due to widespread physician dissatisfaction regarding the revisions. For example, HCFA advocated adding formulas and values to elements in the medical record to ensure consistency in medical review and payment. The AMA House of Delegates, however, continues to reject documentation that requires formulas or counting.

As of this publication, HCFA was determined to develop new guidelines to replace the 1995 and 1997 versions now used by carriers to review claims. The federal agency acknowledges AMA opposition to counting and numerical values, but insists that the formulas are necessary to assure consistent interpretation by Medicare carriers. HCFA plans to use the new framework developed in conjunction with medical professionals as the starting point for the new set of guidelines. Documentation will require counting and numerical values and HCFA has stated that it will test the guidelines and educate physicians and Medicare carriers prior to full implementation. No date has been set, though they could be ready in draft by Spring 1999. Until formal adoption, Medicare carriers are to use either the 1995 or 1997 guidelines, depending upon which set is more advantageous to the physician.

Medicare and Critical Care

Medicare clarified its policy for the use of critical care codes (99291–99292). Critical care includes the care of patients who might not be in a "medical emergency" but who nonetheless require constant physician attention because they are unstable and critically ill, or unstable and critically injured. The care of such patients involves decision-making of high complexity to assess, manipulate, and support circulatory, respiratory, central nervous, metabolic, or other vital system functions to prevent or treat single or multiple vital organ system failure. The management of the patient often requires extensive interpretation of multiple databases and the application of advanced technology.

This expanded definition does not mean that the care of a patient in a critical care, intensive care, or other specialized care unit should be reported with the critical care codes. In such a unit, the

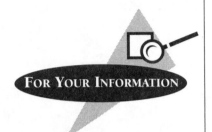

FOR YOUR INFORMATION

HCFA continues to work on the documentation guidelines for evaluation and management services. A draft may be ready by Spring 1999, but until that time physicians are advised to apply either the 1995 or 1997 guidelines. Preference depends on the advantage to the respective physician.

care of a patient who is not unstable and critically injured is reported using the appropriate subsequent hospital care code (99231–99233) or inpatient consultation code (99251–99263).

"Constant Attendance" as a Prerequisite for Use of Critical Care Codes

There are no absolute limits on the amount of critical care services that can be reported per day or per hospital. A physician must be prepared to demonstrate that the service billed meets the definition of critical care. Medicare may request documentation for cases in which it is implausible that the amount of critical care billed was provided (e.g., more than a total of 12 hours of critical care billed by the physician for one or more patients on the same day).

Critical Care and Aftercare Days

Critical care cannot be paid on the day the physician also bills a procedure code with a global surgical period. The exception to this is when the critical care is billed with modifier -25 to indicate that the critical care is a significant, separately identifiable E/M service that is above and beyond the usually pre- and postoperative care associated with the procedure that is performed.

If denials for critical care are occurring, they may relate to a misunderstanding of what services are included or bundled into critical care. Prior to 1993, the CPT definition of critical care bundled a number of fairly significant procedures into the critical care codes, including endotracheal intubation and placement of catheters. At that time, it would have been consistent, with the CPT definition, for Medicare to deny payment for those procedures when they were billed on the same date as the critical care codes. However, beginning in 1993 the CPT definition of critical care was revised, and HCFA assigned relative value units to the critical care codes to be consistent with the revised definition.

Hospital Observation Services

A physician may report the hospital observation codes (99217–99220) when (1) a physician who admits the patient to hospital observation and is responsible for the patient's care during the stay in observation, or (2) a physician who does not have inpatient admitting privileges but it authorized to admit a patient to observation. The physician should report only the initial hospital care code when a patient is admitted to the hospital on the same day the patient was admitted for observation (99234–99236). The care code should include the services related to observation services provided. These codes are covered by a global surgical fee unless the attending physician appends modifier -57 for consultation that leads to the surgery.

Physicians reporting observation codes must maintain an observation record with dated and timed admitting orders, nursing notes, and progress notes prepared by the physician while the patient was in observation status.

Only the observation care code may be reported if the patient is discharged on the same day the patient was admitted to observation status. For patients remaining in observation status after the first night's count and discharged the next day, the physician must report 99217.

The physician must report an initial hospital visit for any E/M services provided when a patient is admitted to inpatient status from observation status on the same day. Medicare payment for the initial hospital visit includes all services provided by that physician on the date of admission, regardless of site of service.

Typically, the global surgical fee includes payment for hospital observation services and any additional payments can be made only if (1) the hospital observation services can be reported

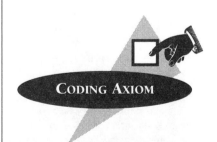

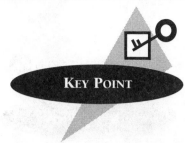

HCFA has revised their policy to permit the physician to bill the patient for the noncovered part of the visit. To bill for this service properly you must:

- Determine your usual fee for the noncovered, routine physical examination

- Determine your fee for the covered portion of the examination (nonparticipating physicians use their limiting charge)

- Bill the covered portion using the appropriate E/M visit code (99201–99215) and charge (nonparticipating physicians use their limiting charge)

- Bill the balance (the difference between the noncovered and covered fees) using the preventive medicine codes (99381–99397)

- When a service is not reasonable or necessary, a beneficiary may have liability waived. The beneficiary will be liable, however, if the beneficiary has received in advance written notice of noncoverage. This is called an advanced beneficiary notice (ABN).

Consultation (Clinical Pathology)

Note the following guidelines for Medicare and consultations:

1. The clinical pathology consultation must be requested by the patient's attending physician and there must be specific documentation in the medical record.

2. The clinical pathology consultation must relate to test results that lie outside the clinically significant normal or expected range in view of the patient's condition.

3. The results of the clinical pathology consultation must result in a written narrative report, which is included in the patient's medical record.

4. Require the "exercise of medical judgment" by the consulting physician.

5. Routine conversations a laboratory director may have with an attending physician about test orders or results are not a consultation unless the four preceding requirements are met.

with modifier -24, -25, or -57; and (2) the observation services provided by the surgeon meet all criteria for the code reported.

Consultations

For a service to qualify as a consultation, there must be a formal request made by the attending physician. Also, the purpose of the request must be to obtain an opinion or advice regarding the evaluation and/or management of a specific problem.

Services provided by a physician who was "recommended" to a patient by his or her family doctor do not qualify as a consultation. This would include a situation in which a patient desires an additional physician or a specialist and seeks a referral from the doctor. Additionally, a service performed solely on the basis of a "request for consultation" by the patient does not constitute a consultation.

Prolonged Services

Under Medicare rules, physician standby services (99360) are considered hospital services and are not payable under the physician fee schedule. No RVUs are assigned to 99360.

CARE PLAN OVERSIGHT SERVICES

Home Health Agencies

According to Medicare guidelines, a home health beneficiary must be confined to the home and under the care of a physician who has established a care plan that is periodically reviewed. Or, the beneficiary must demonstrate the need for skilled nursing care, or physical, speech-language, and occupational therapy.

Home health agencies are responsible for services that include part-time or intermittent skilled nursing care, part-time home health aide services, medical supplies, durable medical equipment, and medical social services. Speech-language, occupational and physical therapy may be provided as specified in the patient's care plan.

Hospice

Medicare covers hospice services for two initial 90-day periods followed by an unlimited number of subsequent 60-day periods. A physician must certify that the patient has a terminal illness with a prognosis that the individual's life expectancy is six months or less. A person who is discharged from hospice care because he or she is no longer terminally ill may use the same services later if the patient again develops a terminal illness.

Reimbursement

Medicare does not allow separate payments for case management services a physician provides to patients in a nursing facility or under home health or hospice care. The physician is paid according to a global fee. The exception for payment applies to therapy provided on a recurring basis as part of the care plan. These services are billed to the Part B carrier and reimbursed according to the fee schedule. Assignment is mandatory.

Preventive Medicine Services

Medicare policy dictates that when a physician schedules both a routine physical examination (preventive service) and a Medicare-covered service (E/M service) during the same office visit, the covered service is payable but the routine service is not. Under Medicare policy, you are not required to give the beneficiary written advance notice of noncoverage.

ANESTHESIA

Physician anesthesia services are included under the physician fee schedule but are paid under a different payment methodology. The methodology uses a separate conversion factor and allowable base and time units. Physician anesthesia services do not have practice expense and malpractice expense RVUs.

Medicare pays for medical and surgical services furnished by an anesthesiologist if rebundling provisions do not preclude separate payment. The services may be furnished in conjunction with the anesthesia procedure or as single services, e.g., during the day of or the day before the anesthesia service. These services include the insertion of a Swan Ganz catheter, the insertion of central venous pressure lines, emergency intubation, and critical care visits.

Medicare and Multiple Anesthesia Procedures

Medicare pays for anesthesia services associated with multiple surgical procedures or multiple bilateral procedures. Payment is determined based on the base unit of the anesthesia procedure with the highest base unit value and time units based on the actual anesthesia time of the multiple procedures.

Most anesthesiologists utilize base units from the ASA *Relative Value Guide*; other relative value guides may differ significantly in the amount of base units — as much as three or more units difference — in the same codes. How this affects reimbursement depends upon how time units and other factors are calculated in a given area.

Medicare Policy for Time Units

Currently, Medicare calculates one anesthesia time unit equivalent to 15 minutes when a physician personally performs an anesthesia procedure. Less than 15 minutes of anesthesia, in total or as part of the total anesthesia time, is converted to a fraction of 1 time unit (e.g., 12 minutes of anesthesia equals .8 time units).

For services furnished in 1997, both the physician medical direction allowance and the medically directed CRNA allowance has been calculated at 52.5 percent of the allowance that was recognized if an anesthesiologist performs the procedure.

Time units involve the continuous presence of the physician (or of the medically directed qualified anesthetist or resident) and start when the anesthesiologist begins preparing the patient for anesthesia care. Time units end when the anesthesiologist (or medically directed CRNA) is no longer in personal attendance and the patient may be safely placed under postoperative care.

Medicare Policy for Modifying Units

Medicare does not allow additional unit values for physical status modifiers or qualifying circumstances (OBRA '89). Other ASA/CPT anesthesia modifiers are usually recognized by Medicare carriers, but no additional value is allowed.

SURGERY

Global Surgery and Medicare Preoperative Care

The surgeon's initial evaluation or consultation to determine the necessity for major surgery is not considered part of the global payment; a separate allowance is made. Modifier -57 has been created to identify when the surgical decision is made. Once decided, preoperative visits for care of the surgical problem, other than the initial evaluation, are usually included in the surgical

KEY POINT

The following anesthesia modifiers are currently recognized by HCFA:

-AA Anesthesia services performed personally by anesthesiologist

-AB Medical direction of own employee(s) by anesthesiologist (not more than four employees)

-AC Medical direction of other than own employee(s) by anesthesiologist (not more than four individuals)

-AD Medical supervision by a physician: more than four concurrent anesthesia procedures

-AE Direction of residents in furnishing not more than two concurrent anesthesia services — attending physician relationship met

-AF Anesthesia complicated by total body hypothermia

-AG Anesthesia for emergency surgery on a patient who is moribund or who has an incapacitating systemic disease that is a constant threat to life (may warrant additional charge)

-QK Medical direction of two, three, or four concurrent anesthesia procedures involving qualified individuals

-QS Monitored anesthesiology care services (CRNA or physician; informational only)

-QX CRNA with medical direction by physician

-QZ CRNA without medical direction by physician

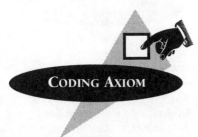

Medicare's policy defines the postoperative period for nearly all major surgical services as 90 days following the date of surgery. Minor surgeries have either a zero or 10-day postoperative follow-up period.

package. Preoperative visits for care of the surgical problem other than the initial evaluation beginning one day prior to surgery, regardless of location, are included in the surgical fee.

Postoperative Care

Medicare's position on unrelated problems is unchanged. When a patient is seen during the postoperative period for an unrelated problem, services such as the following are paid separately:

- Services of other physicians except where there is an agreed upon transfer of care. This agreement may be in the form of a letter or an annotation in the discharge summary, hospital record, or ASC record.

- Visits unrelated to the diagnosis for which the surgical procedure is performed, unless the visits occur due to complications of the surgery.

- Treatment for the underlying condition or an added course of treatment that is not part of normal recovery from surgery.

- Diagnostic tests and procedures, including diagnostic radiological procedures.

- Clearly distinct surgical procedures during the postoperative period that are not re-operations or treatment for complications. (A new postoperative period begins with the subsequent procedure.) This includes procedures done in two or more parts for which the decision to stage the procedure is made prospectively or at the time of the first procedure. Examples of this are procedures to diagnose and treat epilepsy (61533, 61534–61536, 61539, 61541, and 61543), which may be performed in succession within 90 days of each other.

- Treatment for postoperative complications that requires a return trip to the operating room (OR). An OR in this instance is defined as a place of service specifically equipped and staffed for the sole purpose of performing procedures. The term includes a cardiac catheterization suite, laser suite, treatment room, recovery room, or an intensive care unit (unless the patient's condition was so critical that there is insufficient time for transportation to an OR).

- If a less extensive procedure fails, and a more extensive procedure is required, the second procedure is payable separately.

- Certain services performed in a physician's office requiring use of a surgical tray. Splints and casting supplies are also payable separately under the reasonable charge payment methodology.

- Immunosuppressive therapy for organ transplants.

- Critical care services (99291 and 99292) unrelated to the surgery when a seriously injured or burned patient is critically ill and requires constant attendance of the physician.

Complications

Medicare allows reimbursement for postoperative complications requiring a return trip to the operating room. These services are denoted with modifier -78 *Return to the operating room for a related procedure during the postoperative period.* The payment level for these "re-operations" for complication is set at the value of the intra-operative portion of the procedure described by the CPT code. If there is no code, payment cannot exceed 50 percent of the intra-operative portion of the service originally performed.

Medicare and Minor Procedures

"Starred" procedures as well as some diagnostic and therapeutic endoscopy procedures are included in this list

Same-Day Evaluation or Consultation

Same-day services are included unless they are unrelated to, or can be identified separately from, the procedure.

Postoperative Care

Minor surgeries have either a zero- or a 10-day postoperative follow-up period. Those with 10-day periods include all services related to the recovery from surgery. Other services during that period, whether for the underlying condition or for an unrelated condition, are paid separately.

Medicare Endoscopy

Special payment rules apply when multiple endoscopy procedures are rendered at the same session. HCFA has identified "families" of related endoscopies and has developed a "base" endoscopy for each family.

Payment for multiple related endoscopies is determined as follows: 100 percent for the primary endoscopy plus the difference between the Medicare Fee Schedule amount for the next highest procedure and the base endoscopy amount. No payment is made for a secondary procedure if the base procedure has a higher value. This payment adjustment applies only when the related multiple procedures are performed through the same orifice. Medicare will not pay for any portion of a diagnostic procedure when it is reimbursing for other secondary surgical procedures performed through the same orifice and at the same time.

Special reimbursement rules apply to multiple endoscopic procedures. The payment for multiple procedures depends upon the endoscopic procedures performed on one day.

"Stand alone" endoscopy procedures (procedures that do not have a base code) and single endoscopy procedures from several different code families are reimbursed under the multiple surgery guidelines at 100 percent for the first endoscopy procedure, 50 percent for the second through fifth procedures. Subsequent procedures are "by report."

Example Medicare's payment rules

In the course of performing a fiberoptic colonoscopy (45378), a physician performs a biopsy on a lesion (45380) and removes a polyp (45385) from a different part of the colon. The physician reports 45380 and 45385. Codes 45380 and 45385 both have the value of the diagnostic colonoscopy (45378) built in. Rather than paying 100 percent for the highest valued procedure (45385) and 50 percent for the next (45380), the full value of the higher valued endoscopy (45385) is paid, plus the difference between the next highest endoscopy (45380) and the base endoscopy (45378).

Assume the following fee schedule amounts for these codes:

45385	=	$374.56 (Not on base list, pay at full value)
45378	=	$255.40
Plus		
45380	=	$285.98
		$ 30.58

(On base list, pay difference between 45378 and 45380)
Total payment　　　= $405.14
(Full value for 45385 plus difference between 45378 and 45380)

Medicare's Supply Policy

Medicare makes no special allowance for supplies routinely furnished in the course of patient care in the office. Included are supplies used in laceration repairs and when administering chemotherapy. Chemotherapy drugs, however, are not considered routine supplies. Splints, casting supplies, and surgical dressings are allowed separately.

Exceptions are made for certain expensive, and mostly disposable, supplies used in the performance of facility-based procedures in a physician's office. Offices should obtain a copy of the facility-based national list, including bunion correction, endoscopy (esophagus, upper GI, and operative upper GI), colonoscopy, and several others. When the physician performs one of these procedures in the office, report A4550.

Medicare's reimbursement for A4550 is limited and does not offer much of a financial advantage to the physician. In deciding whether to provide these services, consider the convenience factor as well as the proportions of your practice that are Medicare and non-Medicare. Private payors may be more liberal in their allowance for surgical supplies.

Physicians may receive separate reimbursement for A4263 *Permanent, long-term, nondissolvable lacrimal duct implant, each* when reported with 68761.

Reimbursement may also be made for A4300 *Implantable access portal/catheter* (venous, arterial, epidural, or peritoneal) when reported with 36533.

Medicare's Policy Claims for Multiple Surgeries

Cosurgeons, surgical teams, or assistants at surgery may participate in performing multiple surgeries on the same patient on the same day.

Medicare will pay the lesser of the actual charge or 100 percent of the fee schedule amount for the highest priced procedure. Payment for the second through fifth procedures is based on the lesser of the actual charge or 50 percent of the fee schedule amount. Surgical procedures beyond the fifth procedure continue to be "by report" and payments based on documentation of the services performed.

Medicare and Starred Procedures

Medicare generally views starred procedures as minor surgeries which are not traditionally paid using a global surgery policy. Medicare does not recognize the CPT starred procedure.

Medicare and Surgical Destruction

Medicare recognizes the use of lasers for many medical indications. In the absence of a specific noncoverage instruction, and where a laser has been approved for marketing by the Food and Drug Administration, the contractor must determine whether a laser procedure is reasonable and necessary and, consequently, covered.

RADIOLOGY

Medicare Bilateral Radiology Procedures

Under Medicare, the bilateral concept and payment for radiology procedures are not subject to the special payment rules for bilateral surgeries (paid at 150 percent). A different bilateral concept is applied to radiology.

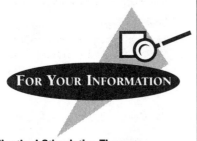

FOR YOUR INFORMATION

Electical Stimulation Therapy
The cost of treatment to promote healing of open wounds by means of electical stimulation therapy qualifies for Medicare reimbursement.

Bilateral Codes

Bilateral payment may be inappropriate for codes because: (1) of physiology or anatomy, or (2) the code description specifically states that it is a unilateral procedure and there is an existing code for the bilateral procedure.

Billing for a Purchased Technical Component

Medicare law does not allow a provider to mark up the cost of a purchased diagnostic test. Accordingly, when physicians bill for diagnostic tests they did not perform or supervise, Medicare pays the lower of (1) the actual acquisition cost including any discount, or (2) the physician fee schedule amount for the test. The billing physician must identify the supplier, the supplier's provider number, and the amount the supplier charged. No payment may be made to the physician without this information unless the statement "No purchased tests are included" is noted on the claims. Most Medicare carriers have local Level III modifiers (available from your carrier) assigned to designate this situation.

PATHOLOGY AND LABORATORY

Laboratory Tests

When a group of laboratory tests is performed on automated equipment, it is generally called "multichannel testing." Groups of automated tests are classified as "panels" or "profiles." The Pathology and Laboratory section of the CPT provided, under "automated, multichannel tests," a list of 19 chemistry tests that were frequently performed on automated equipment, and HCFA identified three additional, related tests. When these tests were performed as groups or in combinations ("profiles"), codes were assigned to the group to reflect the number of tests actually performed (CPT Codes 80002–80019, HCPCS Codes G0058–G0060). In addition, the CPT lists "Organ or Disease Oriented Panels." The tests listed under each panel (e.g., Lipid Panel, Code 80061) identify the defined components of that panel.

The 1998 edition of the CPT manual eliminated the multichannel test codes and replaced them with three new and one revised Organ or Disease Oriented laboratory panels: the electrolyte panel (CPT 80051), the hepatic function panel (CPT 80058), the basic metabolic panel (CPT 80049), and the comprehensive metabolic panel (CPT 80054).

According to HCFA guidelines for claims processing, "any and all automated tests must be paid as a panel, but still retain their individual identity for duplicate detection and medical necessity review." Frequency of the tests are limited by coverage policy (statutory limit or because it is never medically necessary to conduct a particular test on the same individual beyond a certain frequency). In other words, most tests will be covered only if required because of a specific patient complaint, symptom, or diagnosis.

Revised Codes Raise Concerns

Carriers and laboratories have raised several issues since the establishment of new and revised test codes, and how they affect reimbursement. For example:

1. Unbundling was one of the core issues. "Unbundling" is essentially the separate billing of multiple procedure codes for a group of procedures covered by a single, comprehensive code. The concern was that a physician could order the group of tests with one check, but then the laboratory would "unbundle" the tests and bill them under separate codes (receiving more reimbursement).

KEY POINT

Consultation (Clinical Pathology)
Note the following guidelines for Medicare and consultations:

1. The clinical pathology consultation must be requested by the patient's attending physician and there must be specific documentation in the medical record.

2. The clinical pathology consultation must relate to test results that lie outside the clinically significant normal or expected range in view of the patient's condition.

3. The results of the clinical pathology consultation must result in a written narrative report, which is included in the patient's medical record.

4. Require the "exercise of medical judgment" by the consulting physician.

5. Routine conversations a laboratory director may have with an attending physician about test orders or results are not a consultation unless the four preceding requirements are met.

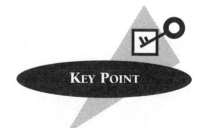

KEY POINT

The CLIA number must be included on each HCFA-1500 claim for laboratory services performed by any laboratory providing the tests covered by CLIA. Claims without CLIA numbers are rejected, and claims are not paid.

The waived tests requiring CLIA certification are:

- Dip stick or tablet reagent urinalysis (nonautomated) for bilirubin, glucose, hemoglobin, ketones, leukocytes, nitrite, pH, protein, specific gravity, or urobilinogen

- Fecal occult blood

- Ovulation tests — visual color comparison tests

- Urine pregnancy tests — visual color comparison tests

- Erythrocyte sedimentation rate (nonautomated)

- Hemoglobin by copper sulfate method

- Spun microhematocrit

- Glucose, blood by glucose monitoring device(s) cleared by the FDA specifically for home use

- Total serum cholesterol

- Glucose tolerance testing

- Blood count, hemoglobin

- Sedimentation rate

- Bacterial culture

- Strep screen

- HDL cholesterol

- Triglycerides

- Microalbumin

- Quantitative glucose

2. Duplicate billing — a laboratory bills for both a panel and for an individual test included in the panel or for overlapping panels. According to guidelines, if a physician orders two of the new clinically relevant panels that overlap, the laboratory will be required to "unbundle" one of the panels and bill only for the tests that are not duplicative

3. Advance Beneficiary Notices (ABN). Laboratory representatives said that the laboratories are not in a position to know whether a test will exceed a frequency limit for a particular patient since a test may have previously been performed by another laboratory. According to rules, the provider may be held responsible for payment in the absence of an ABN.

Anticipate New Coverage Guidelines

HCFA is now developing a new rule for Medicare coverage of lab tests due to the issues and requirements of the Balanced Budget Act of 1997. The BBA requires a national policy that establishes uniformity in diagnostic testing payable under Part B. Provisions in the policy must include:

- Beneficiary information submitted with each claim or order for laboratory tests

- Medical necessity

- Appropriate use of procedure codes in billing for a laboratory test, including the unbundling of laboratory services

- The medical documentation with section 1833(e) of the Social Security Act.

- Limitation on frequency of coverage for the same tests performed on the same individual

CLIA REGULATIONS

CLIA regulations define laboratory testing in relation to laboratory certification and accreditation, proficiency testing, quality assurance, personnel standards, and program administration. There are also specific cytology requirements. Laboratory tests are classified as waived, moderately complex, and highly complex. Obviously, changes to pathology and laboratory codes, and the BBA requirements, will show their affect on CLIA regulations. As mentioned in the previous section, automated panels — among other issues — complicate the reporting, monitoring, and coverage of diagnostic tests. Until a new rule is in place, the following sections still apply.

Waived Tests

The waived tests listed in the margin require CLIA certification but are not subject to routine inspection. Laboratories performing only these tests may request a certificate of waiver. This certification is issued to providers who only perform one or more of the following simple procedures: 80061, 81002, 81025, 82044, 82270, 82273, 82465, 82947, 82950, 82951, 82952, 82962, 82985, 83026, 83718, 83986, 84478, 84830, 85013, 85014, 85018, 85651, 86318, 86588, and 87072. Modifier -QW should always be appended to these codes to indicate they are a CLIA waived test.

Moderately Complex Tests

Tests of moderate complexity require limited manual intervention, or are automated procedures that do not require operator intervention during the analytic process. This category accounts for approximately 75 percent of all laboratory procedures. For CLIA certification, each laboratory performing moderately complex tests must have a laboratory director, a technical supervisor, a clinical consultant, and testing personnel.

Highly Complex Tests

Most all other laboratory procedures fall into the high complexity category, including all tests pertaining to cytogenetics, histopathology, histocompatibility, and cytology. Regulations and personnel standards for highly complex tests are much more rigorous than for the other categories. Each laboratory must have a laboratory director, technical supervisor for each specialty or subspecialty, general supervisor, clinical consultant, and testing personnel. Separate regulations that apply to cytology laboratories allow limited grandfathering of testing personnel and generally require personnel to be cytotechnologists.

Microscopy Unregulated Tests

A new, largely unregulated category for physician-performed microscopy procedures was recently approved. While the following moderately complex tests are not waived procedures, they do not require routine inspection because no effective quality-control measures currently apply: 81000, 81015, 81020, 89190, G0026, G0027, Q0111, Q0112, Q0113, Q0114, Q0115.

MEDICINE

Medicare and Therapeutic Services

Placement of intracoronary stents is covered by Medicare. Two codes report percutaneous placement of an intracoronary stent(s): 92980 and 92981. These codes include the work of angioplasty or atherectomy on the vessel(s) in which the stent is placed. If additional vessels are treated without stent placement, 92984 and/or 92986 should be used.

Medicare and Cardiovascular Stress Tests

Physicians were instructed by HCFA in 1993 to use 93015-26 to report the physician supervision and performance of interpretation for cardiovascular stress tests. The 1994 Medicare Fee Schedule "deleted" the professional component (which represented the physician supervision, interpretation, and report) of 93015. Code 93016 represents the physician supervision only of a cardiovascular stress test, and 93018 represents the physician interpretation and report of a cardiovascular stress test.

Medicare will continue to consider whether there are efficiencies in the provision of nonsurgical procedures which should result in reduced payment when more than one service category is provided on the same day to a beneficiary. See the October 31, 1997 *Federal Register* for a discussion of the level of supervision requirements.

Injections

Medicare bundles the administration of the medication into the E/M service, but it allows separate payment for the drug. Each Medicare and Medicaid carrier has individual requirements for the use of HCPCS Level II codes to describe the drug administered. Some carriers require the use of the CPT code and the HCPCS Level II J code, while others use only the J code and require a local modifier to designate the method of administration.

Dialysis

Medicare's policy for home glucose monitors no longer requires a patient to be "subject to poor diabetic control" in order to be eligible for Medicare coverage. In addition, the revised policy also allows any responsible individual, not just a family member, to be trained to use the equipment and monitor the patient if the patient is not able to do so.

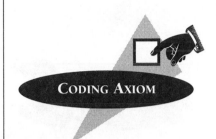

CODING AXIOM

When a physician supervises the cardiovascular stress test and provides an interpretation and report, the physician may report and be paid for both 93016 and 93018.

Ophthalmic Services

Modifier -50 is not applicable to visual field testing because the codes are listed as unilateral or bilateral. Medical diagnostic evaluation is included in these tests and should not be reported separately. Some codes, such as 92225 and 92226, are unilateral.

Medicare does not cover 92015. Coverage is denied as a "noncovered service" rather than being "medically unnecessary." This distinguishing factor does allow billing patients directly for this service.

Bilateral Versus Unilateral

According to the *Federal Register* Vol. 58, No. 230, the relative value units for ophthalmology services "are based on the assumptions that the codes describe bilateral services." When the diagnostic service is performed on only one eye, use modifier -52 to identify a reduced service.

Medicare and Monitors

Conventional tape type monitors and real-time devices which use data compression techniques to produce a full-disclosure printout are used for long-term ECG monitoring. To be reimbursed by Medicare, such monitoring needs to be related to a disease process documented by signs and/or symptoms such as palpitations or near syncope. Long-term ECG monitoring for the routine assessment of pacemaker function is not usually reimbursed by Medicare. A monitoring period of up to 24 hours is generally considered adequate to provide essential diagnostic information, and the medical necessity of longer periods must be documented.

Signal averaged electrocardiogram (SAECG) (93278) is a computerized, noninvasive diagnostic method for determining patients at risk for life-threatening ventricular arrhythmias. It is used to identify late potentials, which refers to areas of delayed or fragmented ventricular depolarization. These abnormalities are indicators of a diseased myocardium with the potential of initiating a life-threatening ventricular tachycardia or fibrillation.

Medicare will cover SAECG only in patients who have had a recent myocardial infarction (MI) and who have a documented ventricular ejection fraction (EF) of less than or equal to 40 percent.

HCFA states it has been informed that some suppliers of these types of services have decided that, since their devices provide both pre-symptom memory loop and post-symptom recording, they may report for two codes, e.g., G0006 and G0015, to increase their payments. This is incorrect and represents a duplicate reporting for the services furnished.

All of these devices provide post-symptom recording. Therefore, the codes denoting pre-symptom memory loop (G0004–G0007) also include payment for post-symptom recording. The basis for having G0015 and G0016 is to describe services in which the device used does not have the capacity for pre-symptom memory loop recording.

Payment System Changes for Antigen Therapy

Since implementation of the *Medicare Fee Schedule* in 1992, payment for antigen therapy has been split between the fee schedule and the original reasonable charge system (e.g., the system that requires calculation of customary and prevailing charges based on physicians' actual charging patterns).

While the injection portion of antigen therapy has been paid under the fee schedule, the antigen itself and its preparation has been paid under the reasonable charges system. For CPT codes representing both the injection and antigen, payment for these "complete service" codes has also been based on reasonable charges. Now, due to provisions in the Omnibus Budget Reconciliation

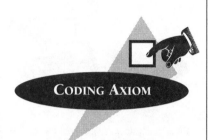

CODING AXIOM

Medicare and many national payors are moving toward the single line entry to identify a bilateral situation. However, careful monitoring will ensure correct reimbursement for both sides. Some payors allow 100 percent for each side if a separate incision is involved. Payors that do not allow 100 percent for the second side usually allow from 50 to 75 percent. Because of the varying allowances, monitor your reimbursement to determine the percentage allowed for the second side. When billing Medicare, special rules apply. If contracts are not specific or a contract is not in force, establish policies for handling balances above third-party payer reimbursements and make patients aware of your policies.

Act of 1993, this payment structure is changed. The antigen/antigen preparation codes and the complete service codes fall under the Medicare Fee Schedule.

The following chart and explaining text, taken from a letter that the HCFA sent to Medicare carriers, depicts changes in the payment system in terms of the CPT codes that report antigen therapy.

Type	Codes	Payment
Injection Codes	95115–95117	Fee schedule
Antigen/antigen prep codes	95144–95170	Fee Schedule

Codes 95145–95149 and 95170 are antigen/antigen preparation codes for stinging/biting insects. All other antigen/antigen preparation services (e.g., dust, pollens, etc.) are reported under the remaining codes: 95144 for single dose vials and 95165 for multiple dose vials.

Other codes not listed above are referred to as "complete service" antigen codes. These codes, 95120–95134, represent both the injection and the antigen/antigen preparation services. No Medicare payment will be made for these codes. This decision, in HCFA's judgment, provides that accurate payment cannot be guaranteed under the complete service codes. Those codes can represent more than one way to deliver antigen services (e.g., through single or multiple dose vials) and one delivery method (e.g., single dose vials) costs more than the other (e.g., multiple dose vials.)

Component Billing

The new payment policy for antigen therapy means that allergists providing both components of the service must now do component billing. They do not have the option of using a complete service code. Instead of using any code in the series 95120–95134, the allergist must, as appropriate, report one of the injection codes (95115 or 95117) and one of the antigen/antigen preparation codes (95145, 95146, 95147, 95148, 95149, 95165, or 95170). Note that 95144, the single dose vial antigen/antigen preparation code, is not listed as one of the components to be reported by an allergist performing a complete service. This is because the code, although its language is not explicit in this regard, is not to be used by allergists providing both the injection and antigen/antigen preparation services. Single dose vials of antigens, which are more costly to produce than multiple dose vials, should be used only when an allergist is preparing extract to be injected by another physician. Medicare will pay an allergist reporting both an injection service and either 95144 or 95165 based on the injection fee plus the fee for 95165, the multiple dose vial code.

Vial Preparation

Requiring physicians to use the above listed antigen/antigen preparation codes has caused some concern among allergists who use treatment boards and who, therefore, do not create vials. The listed antigen/antigen preparation codes all have wording which assumes vial preparation, while the complete service codes, which will not longer be recognized, do not. Allergists who use treatment boards, who formerly used complete service codes, are to use the extract/extract preparation vial codes (e.g., 95145–95149, 95165 and 95170) although they prepare no vials. Therefore, like all other allergists furnishing a complete service, they must report it on a component basis. Treatment board allergists are not expected to use extract/extract preparation 95144, the single dose vial code. They should report the appropriate injection code plus 95165. As noted under our claims processing system, HCFA will pay for the injection plus the amount for 95165, regardless it the physician reports 95144 or 95165.

Payment for Antigen Services

Average payment amounts were derived by using relative value units recommended by the Joint Council of Allergy and Immunology. In CPT the antigen/antigen prep codes require the biller to specify the number of doses reported. HCFA's payment amounts for these codes are calculated on a per dose basis. HCFA will calculate payments by multiplying the per dose allowance by the number of doses reported. When submitting Medicare claims, specify the number of doses in the units field of the HCFA-1500 (paper claims or electronic format). If an allergist has prepared a multidose vial of antigens (e.g., a vial with seven doses), and injects one dose, report the seven doses of antigen and the one injection service. When physician injects the remaining six doses at subsequent times, only injection services are to be reported.

Some individuals have expressed concern about the use of doses in HCFA's payment calculations. They are concerned about the potential for abuse if physicians change their practice patterns by routinely reducing the amounts of antigen that they provide in a "dose" and thereby increase the number of doses they can get from a multidose vial. This would essentially result in Medicare and beneficiaries paying more for the same amount of service/item. HCFA does not expect this kind of behavior change but plans to monitor for dose volume changes.

MEDICARE AND MODIFIERS

-21 Prolonged Evaluation and Management Services

The carrier will determine from review of the records if the services were appropriate. The evaluation and management service (99205, 99215, 99223, 99233, 99245, 99255, 99263, 99285, 99303, or 99313) will be allowed and will include up to 30 minutes of time in excess of the code description. Submit a report with the claim.

-22 Unusual Procedural Services

Use of modifier -22 can be applied to all codes with a global period of 0, 10, or 90 days. It also includes services that are not surgical; for example 90945. Modifier -22 may generate an increased payment amount if the claim is sufficiently documented. An operative report must be submitted with the claim.

-23 Unusual Anesthesia

Modifier -23 is not appropriate with codes that state "without anesthesia" in the code description, nor with codes that report procedures or services usually performed under general anesthesia.Modifier -23 is appropriate with codes that report procedures or services usually performed under local anesthesia.

-24 Unrelated Evaluation and Management Service by the Same Physician During a Postoperative Period

This modifier has no effect on the Medicare payment amount and should be used only with E/M codes. Use modifier -24 to indicate that an E/M service performed during the postoperative period was not related to the original procedure.

-25 Significant, Separately Identifiable Evaluation and Management Service by the Same Physician on the Same Day of the Procedure or Other Service

Modifier -25 is used to report that on the day a procedure was performed, the patient's condition required significant, separately identifiable E/M service above and beyond the usual pre- and postoperative care associated with the procedure.

-26 Professional Component

Modifier -26 affects the amount a provider is paid. The *Medicare Fee Schedule* contains different payment amounts for professional components. See Medicare RBRVS and payment components in the Federal Register.

-32 Mandated Services

Mandated services have no effect on Medicare's payment amount.

-47 Anesthesia by Surgeon

This modifier is not a Medicare covered benefit.

-50 Bilateral Procedure

Comparable HCPCS Level II (Medicare) modifiers are -LT and -RT, but Medicare carriers have been directed to accept either CPT or Level II modifiers.

Bilateral procedures can be billed when the services are provided by the same surgeon, on the same patient, on the same day. Attach modifier -50 to the procedure code as a one-line item to indicate the bilateral nature of the surgery. Medicare allows payment for both procedures at a total of 150 percent of the usual amount for one procedure (200 percent for x-rays). The physician's fee should reflect this adjustment.

Some codes have the bilateral aspect built into the description. Bilateral codes receive no additional payment and may not be billed with modifier -50.

-51 Multiple Procedures

Multiple surgeries are separate procedures performed by a physician on the same patient at the same operative session or on the same day for which separate payment may be allowed. Co-surgeons, surgical teams, or assistants-at-surgery may participate in performing multiple surgeries on the same patient on the same day.

Multiple surgeries are distinguished from procedures that are components of or incidental to a primary procedure. These intraoperative services, incidental surgeries, or components of more major surgeries are not separately billable.

Medicare pays the lesser of the actual charge or 100 percent of the fee schedule amount for the highest priced procedure. Payment for the second highest valued procedure is based on the lesser of the actual charge or 50 percent of the fee schedule amount. Payment for the third to fifth highest valued procedure(s) is based on the lesser of the actual charges or 50 percent of the fee schedule amount. Surgical procedures beyond the fifth procedure continue to be "by report" and payment, if any, is based on documentation of the services performed.

-52 Reduced Services

Modifier -52 should be billed to Medicare when appropriate. However, for exams that are considered global, this modifier is informational only and does not affect payment amount. For other situations, such as aborted procedures, a reduction in payment may occur. Under these circumstances, the service provided can be identified by its usual procedure code with modifier -52 attached. Documentation should be furnished explaining the reduction.

-53 Discontinued Procedure

Under certain circumstances, the physician may elect to terminate a surgical or diagnostic procedure. Due to extenuating circumstances or those that threaten the well-being of the patient, it may be necessary to indicate that a surgical or diagnostic procedure was started but discontinued. Effective January 1, 1997, the following documentation is required for processing: operative report, reason for termination, services actually performed, supplies actually provided, time spent in (preoperative, operative, and postoperative) services, time and supplies necessary for complete procedure, and CPT code for the completed procedure. These services will be medically reviewed and reimbursed dependent on the information documented. Code 45378, colonoscopy, is the only code not subject to carrier review when billed with modifier -53.

-54   Surgical Care Only
Payment will be limited to the amount allotted to the preoperative and intra-operative services only. Use only with surgical codes. Medicare has split global surgery package relative values into preoperative, intra-operative, and postoperative percentages. The percentages are necessary to calculate fees when different physicians provide separate phases of care. This information is part of the *Medicare Fee Schedule* database and is available from your Medicare carrier.

-55   Postoperative Management Only
Payment will be limited to the amount allotted for postoperative services only. (See Medicare modifier -54 for information on Medicare's split global surgery package). If more than one physician bills for the postoperative care, apportion the postoperative percentage according to the number of days each physician was responsible for the patient's care.

-56   Preoperative Management Only
Medicare does not recognize the use of modifier -56.

-57   Decision For Surgery
Modifier -57 should be used only in cases in which the decision for surgery was made during the preoperative period (the day before and the day of) a major surgical procedure (procedures with 90 days of follow-up).

-58   Staged Procedure or Service by the Same Physician During the Postoperative Period
This modifier does not affect Medicare payment. Use only on surgery codes to indicate a related surgery that is due to a progression of the disease.

-59   Distinct Procedural Service
Under certain circumstances, the physician may need to indicate that a procedure or service was distinct or independent from other services performed on the same day. Modifier -59 is used to identify procedures/services that are not normally reported together, but are appropriate under the circumstances. This may represent a different session or patient encounter, different procedure or surgery, different site or organ system, separate incision/excision, separate lesion, or separate injury (or area of injury in extensive injuries) not normally encountered or performed on the same day by the same physician. However, when another modifier is appropriate it should be used rather than modifier -59. Modifier -59 should only be reported if a more descriptive modifier is not available and modifier -59 best explains the circumstances.

-62   Two Surgeons (Cosurgery)
According to Medicare guidelines, "Cosurgery refers to a single surgical procedure which requires two surgeons. It may also apply when a surgical procedure involves two surgeons performing parts of the procedure simultaneously, e.g., heart transplant, bilateral knee replacements." Cosurgery is allowed at 125 percent of the global procedure amount divided equally between the two surgeons, so each surgeon is allowed 62.5 percent of the global surgery amount. Each surgeon bills the procedure with a modifier -62. No payment is allowed for an assistant surgeon.

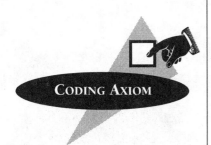

CODING AXIOM

Modifier -57 should not be used with E/M visits furnished during the global period of minor procedures. Use modifier -25 to report a significant, separately identifiable evaluation and management service by the same physician on the day of a procedure.

-66 Surgical Team

Medicare guidelines state, "Team surgery refers to a single procedure which requires more than two surgeons of different specialties. If surgeons of different specialties are each performing a different procedure (with specific CPT codes), multiple surgery rules do not apply. If one of the surgeons performs multiple procedures, the multiple procedure pricing rule applies to that surgeon's services." Each surgeon bills the service with a modifier -66.

Carriers price this type of surgery modification "By Report." Documentation of the medical necessity for team surgeons is required for some surgeries.

-73 Discontinued Outpatient Hospital/Ambulatory Surgery Center (ASC) Procedure Prior to Administration of Anesthesia

Due to extenuating circumstances or those which threaten the well-being of the patient, the physician may cancel a diagnostic or therapeutic service or procedure prior to the administration of anesthesia. When cancellation of the procedure occurs subsequent to the patient's surgical preparation (including sedation and transfer to the room where the procedure is to be performed) but prior to the administration of anesthesia (local, regional, or general), append modifier -73 to the CPT code which would have been reported had the procedure been performed as planned. Modifier -73 applies only to facility reporting and should not be used by the physician. Physician reporting of a discontinued procedure should be reported with modifier -53. The cancellation of a procedure prior to the patient's preparation for surgery and prior to occupation of the surgical/special procedure room should not be reported.

-74 Discontinued Outpatient Hospital/Ambulatory Surgery Center (ASC) Procedure After Administration of Anesthesia

Due to extenuating circumstances or those which threaten the well-being of the patient, the physician may cancel a diagnostic or therapeutic service or procedure subsequent to the administration of anesthesia. When cancellation occurs after the administration of anesthesia (local, regional, general) or after the procedure was started (incision made, intubation started, scope inserted, etc), append modifier -74 to the CPT code which would have been reported had the procedure been performed as planned. Modifer -74 applies only to facility reporting and should not be used by the physician. Physician reporting of a discontinued procedure should be reported with modifier -53.

-76 Repeat Procedure by Same Physician

This modifier does not affect Medicare payment; it is used for informational purposes only.

-77 Repeat Procedure by Another Physician

This modifier does not affect Medicare payment; it is used for informational purposes only.

-78 Return to the Operating Room for a Related Procedure During the Postoperative Period

When an unlisted procedure is billed because no code exists to describe the treatment for complications, base payment on a maximum of 50 percent of the value of the intra-operative services originally performed. If multiple surgeries were originally performed, base payment on no more than 50 percent of the value of the intra-operative services of the surgery for which the complications occurred.

-79 Unrelated Procedure or Service by the Same Physician During the Postoperative Period

This modifier has no effect on the Medicare payment amount. Use only on surgical codes. Payment will not be allowed for this service without use of the modifier.

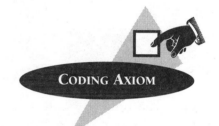

Coding Axiom

Modifier -80: Medicare publishes a list of procedures that specifies procedures where a surgical assist is allowed, procedures where a surgical assist is not allowed and payment will be denied (and the patient cannot be billed for the assistant surgeon charge), and procedures where surgical assist might be allowed upon carrier review.

-80   Assistant Surgeon

Medicare restricts the use of this modifier to the primary procedure performed. Where payment for an assistant surgeon is allowed, payment is based on 16 percent of the fee schedule payment amount.

-81   Minimum Assistant Surgeon

Medicare does not recognize modifier -81.

-82   Assistant Surgeon (when qualified resident surgeon not available)

Refer to modifier -80 above for assistant surgeon guidelines.

-90   Reference (Outside) Laboratory

Do not report this modifier on Medicare claims; the performing laboratory should bill Medicare directly.

-99   Multiple Modifiers

Enter all applicable modifiers when modifier -99 is used. If modifier -99 is entered on multiple line items of a single claim form, all applicable modifiers for each line item containing a -99 modifier should be listed as follows: 1= (mod). The number "1" represents the line item and "mod" represents all modifiers applicable to the referenced line item.

DISCUSSION QUESTIONS

1.   When a physician provides supplies that are not included in the surgical package how should they be coded according to Medicare?

_____

_____

_____

2.   Explain the special Medicare issues involved with critical care codes.

_____

_____

_____

3.   How is payment for multiple related endoscopies determined?

_____

_____

4.   What is the different bilateral concept that is applied to radiology?

_____

_____

_____

5.   How do CLIA regulations affect pathology and laboratory billing?

_____

_____

_____

6. What are the qualifications for reimbursing monitoring devices?

_____

_____

_____

Specialty-Specific Scenarios

The following surgical scenarios are designed by specialty to help make the leap from documentation to correct code choices.

OBJECTIVES

See the practical application of Medicare coding

Identify the special circumstances and rules of specialties

GYNECOLOGY SCENARIO – OUTPATIENT

A 67-year old patient with a long history of vaginitis and candidiasis presents as a new patient to her daughter's gynecologist while visiting for the holidays. She also has a carbuncle of her vagina. The physician does an examination which is primarily limited to her presenting problems — the vaginal carbuncle and candidiasis. The physician irrigates the vagina with a bacteriostatic agent and prescribes appropriate follow-up medications for both conditions. An abbreviated, problem-oriented follow-up history with physical examination is done two days later with demonstrated resolution of both problems. Code the services provided on both days.

21. DIAGNOSIS OR NATURE OF ILLNESS OR INJURY (RELATE ITEMS 1, 2, 3 OR 4 TO ITEM 24E BY LINE)

1. | 616.8   3. |____|
2. | 112.1   4. |____|

24.	A					B	C	D		E
	DATE(S) OF SERVICE					Place of Service	Type of Service	PROCEDURES, SERVICES, OR SUPPLIES (Explain Unusual Circumstances)		DIAGNOSIS CODE
MM	From DD	YY	MM	To DD	YY			CPT / HCPCS	MODIFIER	
12	26	98	12	26	98	3		57150*		1
12	28	98	12	28	98	3		99212		1,2

ICD-9-CM

616.8   Other specified inflammatory disease of cervix, vagina, and vulva

112.1   Candidiasis of vulva and vagina

CPT

57150*   Irrigation of vagina and/or application of medicament for treatment of bacterial, parasitic, or fungoid disease

99212   Office or other outpatient visit for the evaluation and management of an established patient, which requires at least two of these three key components: a problem focused history; a problem focused examination; straightforward medical decision making. Counseling and/or coordination of care with other providers or agencies are provided consistent with the nature of the problem(s) and the patient's and/or family's needs. Usually, the presenting problem(s) are self limited or minor. Physicians typically spend 10 minutes face-to-face with the patient and/or family.

Medicare does not recognize starred procedures. Many starred procedures are included in Medicare's minor surgery rule. Same-day evaluation or consultation services are included unless they are unrelated to, or can be identified separately from, the procedure. Because 57150* *Irrigation of vagina and/or application of medicament for treatment of bacterial, parasitic, or fungoid disease* is a starred procedure and the services are related to the procedure, 99025 *Initial (new*

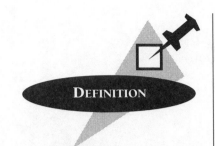

DEFINITION

The **principal diagnosis** is designed and defined as the condition established after study to be chiefly responsible for occasioning the admission of the patient to the hospital for care.

patient) visit when starred surgical procedure constitutes major service at that visit cannot be billed. Because 57150* has zero Medicare follow-up days, the physician may bill for the follow-up office visit. The minor surgery rule for postoperative care specifies that minor surgeries have either a 0- or a 10-day postoperative period. Those with a 10-day period include all services related to the recovery from surgery. Other services during that period, whether for the underlying condition or for an unrelated condition, are paid separately.

RECONSTRUCTIVE SURGERY SCENARIO — INPATIENT AND OUTPATIENT

A 67-year-old male, Medicare patient sustains a closed orbital floor blow-out fracture, and a closed depressed malar fracture, which included the zygomatic arch and malar tripod as a passenger in an head-on traffic accident with another automobile. Per the EMT report, the patient is unconscious upon arrival at the scene of the accident, but regains consciousness in the ambulance on the way to the hospital. He is evaluated by a reconstructive surgeon in the emergency department, and taken to surgery. In the operating room, the surgeon uses an open periorbital approach and bone grafts to treat the orbital floor "blow-out" fracture. Surgery is difficult and takes an additional 90 minutes beyond the normal time for the procedure due to the severity of the fracture. He also performs an open treatment of the depressed malar fracture. Following surgery the patient is admitted as an inpatient to follow his post surgical status as well as his concussion. Code the diagnoses and procedures for the surgeon.

21. DIAGNOSIS OR NATURE OF ILLNESS OR INJURY (RELATE ITEMS 1, 2, 3 OR 4 TO ITEM 24E BY LINE)
1 ∟ 802.6   3 ∟ 850.1
2 ∟ 802.4   4 ∟ E812.1

24.	A						B	C	D		E
	DATE(S) OF SERVICE						Place of Service	Type of Service	PROCEDURES, SERVICES, OR SUPPLIES (Explain Unusual Circumstances)		DIAGNOSIS CODE
	From MM DD YY			To MM DD YY					CPT / HCPCS	MODIFIER	
	5	9	98	5	9	98	23		21395	−22	1,2,3
	5	9	98	5	9	98	23		21360	−51	1,2,3

ICD-9-CM diagnoses — Inpatient

Principal diagnosis

802.6   Orbital floor (blow-out), closed fracture

Secondary diagnosis

802.4   Malar and maxillary bones, closed fracture

850.1   Concussion with brief (less than one hour) loss of consciousness

E812.1   Other motor vehicle traffic accident involving collision with motor vehicle, passenger in motor vehicle other than motorcycle

HCPCS Level I (CPT)

Surgeon

21395-22 Open treatment of orbital floor "blowout" fracture; periorbital approach with bone graft (includes obtaining graft) — Unusual Procedural Services

21360-51 Open treatment of depressed malar fracture, including zygomatic arch and malar tripod — Multiple Procedures

In the main body of this chapter, Medicare's primary and secondary rules are listed. Medicare criteria specifies that payment is secondary when a patient's treatment is covered by automobile no-fault or liability insurance.

The automobile insurance carrier must be billed first to avoid delay caused by first submitting the claim to Medicare and waiting for a denial.

The first fracture listed is the most resource-consuming and thus the principal and primary diagnosis. The malar fracture is listed as a secondary code.

The CPT HCPCS Level I codes are the same for Medicare and for the automobile insurance carrier. Modifier -22 indicates an unusual procedural service and should be reported with 21395. To report increased time and difficulty when billing Medicare, modifier -22 may be applied to any codes with a global period of 0, 10, or 90 days, including services that are not surgical (e.g., 90945). Modifier -22 should also be appended when the claim is submitted to the automobile insurance carrier.

The highest dollar value code is sequenced first. Secondary and subsequent codes should be appended with a -51 modifier when performed at the same operative session and area.

ORTHOPEDIC SURGERY SCENARIO — INPATIENT

A 70-year-old male had a total hip arthroplasty performed one month prior to the current hospital admit. The admission and discharge diagnosis listed in the medical record was "infected total right hip arthroplasty." The patient's hospital course was complicated by an accidental laceration of a vein during surgery for removal of a total hip prosthesis. The lacerated vein was repaired by suture (direct repair) in the operating room at the time of surgery. On postoperative day eight the patient was discharged to a skilled nursing facility. Code the ICD-9-CM diagnoses and HCPCS Level I (CPT) procedures for the Medicare patient.

21. DIAGNOSIS OR NATURE OF ILLNESS OR INJURY (RELATE ITEMS 1, 2, 3 OR 4 TO ITEM 24E BY LINE)						
1. 996.66			3. ___ ___			
2. 998.2			4. ___ ___			

24. A DATE(S) OF SERVICE From MM DD YY	To MM DD YY	B Place of Service	C Type of Service	D PROCEDURES, SERVICES, OR SUPPLIES CPT/HCPCS	MODIFIER	E DIAGNOSIS CODE
10 1 98	10 1 98			27091		1,2

Admission diagnosis
996.66 Infection due to internal orthopedic device, implant, and graft
Discharge diagnoses
Principal diagnosis
996.66 Infection due to internal orthopedic device, implant, and graft
Secondary diagnosis
998.2 Accidental puncture or laceration during a procedure
CPT Procedures
27091 Removal of hip prosthesis; complicated, including total hip prosthesis, methylmethacrylate with or without insertion of spacer

The principal diagnosis is designed and defined as the condition established after study to be chiefly responsible for occasioning the admission of the patient to the hospital for care. The accidental laceration of the vein is a complication of a surgical procedure and is sequenced second. HCPCS Level I (CPT) procedures should be sequenced based on the relative value with the higher dollar value procedure sequenced first.

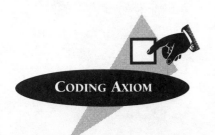

When a physician supervises the cardiovascular stress test and provides an interpretation and report, the physician may report and be paid for both 93016 and 93018.

MEDICAL SPECIALTIES/CARDIOLOGY SCENARIO — OUTPATIENT

A 65-year-old male Medicare beneficiary with a history of angina asks to be worked into the office schedule of a cardiologist. The patient is having tightness in his chest and night sweats. The cardiologist reviews past and present medical history. An extended examination of head, heart, lungs, and abdomen is obtained. As a part of the exam, the cardiologist provides a 12-lead ECG and complete, transthoracic echocardiography with pulsed wave doppler and color flow mapping in the office. The patient is diagnosed with acute angina with an impending MI. He is immediately admitted to the cardiac care unit of the local hospital.

21. DIAGNOSIS OR NATURE OF ILLNESS OR INJURY (RELATE ITEMS 1, 2, 3 OR 4 TO ITEM 24E BY LINE)

1. | 411.1
2. |
3. |
4. |

24.	A DATE(S) OF SERVICE						B Place of Service	C Type of Service	D PROCEDURES, SERVICES, OR SUPPLIES (Explain Unusual Circumstances)		E DIAGNOSIS CODE
	From MM	DD	YY	To MM	DD	YY			CPT / HCPCS	MODIFIER	
	1	9	98	1	9	98	1		99222		1
	1	9	98	1	9	98	1		93307		1
	1	9	98	1	9	98	3		93320		1
	1	9	98	1	9	98	3		93325		1
	1	9	98	1	9	98	3		93005		1

ICD-9-CM

411.1 Intermediate coronary syndrome

CPT

99222 Initial hospital care, per day, for the evaluation and management of a patient, which requires these three key components: a comprehensive history; a comprehensive examination; and medical decision making of moderate complexity. Counseling and/or coordination of care with other providers or agencies are provided consistent with the nature of the problem(s) and the patient's and/or family's needs. Usually, the problem(s) requiring admission are of moderate severity. Physicians typically spend 50 minutes at the bedside and on the patient's hospital floor or unit.

93307 Echocardiography, transthoracic, real-time with image documentation (2D) with or without M-mode recording; complete

93320 Doppler echocardiography, pulsed wave and/or continuous wave with spectral display (List separately in addition to codes for echocardiographic imaging); complete

93325 Doppler echocardiography color flow velocity mapping (List separately in addition to codes for echocardiography)

93005 Electrocardiogram, routine ECG with at least 12 leads; tracing only, without interpretation and report

Report 93320 for pulsed wave Doppler and 93325 for Doppler color flow velocity mapping in addition to the code for the basic echocardiography.

Inform Medicare that the diagnostic services have not been purchased from another entity (non-purchased diagnostic test ruling). Each Medicare carrier has specific rules on this issue.

GENERAL SURGERY SCENARIO

A patient is admitted to the ICU with possible peritonitis. A general surgeon performs a comprehensive history and examination, with medical decision-making of moderate complexity. After reviewing the patient's records and performing the history and examination, the physician makes the diagnosis of an "acute abdomen" and requests that the OR be notified to stand-by for a possible abdominal surgery. The general surgeon writes the history, examination, and findings in the medical record and advises the attending physician of the need for surgery both in writing in the medical record and verbally in a phone conversation. The attending physician asks the general surgeon to assume the care of the patient's acute abdominal problem including the recommended surgery and its associated postoperative follow-up care. Intra-operatively, the general surgeon finds the patient does have generalized peritonitis due to a perforated duodenal ulcer. The surgeon performs a repair of the small intestine perforation by suture.

21. DIAGNOSIS OR NATURE OF ILLNESS OR INJURY (RELATE ITEMS 1, 2, 3 OR 4 TO ITEM 24E BY LINE)

1. | 532.10   3. |___ . ___
2. | 567.2   4. |___ . ___

24.		A					B	C	D		E
			DATE(S) OF SERVICE				Place of Service	Type of Service	PROCEDURES, SERVICES, OR SUPPLIES (Explain Unusual Circumstances)		DIAGNOSIS CODE
	From			To					CPT / HCPCS	MODIFIER	
MM	DD	YY	MM	DD	YY						
5	8	98	5	8	98				44602		1,2
5	8	98	5	8	98				99254	-57	1,2

ICD-9-CM diagnoses codes

Primary diagnosis

532.10   Acute duodenal ulcer with perforation, without mention of obstruction

Secondary diagnosis

567.2   Other suppurative peritonitis

CPT procedure codes

44602   Suture of small intestine (enterorrhaphy) for perforated ulcer, diverticulum, wound, injury or rupture; single perforation

99254-57   Initial inpatient consultation, comprehensive — Decision for surgery

Summary

The primary diagnosis is designated as the code that reflects the current, most significant reason for the services or procedures provided. The most significant reason for the service or procedure was a perforated duodenal ulcer with a complicating diagnosis of peritonitis. The primary procedure was the suture of the perforated ulcer. The consultation is billable to Medicare because the decision for surgery fits the definition of a consultation. Modifier -57 per Medicare should be used only in cases when the decision for surgery was made during the preoperative period (the day before and the day of) of a major surgical procedure (procedures with 90 days of follow-up).

CPT defines a consultation as an opinion or advice regarding evaluation and/or management of a specific problem requested by another physician or appropriate source. Per CPT, the consultant may initiate diagnostic and/or therapeutic services. Any specifically identifiable procedure (e.g., identified with a specific CPT code) performed on or subsequent to the date of the initial consultation should be reported separately. If subsequent to completing a consultation, the consultant assumes responsibility for management of a portion or all of the patient's condition(s), the follow-up consultation codes should not be used.

The documentation per CPT must clearly indicate that the services were initiated at the request of the attending physician or other appropriate source. The need for consultation must be documented in the patient's medical record. The consultant's opinion and any services that were ordered or performed must also be documented in the patient's medical record and communicated to the requesting physician or other appropriate source.

OPHTHALMOLOGY SCENARIO — OUTPATIENT

A new patient schedules an appointment with an ophthalmologist for an eye exam. The patient presents with no complaints regarding her vision and expresses concern regarding glaucoma due to a positive family history of glaucoma (sister, mother). The ophthalmic assistant records the patient's complete personal, general, and ocular history as well as the complete family and social history. A general medical observation is made, and current medications are noted for both general and ocular medications. The doctor notes the patient's current vision with correction at 20/70, O.D., and 20/80 O.S. The lenses are neutralized and the patient's prescription recorded. Gross visual fields are documented and a basic cover test is taken. The tonometry recording was 25 O.D. and 23 O.S. The doctor performed and documented a refraction. A slit lamp exam reveals normal eyelids, conjunctiva, cornea, and anterior chamber, O.U. The exam also reveals clear lenses, O.U. A direct ophthalmoscopy shows that the angles are open, but the disc, O.D. is 0.7 and cupped. The diagnosis is primary open angle glaucoma, O.U. The medical decision is Betoptic lgtt. BID, O.U., visual field that day and recheck in one week. The risks of noncompliance in relation to glaucoma are discussed with the patient who is counseled regarding medications prescribed.

21. DIAGNOSIS OR NATURE OF ILLNESS OR INJURY (RELATE ITEMS 1, 2, 3 OR 4 TO ITEM 24E BY LINE)			
1	365.11	3	V19.1
2	V72.0	4	

24.	A DATE(S) OF SERVICE From MM DD YY	A To MM DD YY	B Place of Service	C Type of Service	D PROCEDURES, SERVICES, OR SUPPLIES (Explain Unusual Circumstances) CPT / HCPCS MODIFIER	E DIAGNOSIS CODE
	3 30 98	3 30 98	11		92004	1,2,3
	3 30 98	3 30 98	11		92015	1,2,3

ICD-9-CM

365.11	Primary open-angle glaucoma
V72.0	Examination of eyes and vision
V19.1	Family history of other eye disorders

CPT

92004	Ophthalmological services: medical examination and evaluation with initiation of diagnostic and treatment program; comprehensive, new patient, one or more visits
92015	Determination of refractive state

The patient presented with no complaints (note Medicare guideline) other than a concern regarding glaucoma. Payment for services by an ophthalmologist is dependent on the purpose of the exam, rather than on the ultimate diagnosis of the patient's condition.

If the patient has a complaint or symptoms of an eye disease or injury, the examination is covered regardless that only eyeglasses were prescribed. However, if the patient desires an exam with no specific complaint, the expenses for the examination would normally not be covered, although the doctor discovered a pathological condition (reference MCM 2320).

PATHOLOGY AND LABORATORY SCENARIO

A blood sample is sent to an outpatient laboratory with a request for the following: albumin, bilirubin (total or direct), calcium, chloride, creatinine, glucose, phosphatase, alkaline, potassium, total protein, sodium, SGOT, and BUN. The request slip includes the patient's name, a diagnosis of history of breast cancer with metastasis to the spine, and her Medicare beneficiary number. Code the service for the outpatient laboratory.

21. DIAGNOSIS OR NATURE OF ILLNESS OR INJURY (RELATE ITEMS 1, 2, 3 OR 4 TO ITEM 24E BY LINE)			
1 ∟ 198.5		3 ∟ ___ ___	
2 ∟ V10.3		4 ∟ ___ ___	

24.	A				B	C	D		E
	DATE(S) OF SERVICE				Place of Service	Type of Service	PROCEDURES, SERVICES, OR SUPPLIES (Explain Unusual Circumstances)		DIAGNOSIS CODE
	From		To				CPT / HCPCS	MODIFIER	
MM	DD	YY	MM	DD	YY				
6	8	98	6	8	98	11		80054		1,2

Primary diagnosis

198.5   Secondary malignant neoplasm bone and bone marrow

Secondary diagnosis

V10.3   Personal history of malignant neoplasm breast

Primary procedure

80054   Comprehensive metabolic panel This panel must include the following: albumin (82040), bilirubin, total OR direct (82250), calcium (82310), chloride (82435), creatinine (82565), glucose (82947), phosphatase, alkaline (84075), potassium (84132), protein, total (84155), sodium (84295), transferase, aspartate amino (AST) (SGOT) (84450), urea nitrogen (BUN) (84520)

Multichannel tests were deleted in 1998 and replaced with automated panel codes. Panel codes specifically identify each test included in the service. The requested laboratory tests are all included in 80054 comprehensive metabolic panel.

RADIOLOGY SCENARIO

A 69-year-old, asymptomatic patient comes in to a freestanding clinic for a screening mammogram prescribed by her gynecologist. Two years have passed since her last mammography. Code the bilateral two view mammogram for the radiologist's portion of the bill.

21. DIAGNOSIS OR NATURE OF ILLNESS OR INJURY (RELATE ITEMS 1, 2, 3 OR 4 TO ITEM 24E BY LINE)
1. V76.12   3.
2.   4.

24.	A DATE(S) OF SERVICE						B Place of Service	C Type of Service	D PROCEDURES, SERVICES, OR SUPPLIES (Explain Unusual Circumstances) CPT / HCPCS MODIFIER	E DIAGNOSIS CODE
	From MM DD YY			To MM DD YY						
	8	1	98	8	1	98	11		76092 −26	1

ICD-9-CM

   V76.12   Other screening mammogram

CPT

   76092-26   Screening mammography — Professional component

Medicare has specific guidelines regarding screening mammograms. They are:

AGE	
30–39	base line only
40–49	one allowed per year for women at high risk
40–49	non-high risk women biannual (23 months must have elapsed)
50–64	one per year (eleven months must have elapsed since last screening)
65 and older	biannual (23 months must have elapsed)

Screening mammography for Medicare should be reported with 76092.

Chapter Review

Standardization of Medicare payment policies is vital to implementation of the *Medicare Fee Schedule*. Payment policies and procedures must be administered in the same manner by all Medicare carriers to affect the goal of Physician Payment Reform: like payment for like services. In the past, Medicare carriers were allowed to interpret rules and regulations set forth by HCFA. In the future, standardization will bring much less individual carrier interpretation. Specific Medicare guidelines apply to many sections of CPT coding.

Appendix 1: MDCs

MDC 1
Diseases and Disorders of the Nervous System (DRGs 1–35)

MDC 2
Diseases and Disorders of the Eye (DRGs 36–48)

MDC 3
Diseases and Disorders of the Ear, Nose, Mouth and Throat (DRGs 49–74, 168–169, 185–187)

MDC 4
Diseases and Disorders of the Respiratory System (DRGs 75–102, 475)

MDC 5
Diseases and Disorders of the Circulatory System (DRGs 103–109, 110–145, 478–479)

MDC 6
Diseases and Disorders of the Digestive System (DRGs 146–167, 170–184, 188–190)

MDC 7
Diseases and Disorders of the Hepatobiliary System and Pancreas (DRGs 191–208, 493–494)

MDC 8
Diseases and Disorders of the Musculoskeletal System and Connective Tissue (DRGs 209–213, 216–220, 223–256, 471, 491, 496–503)

MDC 9
Diseases and Disorders of the Skin, Subcutaneous Tissue and Breast (DRGs 257–284)

MDC 10
Endocrine, Nutritional and Metabolic Diseases and Disorders (DRGs 285–301)

MDC 11
Diseases and Disorders of the Kidney and Urinary Tract (DRGs 302–333)

MDC 12
Diseases and Disorders of the Male Reproductive System (DRGs 334–352)

MDC 13
Diseases and Disorders of the Female Reproductive System (DRGs 353–369)

MDC 14
Pregnancy, Childbirth and the Puerperium (DRGs 370–384, 469)

MDC 15
Newborns and Other Neonates with Conditions Originating in the Perinatal Period (DRGs 385–391, 469–470)

MDC 16
Diseases and Disorders of the Blood and Blood Forming Organs and Immunological Disorders (DRGs 392–399)

MDC 17
Myeloproliferative Diseases and Disorders, and Poorly Differentiated Neoplasms (DRGs 400–414, 473, 492)

MDC 18
Infectious and Parasitic Diseases (Systemic or Unspecified Sites) (DRGs 415–423)

MDC 19
Mental Diseases and Disorders (DRGs 424–432)

MDC 20
Alcohol/Drug Use and Alcohol/Drug Induced Organic Mental Disorders (DRGs 433–437)

MDC 21
Injuries, Poisonings and Toxic Effects of Drugs (DRGs 439–455)

MDC 22
Burns (DRGs 504–511)

MDC 23
Factors Influencing Health Status and Other Contacts with Health Services (DRGs 461–467)

MDC 24
Multiple Significant Trauma (DRGs 484–487)

MDC 25
Human Immunodeficiency Virus Infections (DRGs 488–490)

PRE-MDC
Liver Transplant (DRG 480)
Bone Marrow Transplant (DRG 481)
Tracheostomy (DRGs 482–483)

Appendix 2: DRG Listing

DRG	MDC	Description
1	1	Craniotomy except for trauma, age 18 or older
2	1	Craniotomy for trauma, age 18 or older
3	1	Craniotomy, age 17 or younger
4	1	Spinal procedures
5	1	Extracranial vascular procedures
6	1	Carpal tunnel release
7	1	Peripheral and cranial nerve and other nervous system procedures with CC
8	1	Peripheral and cranial nerve and other nervous system procedures without CC
9	1	Spinal disorders and injuries
10	1	Nervous system neoplasms with CC
11	1	Nervous system neoplasms without CC
12	1	Degenerative nervous system disorders
13	1	Multiple sclerosis and cerebellar ataxia
14	1	Specific cerebrovascular disorders except transient ischemic attack (TIA)
15	1	Transient ischemic attack (TIA) and precerebral occlusions
16	1	Nonspecific cerebrovascular disorders with CC
17	1	Nonspecific cerebrovascular disorders without CC
18	1	Cranial and peripheral nerve disorders with CC
19	1	Cranial and peripheral nerve disorders without CC
20	1	Nervous system infection except viral meningitis
21	1	Viral meningitis
22	1	Hypertensive encephalopathy
23	1	Nontraumatic stupor and coma
24	1	Seizure and headache, age 18 or older, with CC
25	1	Seizure and headache, age 18 or older, without CC
26	1	Seizure and headache, age 17 or younger
27	1	Traumatic stupor and coma, coma longer than an hour
28	1	Traumatic stupor and coma, coma less than an hour, age 18 or older, with CC
29	1	Traumatic stupor and coma, coma less than an hour, age 18 or older, without CC
30	1	Traumatic stupor and coma, coma less than an hour, age 17 or younger
31	1	Concussion, age 18 or older, with CC
32	1	Concussion, age 18 or older, without CC
33	1	Concussion, age 17 or younger
34	1	Other disorders of nervous system with CC
35	1	Other disorders of nervous system without CC
36	2	Retinal procedures
37	2	Orbital procedures
38	2	Primary iris procedures
39	2	Lens procedures with or without vitrectomy
40	2	Extraocular procedures, except orbit, age 18 or older
41	2	Extraocular procedures, except orbit, age 17 or younger
42	2	Intraocular procedures except retina, iris, and lens
43	2	Hyphema
44	2	Acute major eye infections
45	2	Neurological eye disorders
46	2	Other disorders of the eye, age 18 or older, with CC

DRG	MDC	Description	DRG	MDC	Description
47	2	Other disorders of the eye, age 18 or older, without CC	72	3	Nasal trauma and deformity
48	2	Other disorders of the eye, age 17 or younger	73	3	Other ear, nose, mouth, and throat diagnoses, age 18 or older
49	3	Major head and neck procedures	74	3	Other ear, nose, mouth, and throat diagnoses, age 17 and younger
50	3	Sialoadenectomy	75	4	Major chest procedures
51	3	Salivary gland procedures except sialoadenectomy	76	4	Other respiratory system operating room procedures, with CC
52	3	Cleft lip and palate repair	77	4	Other respiratory system operating room procedures, without CC
53	3	Sinus and mastoid procedures, age 18 or older	78	4	Pulmonary embolism
54	3	Sinus and mastoid procedures, age 17 or younger	79	4	Respiratory infections and inflammations, age 18 or older, with CC
55	3	Miscellaneous ear, nose, mouth, and throat procedures	80	4	Respiratory infections and inflammations, age 18 or older, without CC
56	3	Rhinoplasty	81	4	Respiratory infections and inflammations, age 17 or younger
57	3	Tonsillectomy and adenoidectomy procedures, except tonsillectomy and/or adenoidectomy only, age 18 or older	82	4	Respiratory neoplasms
58	3	Tonsillectomy and adenoidectomy procedures, except tonsillectomy and/or adenoidectomy only, age 17 or younger	83	4	Major chest trauma with CC
			84	4	Major chest trauma without CC
59	3	Tonsillectomy and/or adenoidectomy only, age 18 or older	85	4	Pleural effusion with CC
			86	4	Pleural effusion without CC
60	3	Tonsillectomy and/or adenoidectomy only, age 17 or younger	87	4	Pulmonary edema and respiratory failure
61	3	Myringotomy with tube insertion, age 18 or older	88	4	Chronic obstructive pulmonary disease (COPD)
			89	4	Simple pneumonia and pleurisy, age 18 or older, with CC
62	3	Myringotomy with tube insertion, age 17 or younger	90	4	Simple pneumonia and pleurisy, age 18 or older, without CC
63	3	Other ear, nose, mouth, and throat operating room procedures	91	4	Simple pneumonia and pleurisy, age 17 or younger
64	3	Ear, nose, mouth, and throat malignancy	92	4	Interstitial lung disease with CC
65	3	Dysequilibrium	93	4	Interstitial lung disease without CC
66	3	Epistaxis	94	4	Pneumothorax with CC
67	3	Epiglottitis	95	4	Pneumothorax without CC
68	3	Otitis media and upper respiratory infection, age 18 or older, with CC	96	4	Bronchitis and asthma, age 18 or older, with CC
69	3	Otitis media and upper respiratory infection, age 18 or older, without CC	97	4	Bronchitis and asthma, age 18 or older, without CC
70	3	Otitis media and upper respiratory infection, age 17 or younger	98	4	Bronchitis and asthma, age 17 or younger
			99	4	Respiratory signs and symptoms with CC
71	3	Laryngotracheitis	100	4	Respiratory signs and symptoms without CC

DRG	MDC	Description	DRG	MDC	Description
101	4	Other respiratory system diagnoses with CC	126	5	Acute and subacute endocarditis
102	4	Other respiratory system diagnoses without CC	127	5	Heart failure and shock
103	5	Heart transplant	128	5	Deep vein thrombophlebitis
104	5	Cardiac valve and other major cardiothoracic procedures with cardiac catheterization	129	5	Cardiac arrest, unexplained
			130	5	Peripheral vascular disorders with CC
105	5	Cardiac valve and other major cardiothoracic procedures without cardiac catheterization	131	5	Peripheral vascular disorders without CC
			132	5	Atherosclerosis with CC
106	5	Coronary bypass with percutaneous transluminal coronary angioplasty (PTCA)	133	5	Atherosclerosis without CC
			134	5	Hypertension
107	5	Coronary bypass with cardiac catheterization	135	5	Cardiac congenital and valvular disorders, age 18 or older, with CC
108	5	Other cardiothoracic procedures	136	5	Cardiac congenital and valvular disorders, age 18 or older, without CC
109	5	Coronary bypass without cardiac catheterization			
110	5	Major cardiovascular procedures with CC	137	5	Cardiac congenital and valvular disorders, age 17 or younger
111	5	Major cardiovascular procedures without CC			
112	5	Percutaneous cardiovascular procedures	138	5	Cardiac arrhythmia and conduction disorders with CC
113	5	Amputation for circulatory system disorders except upper limb and toe	139	5	Cardiac arrhythmia and conduction disorders without CC
114	5	Upper limb and toe amputation for circulatory system disorders	140	5	Angina pectoris
			141	5	Syncope and collapse with CC
115	5	Permanent cardiac pacemaker implant with acute MI, heart failure, or shock, or AICD lead or general procedure	142	5	Syncope and collapse without CC
			143	5	Chest pain
			144	5	Other circulatory system diagnoses with CC
116	5	Other permanent cardiac pacemaker implant or PTCA with coronary arterial stent	145	5	Other circulatory system diagnoses without CC
			146	6	Rectal resection with CC
117	5	Cardiac pacemaker revision except device replacement	147	6	Rectal resection without CC
			148	6	Major small and large bowel procedures with CC
118	5	Cardiac pacemaker device replacement	149	6	Major small and large bowel procedures without CC
119	5	Vein ligation and stripping			
120	5	Other circulatory system operating room procedures	150	6	Peritoneal adhesiolysis with CC
			151	6	Peritoneal adhesiolysis without CC
121	5	Circulatory disorders with acute MI and major complications, discharged alive	152	6	Minor small and large bowel procedures with CC
122	5	Circulatory disorders with acute MI without major complications, discharged alive	153	6	Minor small and large bowel procedures without CC
123	5	Circulatory disorders with acute MI, expired			
124	5	Circulatory disorders except acute MI, with cardiac catheterization and complex diagnosis	154	6	Stomach, esophageal and duodenal procedures, age 18 or older, with CC
125	5	Circulatory disorders except acute MI, with cardiac catheterization without complex diagnosis			

DRG	MDC	Description	DRG	MDC	Description
155	6	Stomach, esophageal and duodenal procedures, age 18 or older, without CC	182	6	Esophagitis, gastroenteritis, and miscellaneous digestive disorders, age 18 or older, with CC
156	6	Stomach, esophageal and duodenal procedures, age 17 or younger	183	6	Esophagitis, gastroenteritis, and miscellaneous digestive disorders, age 18 or older, without CC
157	6	Anal and stomal procedures with CC	184	6	Esophagitis, gastroenteritis, and miscellaneous digestive disorders, age 17 or younger
158	6	Anal and stomal procedures without CC			
159	6	Hernia procedures except inguinal and femoral, age 18 or older, with CC	185	3	Dental and oral disease except extractions and restorations, age 18 or older
160	6	Hernia procedures except inguinal and femoral, age 18 or older, without CC	186	3	Dental and oral disease except extractions and restorations, age 17 or younger
161	6	Inguinal and femoral hernia procedures, age 18 or older, with CC	187	3	Dental extractions and restorations
162	6	Inguinal and femoral hernia procedures, age 18 or older, without CC	188	6	Other digestive system diagnoses, age 18 or older, with CC
163	6	Hernia procedures, age 17 and younger	189	6	Other digestive system diagnoses, age 18 or older, without CC
164	6	Appendectomy with complicated principal diagnosis with CC	190	6	Other digestive system diagnoses, age 17 or younger
165	6	Appendectomy with complicated principal diagnosis without CC	191	7	Pancreas, liver, and shunt procedures, with CC
166	6	Appendectomy without complicated principal diagnosis with CC	192	7	Pancreas, liver, and shunt procedures, without CC
167	6	Appendectomy without complicated principal diagnosis without CC	193	7	Biliary tract procedures except only cholecystectomy, with or without common duct exploration, with CC
168	3	Mouth procedures with CC	194	7	Biliary tract procedures except only cholecystectomy, with or without common duct exploration, without CC
169	3	Mouth procedures without CC			
170	6	Other digestive system operating room procedures with CC	195	7	Cholecystectomy with common duct exploration, with CC
171	6	Other digestive system operating room procedures without CC	196	7	Cholecystectomy with common duct exploration, without CC
172	6	Digestive malignancy with CC	197	7	Cholecystectomy except by laparoscope without common duct exploration, with CC
173	6	Digestive malignancy without CC	198	7	Cholecystectomy except by laparoscope without common duct exploration, without CC
174	6	Gastrointestinal hemorrhage with CC			
175	6	Gastrointestinal hemorrhage without CC	199	7	Hepatobiliary diagnostic procedure for malignancy
176	6	Complicated peptic ulcer	200	7	Hepatobiliary diagnostic procedure for non-malignancy
177	6	Uncomplicated peptic ulcer with CC			
178	6	Uncomplicated peptic ulcer without CC	201	7	Other hepatobiliary or pancreas operating room procedures
179	6	Inflammatory bowel disease			
180	6	Gastrointestinal obstruction with CC	202	7	Cirrhosis and alcoholic hepatitis
181	6	Gastrointestinal obstruction without CC	203	7	Malignancy or hepatobiliary system or pancreas

DRG	MDC	Description	DRG	MDC	Description
204	7	Disorders of pancreas except malignancy	228	8	Major thumb or joint procedures, or other hand or wrist procedures, with CC
205	7	Disorders of liver except malignancy, cirrhosis, alcoholic hepatitis, with CC	229	8	Hand or wrist procedures, except major joint procedures, without CC
206	7	Disorders of liver except malignancy, cirrhosis, alcoholic hepatitis, without CC	230	8	Local excision and removal of internal fixation devices of hip and femur
207	7	Disorders of the biliary tract with CC	231	8	Local excision and removal of internal fixation devices, except hip and femur
208	7	Disorders of the biliary tract without CC	232	8	Arthroscopy
209	8	Major joint and limb reattachment procedures of lower extremity	233	8	Other musculoskeletal system and connective tissue operating room procedures with CC
210	8	Hip and femur procedures exept major joint, age 18 or older, with CC	234	8	Other musculoskeletal system and connective tissue operating room procedures without CC
211	8	Hip and femur procedures exept major joint, age 18 or older, without CC	235	8	Fractures of femur
			236	8	Fractures of hip and pelvis
212	8	Hip and femur procedures exept major joint, age 17 or younger	237	8	Sprains, strains, and dislocations of hip, pelvis, and thigh
213	8	Amputation for musculoskeletal system and connective tissue disorders	238	8	Osteomyelitis
214	8	No Longer Valid	239	8	Pathological fractures and musculoskeletal and connective tissue malignancy
215	8	No Longer Valid			
216	8	Biopsies of musculoskeletal system and connective tissue	240	8	Connective tissue disorders with CC
			241	8	Connective tissue disorders without CC
217	8	Wound debridement and skin graft, except hand, for musculoskeletal and connective tissue disorders	242	8	Septic arthritis
			243	8	Medical back problems
			244	8	Bone diseases and specific arthropathies with CC
218	8	Lower extremity and humerus procedures except hip, foot, and femur, age 18 or older, with CC	245	8	Bone diseases and specific arthropathies without CC
219	8	Lower extremity and humerus procedures except hip, foot, and femur, age 18 or older, without CC	246	8	Nonspecific arthropathies
			247	8	Signs and symptoms of musculoskeletal system and connective tissue
220	8	Lower extremity and humerus procedures except hip, foot, and femur, age 17 or younger	248	8	Tendonitis, myositis, and bursitis
221	8	No Longer Valid	249	8	Aftercare, musculoskeletal system, and connective tissue
222	8	No Longer Valid			
223	8	Major shoulder/elbow procedures, or other upper extremity procedures, with CC	250	8	Fractures, sprains, strains, and dislocations of forearm, hand, or foot, age 18 or older, with CC
224	8	Shoulder, elbow, or forearm procedures except major joint procedures, without CC	251	8	Fractures, sprains, strains, and dislocations of forearm, hand, or foot, age 18 or older, without CC
225	8	Foot procedures			
226	8	Soft tissue procedures with CC	252	8	Fractures, sprains, strains, and dislocations of forearm, hand, or foot, age 17 or younger
227	8	Soft tissue procedures without CC			

DRG	MDC	Description
253	8	Fractures, sprains, strains, and dislocations of upper arm and lower leg, except foot, age 18 or older, with CC
254	8	Fractures, sprains, strains, and dislocations of upper arm and lower leg, except foot, age 18 or older, without CC
255	8	Fractures, sprains, strains, and dislocations of upper arm and lower leg, except foot, age 17 or younger
256	8	Other musculoskeletal system and connective tissue diagnoses
257	9	Total mastectomy for malignancy, with CC
258	9	Total mastectomy for malignancy, without CC
259	9	Subtotal mastectomy for malignancy with CC
260	9	Subtotal mastectomy for malignancy without CC
261	9	Breast procedure for non-malignancy except biopsy and local excision
262	9	Breast biopsy and local excision for non-malignancy
263	9	Skin graft and/or debridement for skin ulcer or cellulitis, with CC
264	9	Skin graft and/or debridement for skin ulcer or cellulitis, without CC
265	9	Skin graft and/or debridement except for skin ulcer or cellulitis, with CC
266	9	Skin graft and/or debridement except for skin ulcer or cellulitis, without CC
267	9	Perianal and pilonidal procedures
268	9	Skin, subcutaneous tissue, and breast plastic procedures
269	9	Other skin, subcutaneous tissue, and breast procedures with CC
270	9	Other skin, subcutaneous tissue, and breast procedures without CC
271	9	Skin ulcers
272	9	Major skin disorders with CC
273	9	Major skin disorders without CC
274	9	Malignant breast disorders with CC
275	9	Malignant breast disorders without CC
276	9	Nonmalignant breast disorders
277	9	Cellulitis, age 18 or older, with CC
278	9	Cellulitis, age 18 or older, without CC
279	9	Cellulitis, age 17 or younger
280	9	Trauma to the skin, subcutaneous tissue, and breast, age 18 or older, with CC
281	9	Trauma to the skin, subcutaneous tissue, and breast, age 18 or older, without CC
282	9	Trauma to the skin, subcutaneous tissue, and breast, age 17 or younger
283	9	Minor skin disorders with CC
284	9	Minor skin disorders without CC
285	10	Amputation of lower limb for endocrine, nutritional, and metabolic disorders
286	10	Adrenal and pituitary procedures
287	10	Skin grafts and wound debridement for endocrine, nutritional, and metabolic disorders
288	10	Operating room procedures for obesity
289	10	Parathyroid procedures
290	10	Thyroid procedures
291	10	Thyroglossal procedures
292	10	Other endocrine, nutritional, and metabolic operating room procedures with CC
293	10	Other endocrine, nutritional, and metabolic operating room procedures without CC
294	10	Diabetes, age 36 or older
295	10	Diabetes, age 35 or younger
296	10	Nutritional and miscellaneous metabolic disorders, age 18 or older, with CC
297	10	Nutritional and miscellaneous metabolic disorders, age 18 or older, without CC
298	10	Nutritional and miscellaneous metabolic disorders, age 17 and younger
299	10	Inborn errors of metabolism
300	10	Endocrine disorders with CC
301	10	Endocrine disorders without CC
302	11	Kidney transplant
303	11	Kidney, ureter, and major bladder procedures for neoplasm
304	11	Kidney, ureter, and major bladder procedures for non-neoplasms, with CC

DRG	MDC	Description
305	11	Kidney, ureter, and major bladder procedures for non-neoplasms, without CC
306	11	Prostatectomy with CC
307	11	Prostatectomy without CC
308	11	Minor bladder procedures with CC
309	11	Minor bladder procedures without CC
310	11	Transurethral procedures with CC
311	11	Transurethral procedures without CC
312	11	Urethral procedures, age 18 or older, with CC
313	11	Urethral procedures, age 18 or older, without CC
314	11	Urethral procedures, age 17 or younger
315	11	Other kidney and urinary tract operating room procedures
316	11	Renal failure
317	11	Admission for renal dialysis
318	11	Kidney and urinary tract neoplasms with CC
319	11	Kidney and urinary tract neoplasms without CC
320	11	Kidney and urinary tract infections, age 18 or older, with CC
321	11	Kidney and urinary tract infections, age 18 or older, without CC
322	11	Kidney and urinary tract infections, age 17 or younger
323	11	Urinary stones with CC, and/or ESW lithotripsy
324	11	Urinary stones without CC
325	11	Kidney and urinary tract signs and symptoms, age 18 or older, with CC
326	11	Kidney and urinary tract signs and symptoms, age 18 or older, without CC
327	11	Kidney and urinary tract signs and symptoms, age 17 or younger
328	11	Urethral stricture, age 18 or older, with CC
329	11	Urethral stricture, age 18 or older, without CC
330	11	Urethral stricture, age 17 or younger
331	11	Other kidney and urinary tract diagnoses, age 18 or older, with CC
332	11	Other kidney and urinary tract diagnoses, age 18 or older, without CC
333	11	Other kidney and urinary tract diagnoses, age 17 or younger
334	12	Major male pelvic procedures with CC
335	12	Major male pelvic procedures without CC
336	12	Transurethral prostatectomy with CC
337	12	Transurethral prostatectomy without CC
338	12	Testes procedures for malignancy
339	12	Testes procedures for non-malignancy, age 18 or older
340	12	Testes procedures for non-malignancy, age 17 or younger
341	12	Penis procedures
342	12	Circumcision, age 18 or older
343	12	Circumcision, age 17 or younger
344	12	Other male reproductive system operating room procedures for malignancy
345	12	Other male reproductive system operating room procedures except for malignancy
346	12	Malignancy of male reproductive system, with CC
347	12	Malignancy of male reproductive system, without CC
348	12	Benign prostatic hypertrophy with CC
349	12	Benign prostatic hypertrophy without CC
350	12	Inflammation of the male reproductive system
351	12	Male sterilization
352	12	Other male reproductive system diagnoses
353	13	Pelvic evisceration, radical hysterectomy, and radical vulvectomy
354	13	Uterine and adnexa procedures for non-ovarian/adnexal malignancy, with CC
355	13	Uterine and adnexa procedures for non-ovarian/adnexal malignancy, without CC
356	13	Female reproductive system reconstructive procedures
357	13	Uterine and adnexa procedures for ovarian or adnexal malignancy
358	13	Uterine and adnexa procedures for nonmalignancy with CC
359	13	Uterine and adnexa procedures for nonmalignancy without CC
360	13	Vagina, cervix, and vulva procedures

DRG	MDC	Description	DRG	MDC	Description
361	13	Laparoscopy and incisional tubal interruption	387	15	Prematurity with major problems
362	13	Endoscopic tubal interruption	388	15	Prematurity without major problems
363	13	D and C, conization, and radio implant for malignancy	389	15	Full-term neonate with major problems
			390	15	Neonates with other significant problems
364	13	D and C, conization, except for malignancy	391	15	Normal newborn
365	13	Other female reproductive system operating room procedures	392	16	Splenectomy, age 18 or older
			393	16	Splenectomy, age 17 or younger
366	13	Malignancy of female reproductive system, with CC	394	16	Other operating room procedures of the blood and blood forming organs
367	13	Malignancy of female reproductive system, without CC	395	16	Red blood cell disorders, age 18 or older
368	13	Infections, female reproductive system	396	16	Red blood cell disorders, age 17 or younger
369	13	Menstrual and other female reproductive system disorders	397	16	Coagulation disorders
			398	16	Reticuloendothelial and immunity disorders with CC
370	14	Cesarean section with CC	399	16	Reticuloendothelial and immunity disorders without CC
371	14	Cesarean section without CC			
372	14	Vaginal delivery with complicating diagnoses	400	17	Lymphoma and leukemia with major operating room procedure
373	14	Vaginal delivery without complicating diagnoses	401	17	Lymphoma and nonacute leukemia with other operating room procedure, with CC
374	14	Vaginal delivery with sterilization and/or D and C	402	17	Lymphoma and nonacute leukemia with other operating room procedure, without CC
375	14	Vaginal delivery with operating room procedure except sterilization and/or D and C	403	17	Lymphoma and nonacute leukemia, with CC
			404	17	Lymphoma and nonacute leukemia, without CC
376	14	Postpartum and postabortion diagnoses without operating room procedures	405	17	Acute leukemia without major operating room procedure, age 17 or younger
377	14	Postpartum and postabortion diagnoses with operating room procedures	406	17	Myeloproliferative disorders or poorly differentiated neoplasms with major operating room procedures, with CC
378	14	Ectopic pregnancy			
379	14	Threatened abortion	407	17	Myeloproliferative disorders or poorly differentiated neoplasms with major operating room procedures, without CC
380	14	Abortion without D and C			
381	14	Abortion with D and C, aspiration curettage, or hysterotomy	408	17	Myeloproliferative disorders or poorly differentiated neoplasms with other operating room procedures
382	14	False labor			
383	14	Other antepartum diagnoses with medical complications	409	17	Radiotherapy
384	14	Other antepartum diagnoses without medical complications	410	17	Chemotherapy without acute leukemia as secondary diagnosis
385	15	Neonates, died or transferred to another acute care facility	411	17	History of malignancy without endoscopy
386	15	Extreme immaturity or respiratory distress syndrome, neonate	412	17	History of malignancy with endoscopy

DRG	MDC	Description
413	17	Other myeloproliferative disorders or poorly differentiated neoplasm diagnosis with CC
414	17	Other myeloproliferative disorders or poorly differentiated neoplasm diagnosis without CC
415	18	Operating room procedure for infectious and parasitic diseases
416	18	Septicemia, age 18 or older
417	18	Septicemia, age 17 or younger
418	18	Postoperative and post-traumatic infections
419	18	Fever of unknown origin, age 18 or older, with CC
420	18	Fever of unknown origin, age 18 or older, without CC
421	18	Viral illness, age 18 or older
422	18	Viral illness and fever of unknown origin, age 17 or younger
423	18	Other infectious and parasitic diseases diagnoses
424	19	Operating room procedure with principal diagnoses of mental illness
425	19	Acute adjustment reaction and disturbances of psychosocial dysfunction
426	19	Depressive neuroses
427	19	Neuroses, except depressive
428	19	Disorders of personality and impulse control
429	19	Organic disturbances and mental retardation
430	19	Psychoses
431	19	Childhood mental disorders
432	19	Other mental disorder diagnoses
433	20	Alcohol/drug abuse or dependence, left against medical advice
434	20	Alcohol/drug abuse or dependence, detoxification, or other symptomatic treatment, with CC
435	20	Alcohol/drug abuse or dependence, detoxification, or other symptomatic treatment, without CC
436	20	Alcohol/drug dependence with rehabilitation therapy
437	20	Alchohol/drug dependence, combined rehabilitation, and detoxification therapy
438		No Longer Valid
439	21	Skin grafts for injuries
440	21	Wound debridements for injuries
441	21	Hand procedures for injuries
442	21	Other operating room procedures for injuries, with CC
443	21	Other operating room procedures for injuries, without CC
444	21	Traumatic injury, age 18 or older, with CC
445	21	Traumatic injury, age 18 or older, without CC
446	21	Traumatic injury, age 17 or younger
447	21	Allergic reactions, age 18 or older
448	21	Allergic reactions, age 17 or younger
449	21	Poisoning and toxic effects of drugs, age 18 or older, with CC
450	21	Poisoning and toxic effects of drugs, age 18 or older, without CC
451	21	Poisoning and toxic effects of drugs, age 17 or younger
452	21	Complications of treatment, with CC
453	21	Complications of treatment, without CC
454	21	Other injury, poisoning, and toxic effect diagnosis, with CC
455	21	Other injury, poisoning, and toxic effect diagnosis, without CC
456		No Longer Valid
457		No Longer Valid
458		No Longer Valid
459		No Longer Valid
460		No Longer Valid
461	23	Operating room procedures with diagnoses of other contact with health services
462	23	Rehabilitation
463	23	Signs and symptoms with CC
464	23	Signs and symptoms without CC
465	23	Aftercare with history of malignancy as secondary diagnosis
466	23	Aftercare without history of malignancy as secondary diagnosis

DRG	MDC	Description
467	23	Other factors influencing health status
468	All	Extensive operating room procedure unrelated to principal diagnosis
469	14	Principal diagnosis invalid as discharge diagnosis
470	15	Ungroupable
471	8	Bilateral or multiple major joint procedures of lower extremity
472		No Longer Valid
473	17	Acute leukemia without major operating room procedure, age 18 or older
474		No Longer Valid
475	4	Respiratory system diagnosis with ventilator support
476	All	Prostatic operating room procedure unrelated to principal diagnosis
477	All	Non-extensive operating room procedure unrelated to principal diagnosis
478	5	Other vascular procedures with CC
479	5	Other vascular procedures without CC
480	All	Liver transplant
481	All	Bone marrow transplant
482	All	Tracheostomy for face, mouth, and neck diagnoses
483		Tracheostomy, except for face, mouth, and neck diagnoses
484	24	Craniotomy for multiple significant trauma
485	24	Limb reattachment, hip and femur procedure, for multiple significant trauma
486	24	Other operating room procedures for multiple significant trauma
487	24	Other multiple significant trauma
488	25	HIV with extensive operating room procedure
489	25	HIV with major related condition
490	25	HIV with or without other related condition
491	8	Major joint and limb reattachment procedures of upper extremity
492	17	Chemotherapy with acute leukemia as secondary diagnosis
493	7	Laparoscopic cholecystectomy without common duct exploration, with CC
494	7	Laparoscopic cholecystectomy without common duct exploration, without CC
495	All	Lung transplant
496	8	Combined anterior/posterior spinal fusion
497	8	Spinal fusion with CC
498	8	Spinal fusion without CC
499	8	Back and neck procedures except spinal fusion with CC
500	8	Back and neck procedures except spinal fusion without CC
501	8	Knee procedure with principal diagnosis of infection, with CC
502	8	Knee procedure with principal diagnosis of infection, without CC
503	8	Knee procedures without principal diagnosis of infection
504	22	Extensive third degree burn with skin graft
505	22	Extensive third degree burn without skin graft
506	22	Full thickness burn with skin graft or inhalation injury with CC or significant trauma
507	22	Full thickness burn with skin graft or inhalation injury without CC or significant trauma
508	22	Full thickness burn without skin graft or inhalation injury with CC or significant trauma
509	22	Full thickness burn without skin graft or inhalation injury without CC or significant trauma
510	22	Non-extensive burns with CC or significant trauma
511	22	Non-extensive burns without CC or significant trauma

Appendix 3: 3-Digit ICD·9

Three-digit ICD-9-CM codes are used to identify a condition or disease only when a fourth or fifth digit is not available. The following are the only ICD-9-CM codes that are valid without further specificity:

024	Glanders
025	Melioidosis
035	Erysipelas
037	Tetanus
042	Human Immunodeficiency Virus (HIV) Infection
048	Other enterovirus diseases of central nervous system
061	Dengue
064	Viral encephalitis transmitted by other and unspecified arthropods
071	Rabies
075	Infectious mononucleosis
080	Louse-borne [epidemic] typhus
096	Late syphilis, latent
101	Vincent's angina
118	Opportunistic mycoses
124	Trichinosis
129	Intestinal parasitism, unspecified
135	Sarcoidosis
138	Late effects of acute poliomyelitis
179	Malignant neoplasm of uterus, part unspecified
181	Malignant neoplasm of placenta
185	Malignant neoplasm of prostate
193	Malignant neoplasm of thyroid gland
217	Benign neoplasm of breast
220	Benign neoplasm of ovary
226	Benign neoplasm of thyroid gland
243	Congenital hypothyroidism
260	Kwashiorkor
261	Nutritional marasmus
262	Other severe protein-calorie malnutrition
267	Ascorbic acid deficiency
311	Depressive disorder, not elsewhere classified
316	Psychic factors associated with diseases classified elsewhere
317	Mild mental retardation
319	Unspecified mental retardation
325	Phlebitis and thrombophlebitis of intracranial venous sinuses
326	Late effects of intracranial abscess or pyogenic infection
340	Multiple sclerosis
347	Cataplexy and narcolepsy
390	Rheumatic fever without mention of heart involvement
393	Chronic rheumatic pericarditis
412	Old myocardial infarction
430	Subarachnoid hemorrhage
431	Intracerebral hemorrhage
436	Acute, but ill-defined, cerebrovascular disease
452	Portal vein thrombosis
460	Acute nasopharyngitis [common cold]
462	Acute pharyngitis
463	Acute tonsillitis
470	Deviated nasal septum
475	Peritonsillar abscess
481	Pneumococcal pneumonia [Streptococcus pneumoniae pneumonia]
485	Bronchopneumonia, organism unspecified
486	Pneumonia, organism unspecified
490	Bronchitis, not specified as acute or chronic
494	Bronchiectasis
496	Chronic airway obstruction, not elsewhere classified
500	Coal workers' pneumoconiosis
501	Asbestosis
502	Pneumoconiosis due to other silica or silicates

503	Pneumoconiosis due to other inorganic dust
504	Pneumonopathy due to inhalation of other dust
505	Pneumoconiosis, unspecified
514	Pulmonary congestion and hypostasis
515	Postinflammatory pulmonary fibrosis
541	Appendicitis, unqualified
542	Other appendicitis
566	Abscess of anal and rectal regions
570	Acute and subacute necrosis of liver
585	Chronic renal failure
586	Renal failure, unspecified
587	Renal sclerosis, unspecified
591	Hydronephrosis
600	Hyperplasia of prostate
605	Redundant prepuce and phimosis
630	Hydatidiform mole
631	Other abnormal product of conception
632	Missed abortion
650	Normal delivery
677	Late effect of complication of pregnancy, childbirth, and the puerperium
683	Acute lymphadenitis
684	Impetigo
700	Corns and callosities
725	Polymyalgia rheumatica
734	Flat foot
769	Respiratory distress syndrome
797	Senility without mention of psychosis
920	Contusion of face, scalp, and neck except eye(s)
931	Foreign body in ear
932	Foreign body in nose
936	Foreign body in intestine and colon
937	Foreign body in anus and rectum
938	Foreign body in digestive system, unspecified
981	Toxic effect of petroleum products
986	Toxic effect of carbon monoxide
990	Effects of radiation, unspecified
V08	Asymptomatic human immunodeficiency virus (HIV) infection status
V51	Aftercare involving the use of plastic surgery

Appendix 4: ICD-9 Coding

The differences and similarities of diagnostic coding rules are explained in this chart and in the introduction. The most important factor in ICD-9-CM coding, whether outpatient or inpatient, is understanding the rules. Correct sequencing and reporting of diagnostic codes must be the goal for all coders.

General Diagnostic Coding

- Consult main terms in Volume 2 (alphabetic index) first then verify the code in Volume 1 (tabular).

- Assign codes to the highest level of specificity. Use fourth and fifth digits when available. Be as specific as possible in describing the patient's condition, illness, or disease.

- Do not add to or subtract from the statements made by the provider. Request further information to clarify an issue.

- For outpatient services, identify the acute conditions of emergency situations, such as coma, loss of consciousness, hemorrhage, etc. For inpatient services, list what the conditions are "due to" (e.g., coma, due to subdural hemorrhage).

- To code poisonings, list the poison code first, manifestation code second, and E code third. To code an adverse effect of a drug in therapeutic use, code the manifestation first and the E code second.

- When coding neoplasms, list the primary site first and the secondary site second if a primary site is still present. This changes when the treatment or workup is aimed solely at the secondary site, in which case the secondary site is sequenced first.

- For multiple injuries, the most severe injury as designated by the physician is always coded first. If injuries are equal in severity, use the code for which definitive treatment was provided as the primary or principal diagnosis.

- Identify how injuries occurred. Always list every pertinent E (external cause) code.

- Identify causes of infection (004.0 *Shigella dysenteriae*) as secondary codes.

- Do not use an unspecified code unless there is no other information and the physician cannot clarify the condition.

- Use a V code for postoperative care, followed by the preoperative condition, unless the condition is no longer present. For inpatient coding always make sure the principal diagnosis is a valid code by consulting the principal diagnosis exclusion list in the Diagnosis Related Groups Definition Manual.

- While many diagnostic codes are specific to an individual condition or disease, others are more general. A general code may encompass many similar conditions and still be a valid code. Because some codes are more general it may be necessary to inform providers that a more specific code for a disease or condition is not always available.

Outpatient Diagnostic Coding

- Code the primary diagnosis first — the current and the most significant reason for the services or procedures provided.

- List all secondary and subsequent codes, coexisting conditions, or conditions developing that pertain to the treatment of the patient.

- Rule-out, possible, probable, suspected, and questionable conditions are not used for outpatient coding.

- Code symptoms rather than rule-out statements if no definitive diagnosis can be made at the visit.

- Report encounters for circumstances other than disease or injury (eg, general medical exam, screening mammogram) with the appropriate V-code.

- Assign each medical service and surgical procedure a corresponding diagnostic code.

- Distinguish between acute and chronic conditions when appropriate. Code chronic complaints only when treatment is provided for the condition. If both an acute and a chronic condition are present and are treated, code the acute condition first and the chronic condition second.

- List commonly used codes on your charge ticket, including the numerical designator and an accurate ICD-9-CM written description. Allow ample room for write-ins. When possible, code from the medical record to ensure that the physician's diagnosis is clearly documented.

- Revise your billing forms periodically to include only accurate and complete ICD-9-CM codes.

- Exercise caution when coding pre-existing conditions.

Inpatient Diagnostic Coding

- List the principal diagnosis first — the main reason the patient was admitted to the hospital after study.

- Code all co-existing conditions or conditions that develop as second and subsequent diagnoses.

- Code a complication that was the reason for the admission as the principal diagnosis.

- Code a complication that occurred during the hospitalization as a secondary code.

- Code an acute condition first and a chronic condition second when both are present, such as acute and chronic asthma.

- Sequence contrasting or comparative diagnoses, based on the circumstances of the admission.

- When a symptom is followed by contrasting/comparative diagnoses, sequence the symptom first. Contrasting/comparative diagnoses are reported secondarily as suspected conditions.

- Code the residual problem of a late effect first, then the late effect code. There is no time limit on late effect codes. Residual effects can occur early or months or years later.

- Code probable, possible, rule-out, and suspected conditions as if they exist, until they are ruled out. The only exception is HIV infection which is coded only when confirmed.

- For two or more diagnoses of equal importance, list the principal diagnosis as the one for which definitive treatment was provided, either surgical or nonsurgical. If no definitive procedure was performed, the most resource-intensive diagnosis becomes the principal diagnosis.

- When a disease is listed with a condition (e.g., cerebrovascular disease with hypertension), list the disease first and the condition second.

- Code what a symptom or condition is "due to." Do not code the symptom or condition.

- Code only those conditions that are significant and pertinent to the current hospital stay, including conditions affecting the management of the patient, conditions for which treatment is performed, or conditions that lengthen the stay.

- Code symptoms if no definitive diagnosis can be made. Use rule-out statements instead of symptoms unless the symptom is the only diagnosis listed.

Appendix 5: DRG Tree

Major Diagnostic Category 6
Diseases and Disorders of the Digestive System

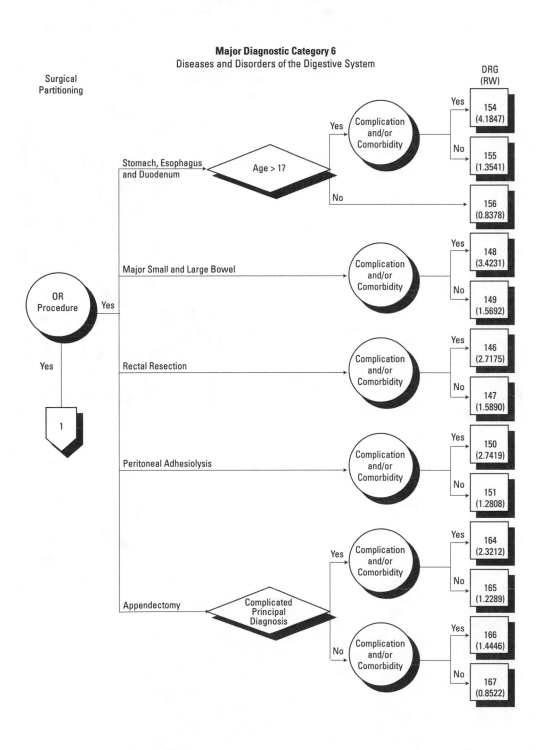

Major Diagnostic Category 6
Diseases and Disorders of the Digestive System

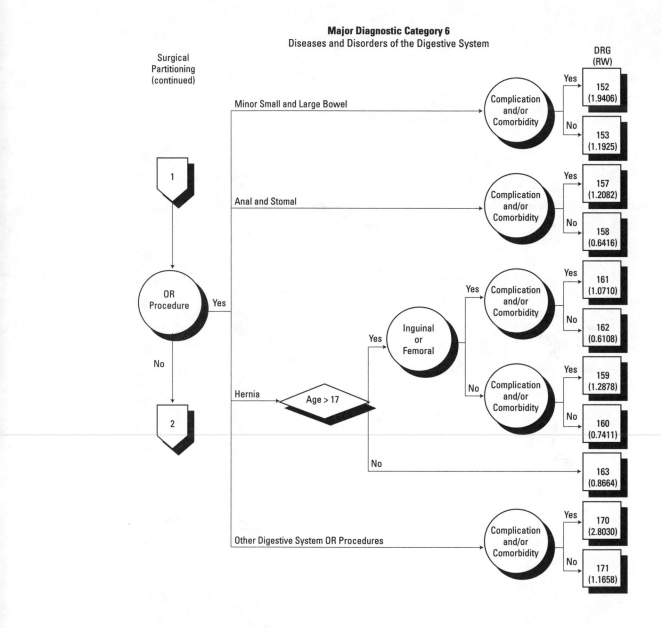

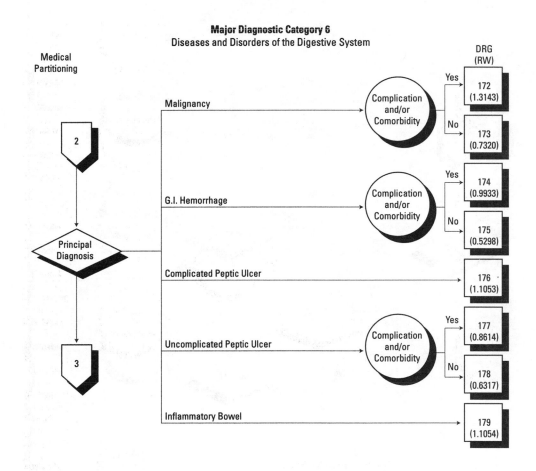

Major Diagnostic Category 6
Diseases and Disorders of the Digestive System

Medical
Partitioning

DRG
(RW)

Major Diagnostic Category 6
Diseases and Disorders of the Digestive System

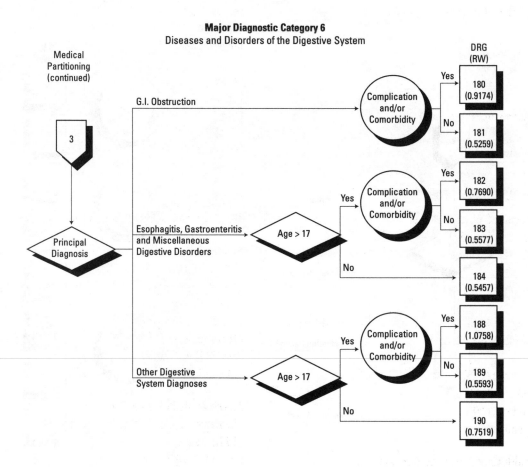

Appendix 6: Addresses

American Academy of Insurance Medicine
PO Box 59811
Potomac, MD 20859-9811
(301) 365-3572
http://www.aaimedicine.org

American Academy of Procedural Coders (AAPC)
145 W. Crystal Ave.
Salt Lake City, UT 84115
(800) 626-CODE (2633)
http://www.aapc.com

American Association of Health Plans
1129 20th Street Nw, Suite 600
Washington, DC 20036-3421
(202) 778-3200
http://www.aahp.org

American College of Physicians — American Society of Internal Medicine (ACP-ASIM)
Headquarters:
190 N. Independence Mall West
Philadelphia, PA 19106-1572
(800) 523-1546 ext. 2600
http://www.acponline.org

Agency for Health Care Policy and Research (AHCPR)
2191 East Jefferson Street
Rockville, MD 20852
(301) 594-8364
http://www.ahcpr.gov

American Health Information Management Association (AHIMA)
919 N. Michigan Ave., Suite 1400
Chicago, IL 60611
(312) 787-2672
http://www.ahima.org

or

For Certification Exam Information
Attention: AHIMA Examination
Applied Measurement Professionals, Inc.
8310 Nieman Rd.
Lenexa, KS 66214
(913) 541-0400
http://www.ahima.org/certification/1999.exams.html

American Hospital Association (AHA)
Coding Advice
Central Office on ICD•9•CM
One North Franklin
Chicago, IL 60606
(312) 422-3000
Fax: (312) 422-4583
(800) 242-2626

American Medical Association (AMA)
The Department of Coding & Nomenclature
515 N. State St.
Chicago, IL 60610-0946
(312) 464-5000
http://www.ama-assn.org

Blue Cross Blue Shield Association
State listings
http://www.bluecares.com

Centers for Disease Control and Prevention
1600 Clifton Rd, NE
Atlanta, GA 30333
(404) 639-3311
http://www.cdc.gov

Health Care Financing Administration (HCFA)
Plans and Providers
7500 Security Blvd.
Baltimore, MD 21244
(410) 786-3000
http://www.hcfa.gov/audience/planprov.htm

Medical Records Institute
567 Walnut Street
PO Box 600770
Newton, MA 02460
(617) 964-3923
Fax: (617) 964-3926
http://www.medrecinst.com

Medicode, Inc
5225 Wiley Post Way, Suite 500
Salt Lake City, Utah 84116
(800) 999-4614
Fax: (801) 536-1009
For specific coding questions:
Medicode Helpline (800) 765-6818
(Calls cost $2.50 per minute for providers)

National Center for Health Statistics (NCHS)
6525 Belcrest Rd.
Hyattsville, MD 20782-2003
(301) 436-8500
http://www.cdc.gov/nchswww

National Committee for Quality Assurance (NCQA)
2000 L Street NW
Suite 500
Washington, DC 20036
(202) 955-3500
Fax: (202) 955-3599
http://www.ncqa.org

National Electronic Biller's Alliance (NEBA)
2226-A Westborough Blvd. #504
South San Francisco, CA 94080
(650) 359-4419
Fax (650) 355-8683
http://www.nebazone.com

National Medical Association
1012 10th Street NW
Washington, DC 20001
(202) 347-1895

US Department of Health and Human Services (HHS)
Office of the Secretary
200 Independence Avenue, SW
Washington, DC 20201
(202) 690-6343
http://www.hhs.gov

US Government Publications
Consumer Information Center
Dept. WWW
Pueblo, CO 81009
(888) 878-3256

or

Consumer Information Center
Room 6-142 (xc)
1800 F Street NW
Washington, DC 20405
(202) 501-1794
http://www.access.gpo.gov

World Health Organization (WHO)
1775 K Street, NW, Suite 430
Washington, DC 20006
(202) 331-9081
http://www.who.int/regions/wdc.html

Appendix 7: Terms

An increasingly complex reimbursement climate means new terminology develops every year. The following glossary includes terms not only used when coding, it includes terms used by major insurers and Medicare.

AAPC – American Academy of Procedural Coders.

AAPCC – Adjusted average per capita cost. HCFA's best estimate of the amount of money it costs to care for Medicare recipients in a given area.

AAPPO – American Association of Preferred Provider Organizations.

Abstractor – A person who selects and extracts data from the medical record to be entered into computer files. The data and coded diagnoses track morbidity and mortality, infectious disease, and index disease. Information may be gathered to track data for departments within the facility, such as quality assurance and utilization review.

Accrual – The amount of money set aside to cover the benefit plan's expenses. Estimated using a combination of data including the claims system and plan's prior history.

ACLS – Advanced Cardiac Life Support. A certification often required of professionals who serve seriously injured or ill patients.

ACR – Adjusted community rate. A calculation of what premium the plan charges to provide Medicare-covered benefits to a group account to allow for greater frequency of use by participants.

ACS contract – *See* ASO

Actuarial assumptions – Characteristics used in calculating the risks and costs of a plan. Assumptions include age, sex, and occupation of enrollees; location; utilization rates; and service costs.

Add-on codes – Procedure performed in addition to the primary procedure and designated with a **+** in CPT. Add-on codes are never reported as stand-alone services. They are reported secondarily in addition to the primary procedure.

Adjudication – The judging of a claim.

ADS – Alternative delivery system. Any method of providing healthcare benefits that differs from traditional indemnity methods.

Adverse selection – The risk of enrolling members who are sicker than assumed and who will utilize more expensive services more frequently.

Age restriction – Limitation of benefits when a patient reaches a certain age.

Age/sex rating – Structuring capitation payments based on members' age and sex.

Aggregate amount – The maximum for which a member is insured for any single event.

AHA – American Hospital Association.

AHIMA – American Health Information Management Association.

ALOS – Average length of stay. A benchmark average used for analysis of utilization.

AMA – American Medical Association.

Ambulatory Surgery – Surgical procedure in which the patient is admitted, treated, and released on the same day.

AMCRA – American Managed Care Review Association.

AMLOS – Arithmetic mean length of stay – Average numbers of days within a given DRG stay in the hospital.

ANA – American Nursing Association.

Anesthesia formula – *See* Standard Anesthesia Formula

Anteroposterior (AP) – Front to back.

Anteroposterior and Lateral – Two projections are included in this examination.

AOA – American Osteopathic Association.

APG – Ambulatory patient group. A reimbursement methodology developed for the Health Care Financing Administration.

Appeal – A request for reconsideration of a negative claim decision.

Appropriateness of care – Term often used to denote proper setting of medical care that best meets the patient's diagnosis.

AP-DRG - All Patient Diagnostic Related Group. 3M HIS made revisions and adjustments to the DRG system, now referred to as the All-Patient DRGs (AP-DRGs). Early features of AP-DRGs included MDC 24, specifically devoted to the human immunodeficiency virus (HIV), as well as restructure of the MDC governing newborns.

APR – Average payment rate. The amount of money the Health Care Financing Administration could pay a Health Maintenance Organization for service to Medicare recipients under a risk contract.

ART – Accredited Record Technician. A certification awarded medical records practitioners.

ASA – American Society of Anesthesiologists publishes the Relative Value Guide with guidelines on anesthesia coding.

ASO – Administrative service only. A contract stipulation between a self-funded plan and an insurance company in which the insurance company assumes no risk and provides administrative services only.

Assignment of benefits – Payment of benefits directly to the provider of the services rather than to the member who received the benefits.

Assignment – An arrangement in which the provider submits the claim on behalf of the patient and is reimbursed directly by the patient's plan. By doing so, the provider agrees to accept what the plan allows.

At risk – A contract between Medicare and a payor or a payor and a provider in which the payor in the case of Medicare and the provider in the case of the payor contracts and gets paid a set amount for care of a patient base. If costs exceed the amount the payor or provider were paid, the patients will still receive care during the term of the contract.

Attained age – The age of the member as of the last birthday.

Auditor – A professional who evaluates a provider's utilization, quality of care, or level of reimbursement.

AWP – 1) Average wholesale price. A pharmaceutical price based on common data that is included in a pharmacy provider contract. 2) Any willing provider. Statutes requiring a provider network to accept any provider who meets the network's usual selection criteria.

Backlog – The queue of claims that have not been adjudicated.

Balance billing – When providers charge the patient the amount not paid by the insurance carrier above the deductible agreed.

Basic coverage – Insurance providing coverage for hospital care.

Basic health services – Benefits all federally qualified HMOs must offer.

Board certification – A certification in a particular specialty based on the physician's expertise and experience.

Boarder baby – 1) A newborn who remains in the nursery following discharge because the mother is still hospitalized; 2) A premature infant who no longer needs intensive care but who remains for observation.

Book of business – A payor's list of clients and contracts.

Bundled – 1) The gathering of several types of health insurance policies under a single payor; 2) The inclusive grouping of codes related to a procedure when submitting a claim.

Business coalition – Employers who form a cooperative to purchase healthcare less expensively.

Cafeteria plan – A benefit by an employer where various services of many payors are offered to members as separate elements in the health care plan.

Cap – Contract maximum.

Capitation – A system in which a set amount of money is received or paid out based on membership rather than on a number of services rendered.

Carrier – Insurance company responsible for processing claims.

Carve-out – 1) Term often used when referring to the integrated plan method of providing coverage to Medicare-eligible employees; 2) Medical benefits for a specific type of care that are not provided by the carrier of the members' insurance (e.g., Mental/Nervous provided by Ajax while Acme carries the medical plan).

Case management – The ongoing review of cases by professionals to assure the most appropriate utilization of services.

Case managers – A medical professional (usually a nurse or social worker) who reviews cases every few days to determine necessity of care and to advise provider on payor's utilization restrictions. Certifies ongoing care.

Catastrophic case management – Also called large case management. A method of review of ongoing cases in which the patient sustains catastrophic or extremely costly medical problems.

Catchment area – The geographical area from which a healthcare organization draws its members.

CCU – Coronary Care Unit. A facility dedicated to patients suffering from heart attack, stroke, or other serious cardiopulmonary problems.

Census – The number and demographics of patients or members.

Certification – Approval by a payor's case manager to continue care for a given number of days or visits.

CHAMPUS – Civilian Health and Medical Program of the Uniformed Services. Federal medical benefits reimbursement program for dependents of military personnel, military retirees, and others.

Cherry picking – Practice of enrolling only healthy individuals and excluding those with existing problems.

Churning — 1) A performance-based reimbursement system emphasizing provider productivity; 2) When a provider sees a patient more than medically necessary with the intent of generating more revenue.

Cineradiography – Movies done by x-ray.

Claim lag – 1) The time between the incurred date of the claim and its submission; 2) the time between the incurred date of the claim and its payment.

Claim manual – The administrative guidelines used by claims processors to adjudicate claims according to company policy and procedure.

Claim – Statement of medical services rendered requesting payment from insurance company or government entity.

Claims manager – Payor's manager who oversees employee who processes routine claims.

Claims reviewer –Payor employee who reviews claims like an auditor, looking at coding, prior authority, contract violations, etc.

CLIA – Clinical Laboratory Improvement Amendments. Requirements set in 1988 CLIA to impose varying levels of federal regulation on clinical procedures, and few laboratories, including those in physician offices, are exempt. Adopted by Medicare and Medicaid, CLIA regulations redefine laboratory testing in regard to laboratory certification and accreditation, proficiency testing, quality assurance, personnel standards, and program administration.

Closed claim – A claim for which all apparent benefits have been paid.

Closed panel – An arrangement in which a managed care organization contracts providers on an exclusive basis, restricting the providers from seeing patients enrolled in other payors' plans.

Closed treatment – A fracture site that is not surgically opened. There are three methods of closed treatment of fractures: without manipulation, with manipulation, and with or without traction.

CMI – Case mix index. Sum of all DRG relative weights, divided by the number of Medicare cases.

CMP – Competitive medical plan. A federal designation allowing plans to obtain eligibility to receive a Medicare risk contract without having to qualify as an HMO.

CMT – Current Medical Terminology. A manual of preferred medical nomenclature published by the American Medical Association prior to Current Procedural Terminology (CPT).

COA – Certificate of authority. A state license to operate as an HMO.

COB – Coordination of benefits. An agreement that prevents double payment for services when the member is covered by two or more sources. The agreement dictates which organization is primarily and secondarily responsible for payment.

COBRA – Consolidated Omnibus Reconciliation Act. Legislation that in part requires employers to offer terminated employees the opportunity to continue buying coverage as part of the employer's group.

Coder – A person who translates documented, written diagnoses and procedures into numeric and alphanumeric codes.

Coding Conventions – Are each space, type face, indentation, and punctuation mark determining how you must interpret ICD-9-CM codes. These "conventions" were developed to help you match correct codes to the diagnoses you encounter.

Cognitive – Being aware by drawing from knowledge, such as judgment, reason, perception, and memory.

Coinsurance – A limitation of the amount payable by the payor to the provider or member for care in traditional plans or in parts of managed care plans. For example, most traditional plans only pay 80% of care costs.

Commercial carriers – For-profit insurance companies issuing health coverage.

Common Working File (CWF) - All beneficiary entitlement information (Part A, Part B, Medicare Secondary Payor, and Health Maintenance Organization), deductible status, and all Part A and Part B claims history are maintained in CWF.

Comorbidity – A pre-existing condition that causes an increase in length of stay by at least one day in around 75 percent of cases. Used in DRG reimbursement.

Community rating – Methodology of state and federal governments that requires qualified HMOs to request the same amount of money for each member in a plan.

Comparative Performance Reports (CPRs) – CPRs annually compare a physician's services and procedures to those of physicians in the same specialty and geographic area.

Complex repair – The repair of wounds requiring reconstructive surgery, complicated wound closure, debridement, skin grafting, or intricate, unusual, and time-consuming techniques to obtain the maximum functional and cosmetic result. Complex repairs include the creation of a defect, (e.g., extending excisions), necessary preparations for repairs, and moderate debridement of complicated lacerations, avulsions, and other wounds.

Complication – A condition that arose during the hospitalization that will prolong the length of the hospital stay by at least one day in approximately 75 percent of the cases.

Component coding – Standardizes the reporting of interventional radiological services. Component coding allows a physician, regardless of specialty, to specifically identify and report those aspects of the service he or she provided, whether the procedural component, the radiological component, or both.

Consultation – A type of service provided by a physician whose opinion or advice regarding evaluation and/or management of a specific problem is requested by another physician or other appropriate source.

Continuity of coverage – Transfer of benefits from one plan to another without a lapse of coverage.

Contrast Material – Usually a radiopaque material that is placed into the body to enable a system or body structure to be visualized. Common terms include: non-ionic and low osmolar contrast media (LOCM), ionic and high osmolar contrast media (HOCM), barium, and gadolinium.

Conversion – Shifting of a member under a group contract to an individual contract.

Conversion factors – National multipliers that convert the geographically adjusted relative value units into Medicare Fee Schedule dollar amounts and applies to all services paid under the MFS.

Coordinated care – *See* managed care.

Copayment – A portion of the medical expense the member must pay out of pocket. In managed care plans, the member pays the copayment while checking in for his or her appointment.

Corridor deductible – A fixed out-of-pocket amount that the member must pay before benefits are available. Also called simply "deductible."

Counseling – A discussion with a patient and/or family concerning one or more of the following areas: diagnostic results, impressions, and/or recommended diagnostic studies; prognosis; risks and benefits of management (treatment) options; instructions for management (treatment) and/or follow-up; importance of compliance with chosen management (treatment) options; risk factor reduction; patient and family education.

Coverage Issues Manual (CIM) – A HCFA publication containing national coverage decisions and which sets forth whether or not specific medical items, services, treatment procedures, or technologies can be paid for under the Medicare program. The CIM is used by Part A Intermediaries, Part B Carriers, and Peer Review Organizations (PROs).

Covered charges – Charges for medical care and supplies that the insurance plan will pay.

Covered person – Any person entitled to benefits under the policy, whether a member or dependent.

CPT - 4 – Current Procedural Terminology, Fourth edition. The American Medical Association's list of five-digit codes used to report medical services. A standard reference for billing.

CPT code – A descriptor of a procedure with a five-digit identifying code number. CPT codes are developed and maintained by the American Medical Association.

CPT modifiers – A descriptor that indicates that a service was altered in some way from the stated CPT description without actually changing the basic definition of the service. Modifiers that apply to each of the six major sections of CPT are listed in the section guidelines. Modifiers can indicate: a service or procedure has both a professional and a technical component, a service or procedure was performed by more than one physician, only part of a service was performed, an adjunctive service was performed, a bilateral procedure was performed, a service or procedure was provided more than once, unusual events occurred, a procedure or service was altered in some way. A complete listing of all modifiers used in CPT coding is located in an appendix of CPT.

Credentialing – Reviewing the medical degrees, licensure, malpractice and any disciplinary record of medical providers for panel and quality assurance purposes.

Critical care – The care of critically ill patients in a variety of medical emergencies that requires the constant attendance of the physician (e.g., cardiac arrest, shock, bleeding, respiratory failure, postoperative complications, critically ill neonate).

Crosswalk – The cross-referencing of CPT codes with ICD-9-CM, anesthesia, dental, or HCPCS codes.

CRT – Cathode ray tube. An old term for the computer used by coders. Refers specifically to the monitor.

CSO – Clinical service organization – Healthcare organization developed by academic medical centers to integrate medical school, faculty practice plan, and hospital

Cutback – Reduction of the amount or type of insurance for a member who attains a specified age or condition (e.g., age 65, retirement).

Daily benefit – A specified maximum benefit payable for room and board charges at a hospital.

Database – The electronic store of utilization information used by payors to pay claims, negotiate contracts, and track utilization and cost of services.

Date of Service – *see* Service date

DAW – Dispense as written. The notation from a physician to a pharmacist requesting that the brand-name medication be given in lieu of a generic medication.

Days per thousand – A standard unit of measurement of utilization determined by calculating the number of hospital days used in a year for each thousand covered lives.

Decapitation – Inadequate capitation.

Decubitus (DEC) – Patient lying on the side.

Deductible – Member's medical services that must be paid out of pocket before the payor begins to pay.

Diagnosis – Determination of condition, disease, or syndrome and its implications.

Diagnostic – Services provided to determine the nature of the member's complaints.

Direct claim payment – A method where members deal directly with the payor rather than submitting claims through the employer.

Direct contract model – A plan that contracts directly with individual private practice physicians rather than through an intermediary.

Discharge plan – A plan submitted by a provider to the case manager as part of the treatment plan that details follow-up care after discharge.

Discharge status – Circumstance of patient at discharge. Examples include "expired,""transferred" to another facility, "left against medical advice."

Diskectomy - The excision of the intervertebral disk material.

DME – Durable medical equipment. Permanent equipment meant for medical treatment.

DOS – Date of service. The date on which care was provided.

DRG – Diagnosis related groups. The method HCFA uses to pay hospitals for Medicare recipients based on a statistical system of classifying any inpatient stay into one of 25 groups. It is a classification scheme whose patient types are defined by patients diagnoses or procedures and in some cases, by the patient's age or discharge status. Each DRG is intended to be medically meaningful and would ordinarily require an approximately equal resource consumption as measured by length of stay and cost.

Drug formulary – *See* Formulary.

DSM-IV – Diagnostic and Statistical Manual of Mental Disorders, Fourth edition. The manual used by mental health workers as the diagnostic coding system for substance abuse and mental health patients.

Dual option – The offering of an HMO and traditional plan by one carrier.

DUR – Drug utilization review. A review to assure prescribed medications medically necessary and appropriate.

E codes – ICD-9-CM codes that describe circumstances of an injury or illness. Their use establishes medical necessity, identifies causes of injury and poisoning, and identifies medications. Their use can also be pivotal in reimbursements from payors such as medical insurance plans, car insurers, home insurers or workers compensation programs. Also known as the Supplementary Classification of External Causes of Injury and Poisoning (E800–E999) The index for the E codes is found in Volume 2, following the Table of Drugs and Chemicals.

E/M codes – Evaluation and management services. E/M codes encompass services that are part of the 90000 series of CPT codes. The codes represent services (e.g., office, emergency department, inpatient visits) that are the most frequently performed by physicians. These codes have been placed, for convenience, at the beginning of CPT.

EAP – Employee assistance program. Short-term counseling offered to members to quickly resolve transient emotional problems and to identify on-going mental or substance abuse problems for subsequent referral. Often limited to a handful of visits.

EdD – Doctor of Education.

EDI – Electronic data interchange. The transference of claims, certifications, quality assurance reviews, and utilization data via computer.

EHO – Emerging healthcare organizations – Hospitals and other providers that are emerging or affiliating.

ELOS – The average number of days of hospitalization required for a given illness or procedure. Base on prior histories of patients who have been hospitalized for the same illness or procedure.

E/M Service Components – The key components in determining the correct level of E/M codes are: history, examination, and medical decision making.

Emergency department – An organized hospital-based facility for the provision of unscheduled episodic services to patients who present for immediate medical attention. The facility must be available 24 hours a day.

Encoder – A software product that helps assign a DRG.

Encounter – Contact with a patient.

Enrollee – A person who subscribes to a specific health plan.

Enrollment – The number of lives covered by the plan.

EOB – Explanation of benefits. A statement mailed to member (and sometimes provider) explaining claim adjudication and payment.

EPO – Exclusive provider organization. Similar to an HMO but the member must remain within the provider network to receive benefits. EPOs are regulated under insurance statutes rather than HMO legislation.

ERISA – Employee Retirement Income Security Act. An act with several provisions protecting both payor and member, including requiring that payors send the member an EOB when a claim is denied.

Established patient – A patient who has received professional services from the physician, or another physician of the same specialty who belongs to the same group practice, within the past three years.

Exclusions – Also called exceptions. Services excluded from a plan's coverage by the employer or payor because of risk or cost.

Experience rating – The designation of a group's previous claims history to help determine premium rates.

External fixation – The use of skeletal pins plus an attaching mechanism for temporary or definitive treatment of acute or chronic bony deformity.

Facility of payment – A contractual relationship that permits the payor to pay someone other than the member or provider.

Fact-oriented V codes – ICD-9-CM codes that do not describe a problem or a service; they simply state a fact. These generally do not serve as an outpatient primary or inpatient principal diagnosis.

FAR – Federal Acquisition Regulations. Regulations of the federal government's acquisition of services.

Federal Register – A government publication listing all changes in regulations and federally-mandated standards, including HCPCS and ICD-9-CM.

Federally qualified HMO – An HMO that meets HCFA guidelines for Medicare reimbursement.

Fee schedule – The maximum fees a plan will pay for services, primarily listed by CPT codes.

FEHBARS –Federal Employee Health Benefits Acquisition Regulations. Federal regulations for acquisition of health services used by government agencies and subcontractors.

FEHBP – Federal Employee Health Benefits Program. Provides health plans to federal workers.

FFS – Fee for service. Situation in which payor pays full charges for medical services.

Formulary – A listing of drugs providers may prescribe as dictated by the plan or Medicare. Prescription of a medication not included in the formulary usually is not reimbursed.

FPP – Faculty practice plan. A form of group practice developed around a teaching program or medical school.

Fragmentation – *See* unbundling.

Fraternal insurance – A cooperative plan provided to members of an association or fraternal group.

Frontal – Face forward.

FTE – Full time employee. The accounting equivalent of one full time employee that includes wages, benefits, and other costs.

Gatekeeper – A practice in which a member's care must be provided by a primary care physician, unless the physician refers the member to a specialist or approves the care provided by a specialist.

GHAA – Group Health Association of America – An HMO trade organization.

Global surgery package – A code denoting a normal surgical procedure with no complications that includes all of the elements needed to perform the procedure.

GMOS — Geometric mean length of stay. A component that figures in the reimbursement calculation for a DRG.

Government mandates – Services mandated by state or federal law. In government claims, the correct use of ICD-9-CM codes is required by law. In 1988, Congress passed the Medicare Catastrophic Coverage Act. Although the act itself was later repealed, the mandate requiring ICD-9-CM codes on all physician-submitted Part B claims was upheld. Medicare's rules changed again in 1996, when it began to reject any claim that did not assign the most specific ICD-9-CM code available.

Grace period – The period after a member has terminated employment for which he or she is still covered.

Group model – An HMO that contracts with a group of providers.

Group practice – A group of providers that shares facilities, resources, and staff, and who may represent a single unit in a managed care network.

Guidelines – Information appearing at the beginning of each of the six major sections of CPT. They also may appear at the beginning of subsections and code ranges. The information contained in the guidelines provides definitions, explanations of terms, and factors relevant to the section.

HCFA – Health Care Financing Administration. The federal agency that oversees all of the money for Medicare. This agency also is responsible for HCPCS, the three-level HCFA Common Procedure Coding System.

HCFA-1500 – A standard claim form usually used by outpatient clinics.

HCPCS – (pronounced "hick-picks") is most accurately used as the acronym for the entire three-level HCFA Common Procedure Coding System. It is also the popular and most commonly used name for the HCPCS/Level II/National Codes—just one part of the larger, three-level HCFA coding system.

HCPCS modifiers – Modifiers should, or in some cases must, be used to identify circumstances that alter or enhance the description of a service or supply. Level II/HCPCS modifiers are two alphabetic digits (AA–ZZ). They are recognized by carriers nationally and are updated annually by HCFA. Level III /Local modifiers are assigned by individual Medicare carriers and are distributed to physicians and suppliers through carrier newsletters. The carrier may change, add, or delete these local modifiers as needed.

Hemilaminectomy - The excision of the right or left lamina, the posterior bony covering of the nerves.

HHS – Health and Human Services. The cabinet department that oversees HCFA, Medicare, and other entities.

HIAA – Health Insurance Association of America. A trade organization for payors.

Hierarchy – The rank or order of codes. Numerical hierarchy plays a key role in ICD-9-CM coding because each digit beyond three adds more detail.

HMO – Health maintenance organization. A health plan that uses primary care physicians as gatekeepers. Emphasis is on preventive care.

Hold harmless – The contractual clause stating that if either party is held liable for malpractice, the other party is absolved.

Home health – Palliative and therapeutic care and assistance in the activities of daily life to home bound Medicare and private plan members.

Hospice – A service program, either inpatient or outpatient, that offers palliative support, counseling, and daily resources to the terminally ill and their family members.

Hospital admission plan – Used to facilitate admission to the hospital and to assure prompt payment to the hospital.

Hospital reimbursement – The payment to an inpatient facility for the costs incurred to treat a patient.

IBNR – Incurred but not reported. The amount of money the payor's plan accrues to forestall unknown medical expenses.

ICD-9-CM – International Classification of Diseases, Ninth Revision, Clinical Modification is a hierarchal listing of codes describing medical conditions.

ICD-10 – International Classification of Diseases, Tenth edition. Classification of diseases by alphanumeric code, used by the World Health Organization but not yet adopted in the United States.

ICD-10-CM – Clinical modification of ICD-10 for use in the United States. Proposed implementation date is October 1, 2001.

ICD-10-PCS – New procedural coding system developed under contract with HCFA by 3M HIS. This is still in the testing phase. Implementation of this procedural coding system or one developed by the AMA is planned for October 1, 2001.

ICF – Intermediate care facility. A step-down facility for patients leaving the hospital but who cannot be discharged to home because of continuing medical needs.

ID card – The wallet card carried by the member providing name, member number, group number, effective dates, deductibles, and other information.

Immediate maternity – Coverage provided for pregnancies that began prior to the date the member became insured.

In plan – Services chosen from a network provider.

Incontestable clause – A provision in a policy that prohibits the plan from disputing coverage for certain conditions after a specified period of time.

Inpatient reimbursement – The payment to a hospital for the costs incurred to treat a patient.

Intermediate repair – A repair performed for wounds and lacerations where one or more of the deeper layers of subcutaneous tissue and non-muscle fascia are repaired in addition to the skin and subcutaneous tissue. Single-layer closure can also be coded as an intermediate repair if the wound is heavily contaminated and requires extensive cleaning or removal of particulate matter.

Internal skeletal fixation – Involves wires, pins, screws, and/or plates placed through or within the fractured area to stabilize and immobilize the injury.

Invalid ICD-9-CM code – A diagnostic. code that is not as specific as it should be because digit(s) are missing. Claims containing invalid ICD-9 codes will be rejected by Medicare and some private payors.

IPA – Individual Practice Association. An organization made up of providers who along with the rest of a group contract with payors at a discounted fee-for-service or capitated rate.

IPO – Individual Practice Organization. See IPA.

IS – Information services. The administrators of the computer systems used by payors and providers.

JCAHO – Joint Commission for the Accreditation of Health Organizations. The primary accrediting body for hospitals, outpatient facilities, and other facilities. This nonprofit organization audits these facilities and was previously known as the Joint Commission for the Accreditation of Hospitals.

JD – Doctor of Jurisprudence. Lawyer.

Key Components – The three components of history, examination, and medical decision making are considered the keys to selecting the correct level of E/M codes. In most cases, all three components must be addressed in the documentation. However, in established, subsequent, and follow-up categories, only two of the three must be met or exceeded for a given code.

Lag study – A report used by plan managers to determine how long claims are pending and how much is paid out each month.

Laminectomy - The removal of the entire lamina on both sides, inclusive of the spinous process.

Laminotomy - The process of creating a hole in the lamina to achieve the required result.

Lapse – A terminated policy.

Late effect – A residual condition occurring after the acute phase of an illness or injury has terminated. The original illness or injury is healed, but a chronic or long-term condition remains.

Lateral (LAT) – Side view.

LCSW – Licensed clinical social worker

Limits – The ceiling for benefits payable under a plan.

Limiting charge – The maximum amount a nonparticipating physician can charge for services to a Medicare patient.

Line of business – Different health plans offered by a larger insurer or insurance broker as a product line.

Lives – The unit of measurement used by plans to determine the number of people covered. Calculated by multiplying the number of members by 2.5.

Local medical review policy – Is carrier specific and is used in the absence of a national coverage policy and is used to make local Medicare medical coverage decisions when needed. Developing local Medicare policy includes creating a draft policy based on review of medical literature, understanding local practice, soliciting comments from the medical community and Carrier Advisory Committee, responding to and incorporating into final local policy comments received, and notifying providers of the policy effective date.

Long-term care facility – A nursing home.

Loss ratio – The ratio between the cost to deliver medical care and the amount of money taken in by the plan.

LPN – Licensed Practical Nurse

LTCF – Long Term Care Facility

LVN – Licensed Vocational Nurse/Licensed Visiting Nurse

MA – Master of Arts degree/Medical Assistant

MAC – Maximum allowable charge. The maximum a pharmacy vendor can charge for something.

Malingering – The feigning of illness, either as the result of intentional deceit or as the result of mental illness.

Managed health care – 1) The concept of managing cases while in progress to assure care is the most appropriate, efficient, and effective; 2) A system of health care meant to manage overall cost; 3) A method of health care where contracted physicians participate in the management of health care costs.

Manipulation – Describes the attempted reduction or restoration of a fracture or joint dislocation to its normal anatomic alignment by the application of manually applied forces.

Maximum allowable charge – Amount set by insurer as highest amount to be charge for particular medical service.

MCE – Medical care evaluation. A part of the quality assurance program that reviews process of medical care.

MCO – Managed care organization. A generic term for EPA, IPO, HMO, and others.

MD – Medical doctor degree. An allopathic, or traditional, physician.

MDCs – Major diagnostic categories – The original DRGs developed at Yale were begun by dividing all possible principal diagnoses into mutually exclusive categories, referred to as Major Diagnostic Categories (MDCs). These broad classification of ICD-9-CM diagnoses are typically grouped by organ system. (See Code It Right's appendix 1 for the current list of MDCs)

ME – Medical Examiner

MEd – Master of Education

Medicaid – Federal-state health insurance for qualified low income people.

Medical loss ratio – *See* loss ratio.

Medical meaningfulness – Patients in the same DRG can be expected to evoke a set of clinical responses which result in a similar pattern of resource use.

Medicare – A national program that provides medical care to the elderly.

Medicare Carriers Manual (MCM) – The manual HCFA provides to Medicare carriers. It contains instructions for processing and payment of Medicare claims, preparing reimbursement forms, billing procedures, and Medicare regulations. As processes and regulations change, HCFA issues revisions to the manual.

Medicare Fee Schedule (MFS) – Slows the rise in cost for services and standardizes payment to physicians regardless of specialty or location. Payments vary through geographic adjustments. Different payment for the same service performed by physicians of different specialties is eliminated. The MFS is based on the Resource Based Relative Value Scale (RBRVS). A national total relative value unit (RVU) is given for each procedure (HCPCs Level I CPT, Level II national codes) provided by a physician. Each total RVU has three components: physician work, practice expense, and malpractice insurance.

Medicare Part A – Coverage includes hospital, nursing home, other inpatient care, and home health. Claims are submitted to intermediaries for reimbursement. Ten regional offices provide the Health Care Financing Administration (HCFA) with a decentralized administration and delivery of Medicare programs. Each regional office manages private insurance companies that contract with the government to process and make payment for Medicare services.

Medicare Part B – Coverage provides payment for physician and outpatient services. Physicians submit their claims to carriers for reimbursement. Ten regional offices provide the Health Care Financing Administration (HCFA) with a decentralized administration and delivery of Medicare programs. Each regional office manages private insurance companies that contract with the government to process and make payment for Medicare services.

Medicare Secondary Payor (MSP) – Medicare becomes secondary when patients are 65 or older and have group health benefits through their own employer or their spouse's. Also covered under the MSP program are patients of any age who have End-Stage Renal Disease (ESRD), are covered by an employer group plan, and are in the first 18 months of treatment. Variables apply to this program.

Medicare supplement – Private insurance coverage that pays costs of services not covered by Medicare.

Medigap policy – As defined by HCFA, is a health insurance policy, or other health benefit plan, offered by a private company to those entitled to Medicare benefits. The policy provides payment for Medicare charges not payable because of deductibles, coinsurance amounts, or other Medicare imposed limitations.

Member months – Total of months each member was covered.

Member services – A payor department that works as a patient advocate to solve problems. The department also works with the patient to take claims appeals to a final committee after all other processes have been exhausted.

Member – A subscriber of a health plan.

Mental health/Substance abuse – A payor term for services rendered to members for emotional problems or chemical dependency.

Mental/Nervous – See Mental health/Substance abuse.

MeSH – Medical Staff-Hospital Organization. Organization that bonds hospital and attending medical staff as a network.

MET – Multiple employer trust. A group of employers which joins together to purchase health insurance on a self-funded approach. This approach lowers cost by preventing an adverse selection by broadening the membership pool.

MEWA – Multiple Employer Welfare Association. See MET.

MHA – Master of Hospital Administration

MIS – Management information system. Hardware and software that facilitates claims management.

Mixed model – An HMO that includes both an open panel and closed panel option.

MLP – Midlevel practitioners. Professionals such as nurse practitioners, nurse midwives, physical therapists, physician assistants, and others who provide medical care but do so with physician input.

Minor procedures – procedure considered by many payors to be part of the package for a primary surgical service.

Modality – A form of imaging. These include x-ray, fluoroscopy, ultrasound, nuclear medicine, duplex Doppler, CT, and MRI. Modality is any physical agent applied to produce therapeutic changes to biologic tissue; includes but is not limited to thermal, acoustic, light, mechanical, or electric energy.

Modifier – *See* CPT modifiers or HCPCS modifiers.

Morbidity rate – Actuarial term describing predicted medical expense rate.

MSN – Master of Science in Nursing

MSW – Master of Social Work

Multiple employer group – A group of employers who contract together to subscribe to a plan, broadening the risk pool and saving money. Different from a multiple employer trust.

NA – Nursing Assistant

NAHMOR – National Association of HMO Regulators.

NAIC – National Association of Insurance Commissioners. An organization of state insurance regulators.

National coverage policy – Outlines Medicare coverage decisions that apply to all states and regions. National coverage policy indicates whether and under what circumstances items/services are covered. These policies are published in HCFA regulations in the Federal Register, contained in HCFA rulings, or issued as program memorandums, manual issuances to Coverage Issues Manual or the Medicare Carriers Manual.

NBICU – Newborn Intensive Care Unit. A special care unit for premature and seriously ill infants.

NCHS – National Center for Health Statistics. This U.S. government agency refines ICD-9-CM every year to reflect advances in medical diagnostics. NCHS holds several hearings a year to consider changes or additions in ICD-9-CM.

NCQA – National Committee on Quality Assurance. The organization that accredits payors' quality assurance programs.

ND – Doctor of Naturopathy

NEC (not elsewhere classifiable) – Indicates that the condition specified does not have a separate more specific listing. This term is used only in Volume 2.

Network model – A plan that contracts with multiple groups of providers, or networks, to provide care.

New patient – Patient who is receiving care from the provider or another physician of the same specialty who belongs to the same group practice for the first time within three years.

Nonspecific code – A catch-all code that specifies the diagnosis as "ill-defined," "other," or "unspecified." A nonspecific code may be a valid choice if no other code closely describes the diagnosis.

NOS (not otherwise specified) – Use an NOS code only when the available information does not permit assignment to a more specific code. NOS is used only in Volume 1.

NPI - National Provider Identifier. HCFA is replacing the UPIN with a national provider identifier (NPI) number. This new identification system applies to all providers in the healthcare industry, including physicians, suppliers, home health agencies, hospitals, and affiliated providers. Planned implementation has been delayed. Check with local medicare carriers for updated information on NPI implementation.

Nurse Practitioner – A specially trained, degreed nurse who assesses, treats, and prescribes medication.

Oblique (OBL) – Slanted view of the object being x-rayed.

Occupational therapy – Therapy meant to help a member who is recovering from a serious illness or injury retain activities of daily life.

OT (outlier threshold) – A component that figures in the reimbursement calculation for a DRG.

Open enrollment period – A period of usually one month annually during which members can revise their medical coverage.

Open panel – An arrangement in which a managed care organization that contracts providers on an exclusive basis is still seeking providers.

Open treatment – Describes a fracture site that is opened surgically for visualization and possible internal fixation.

OPL – Other party liability. In COBs, the decision that the other plan is the primary plan.

Orthotics – Braces and other appliances worn to alleviate a medical condition.

Other specified – A term in ICD-9-CM referring to codes reported when a diagnosis has been made and there is no code identifying it more specifically.

Out of plan – Choosing a provider who is not a member of the preferred provider network.

Out of service area – Medical care received out of the geographic area that may or may not be covered, depending on plan.

Outliers – Medical cases that statistically fall outside of established parameters of length of stay or cost.

Overutilization – Services rendered by providers more frequently than desired by payors.

Paneled – A provider contracted with an HMO.

Par provider – Shorthand for a provider who is participating in the plan.

Partial disability – Inability to perform part of one's job.

Partial payment – A payment to the provider or member in which it is expected that other payments will be made before the claim is closed.

Payor ID – A unique identifier for payors of healthcare claims. All payors will be registered and numbered. This identifier will simplify and improve the processing and administration of healthcare claims.

PAS norms – Professional Acuity Study. Based on a professional activity study performed regularly by the Commission Professional and Hospital Activities and broken out by average length of stay (ALOS) by region.

PBM – Prescription benefit managers – HMO staff who monitor amount and use of drugs prescribed.

PCP – Primary care physician. The physician who makes initial diagnosis and referral and retains control over the patient and utilization of services both in and outside the plan.

Peer review – Evaluation of physician's performance by his or her peers.

PEPM - Per employee per month.

Percutaneous skeletal fixation – Describes fracture treatment that is neither open nor closed. Fixation, such as pins, is placed across the fracture site, usually under x-ray imaging.

Per diem reimbursement – Reimbursement to an institution based on a set rate per day rather than on a charge by charge basis.

PharmD – Doctor of Pharmacy

PhD – Doctor of Philosophy

PHO – Physician-hospital organization. See MeSH

Physician Assistant – A medical professional who receives additional training and can assess, treat, and prescribe medications under a physician's review.

PIN – Physician Identification Number.

Plan manager – Payor employee managing all of the contracts and contract negotiations for one or more specific plans.

PMPM – Per member per month.

PMPY – Per member per year.

Pooling – Health payors' practice of combining risk.

POS – Point of Service. A plan in which members do not have to choose services (HMO vs. traditional) until they need them. Benefits may differ by choice and members may be financially motivated to choose managed care plans.

Posteroanterior (PA) – Back to front.

Posting date –The date a charge is posted to a patient account by the provider. The posting date is frequently not the same as the actual date of service, but usually within five days of the actual date of service. Some providers list the posting date and the actual date of service for a charge.

PPA – Preferred Provider Arrangement. Similar to a PPO.

PPO – Preferred Provider Organization. A plan contracting with providers to provide services on a discounted basis. Members must stay within the plan or pay a greater copay.

PPS – Prospective Payment System. A payment system, such as DRGs, that pays on historical data of case mix and regional differences.

Pre-existing condition – A condition that existed prior to the effective date of the plan. There is often a short-term or permanent limitation to reimbursement for care of this condition.

Precertification – Preadmission certification. The approval of a procedure or hospital stay before the act by a payor employee, who considers the diagnosis, the planned treatment, and expected length of stay.

Presenting problem – A disease, condition, illness, injury, symptom, sign, finding, complaint, or other reason for the patient encounter.

Primary care – First contact and continuing care, including diagnosis and treatment. See PCP.

Primary diagnosis – The code reflecting the current, most significant reason for the services or procedures provided. If the disease or condition has been successfully treated and no longer exists, it is not billable and should not be coded.

Principal diagnosis – The condition established after study to be chiefly responsible for occasioning the admission of the patient to the hospital of care.

Principal procedure – The procedure performed for definitive treatment rather than one performed for diagnostic or exploratory purposes, or was necessary to take care of a complication. If there appears to be two procedures that are prinicipal, then the one most related to the principal diagnosis should be selected as the principal procedure.

PRO – Peer Review Organization. An organization that reviews costs charges in Medicare reimbursement.

Problem-oriented V codes – ICD-9-CM codes that identify circumstances that could affect the patient in the future but are neither a current illness or injury. Use these codes to describe an existing circumstance or problem that may influence future medical care.

Professional association plans – A plan provided by a professional association that affords self-employed professionals (e.g., physicians, CPAs, lawyers) less expensive coverage.

Professional component – A part of a radiology procedure that encompasses all of the physician's work in providing the service, including interpretation and report of the procedure. Costs of education, malpractice insurance, and other expenses incident to maintaining a practice are also included in the professional component.

PTMPY – Per thousand members per year.

QA – Quality assurance. Monitoring and maintenance of established standards of quality for patient care.

QM – Quality management. Monitoring and maintenance of established standards of quality using techniques proposed by Crosby, Demming, and Juran. See TQM.

RBRVS – Resource-based relative value study. A relative value scale originally developed by Harvard for use by HCFA in Medicare. The scale assigns value to procedures based on the resources related rather than based on historical data.

Real-time – Immediate imaging, usually in movement.

Reasonable and customary – The prevailing fees for services in a given geographical area.

Referral – In managed care, the primary care physician's act of sending a member to a specialist within or outside the panel.

Regional Medical Center - A descriptive term for a hospital that provides comprehensive services to a large regional area but that may not be a tertiary care facility. Largely used in the west, where facilities may serve hundreds of square miles.

Rehabilitation – Physical and mental restoration of disabled members.

Reimbursement – Payment of actual charges incurred as a result of accident or illness.

Reinsurance – Insurance purchased by a payor to protect itself from extremely high losses.

Related cases – Procedures with the same diagnosis, same operative area, and same indication.

Relative weight – Assigned weight intended to reflect relative resource consumption associated with each DRG.

Review committee – A multidisciplinary committee that considers denied cases being appealed, catastrophic cases, or fee-for-service cases.

Risk contract – *See* At risk.

Risk factor reduction – The reduction of risk in the pool of members.

Risk manager – The person charged with keeping financial risk low, including malpractice cases.

Risk pool – The pool of people who will be in the insured group, their medical and mental histories, other factors such as age, and their predicted health.

RRA – Registered records administrator. An accreditation for medical records administrators.

Rush charge – A charge for expeditious test results. See Stat charge.

RVS – Relative value study. A guide that shows the relationship between the time, resources, competency, experience, severity, and other factors necessary to perform procedures.

Sanction – Imposition of penalties or exclusion of a provider for infractions such as using services inappropriately, using procedures that are harmful to the patient, and/or using a technique that is inferior in quality. Fraud will also earn a sanction for the provider.

Schedule – The listing of amounts payable for specific procedures.

Second opinion – Another professional's opinion to help determine the necessity of a medical procedure. This is often required by plans before a surgical procedure.

Secondary insurer – In a COB arrangement, the insurer that reimburses for benefits pending after payment by the primary insurer.

Self-insured or self-funded plan – A plan where the risk is assumed by the employer rather than an insurer.

Self-pay patients – Patients who pay for medical care out-of-pocket.

Separate procedures – Services that are commonly carried out as an integral part of a total service, and as such do not warrant a separate identification. These services are noted in CPT with the parenthetical phrase (separate procedure) at the end of the description. When this phrase appears before the semicolon, all indented descriptions that follow are covered by it.

Service date – The date the a charge is incurred for a service.

Service-oriented V codes – ICD-9-CM codes that identify or define examinations, aftercare, ancillary services, or therapy. Use these V codes to describe the patient who is not currently ill but seeks medical services for some specific purpose such as follow-up visits. You can also use this type of V code as a primary diagnosis for outpatient services when the patient has no symptoms that can be coded and screening services are provided.

Service plan – 1) A plan that has contracts with providers but is not a managed care plan; 2) Another name for Blue Cross/Blue Shield plans.

Shadow pricing – Setting rates just below a competitor's rates. This procedure, maximizes profits but raises medical costs.

Simple repair – Is performed when the wound is superficial, e.g., involving partial or full thickness damage to the skin and/or subcutaneous tissues. There is no significant involvement of deeper structures and only simple, primary suturing is required.

Skeletal traction – The application of a force to a limb segment through a wire, pin, screw, or clamp attached to bone.

Skin traction – The application of a force to a limb using felt or strapping applied directly to skin only.

Small subscriber group aggregate – An aggregate of professional associations, small business, or other entities formed to be considered a single, large subscriber group.

SNF – Skilled nursing facility. A facility that cares for long-term patients with acute medical needs.

Specimen – Tissue or tissues submitted for individual and separate attention, requiring individual examination and pathologic diagnosis.

Staff model – An HMO that employs its own providers.

Standard anesthesia formula – Consists of basic value (units) + time units + modifying units (e.g., physical status and qualifying circumstances) + other allowed unit/charges. An abbreviation is B + T + M (basic + time + modifying circumstances). The formula may also include O (other) for other allowed unit charges.

Starred procedure – When a star follows a CPT surgical procedure code, the service listed includes only the surgical procedure, not any associated pre- and postoperative services.

Stat charge – A charge for expeditious test results. See Rush charge.

State insurance commission – The state group that approves insurance certificates for each state and regulate the industry based on statutes.

Steering – The act of providing financial incentives to members to use the managed care provider panel.

Stent – Tube to provide support in a body cavity or lumen.

Stop loss – A form of reinsurance that protects health insurance above a certain limit and minimizes risks for providers.

Subrogation – Recovery of monies or benefits from a third party who is liable for the payment.

Subsidiary "In Addition To" Codes – Services not included as part of the primary procedure. Key phrases are used throughout CPT to indicate that a code is to be used "in addition" to the primary code. Phrases that help identify subsidiary codes include, but are not limited to: each additional, list in addition to, and done at time of other major procedure.

Substantial Comorbidity – A pre-existing condition that will, because of its presence with a specific principle diagnosis, cause an increase in the length of stay by at least one day in approximately 75 percent of the cases.

Substantial Complication – A condition that arises during the hospital stay that prolongs the length of stay by at least one day in approximately 75 percent of the cases.

Subtraction – The removal of an overlying structure in order to better visualize the structure in question. This is done in a series by imposing one x-ray on top of another.

Supplemental health services – Benefits HMOs offer in addition to base services.

Surgical package — A normal, uncomplicated performance of specific surgical services, with the assumption that on average, all surgical procedures of a given type are similar with respect to skill-level, duration, and length of normal follow-up care.

Technical component – A part of a radiology service that includes the provision of the equipment, supplies, technical personnel, and costs attendant to the performance of the procedure other than the professional services.

TEFRA – Tax Equity and Fiscal Responsibility Act. An act that protects the rights of full-time employees to remain on the company's plan to age 69.

Tertiary care facility – A hospital providing specialty care to patients referred from other hospitals because of the severity of their injuries or illnesses.

Therapeutic – An act meant to alleviate a medical or mental condition.

Therapeutic procedures – A manner of effecting change through the application of clinical skills and/or services that attempt to improve function.

Therapeutic services — Are performed for treatment of a specific diagnosis. These services include performance of the procedure, various incidental elements, and normal, related follow-up care.

Third party payor – Payor responsible for claims paid by a health plan or member for claims incurred for which the health plan or member should not have primary liability.

Three-digit diagnostic codes – Are used only when no fourth or fifth digit is available. There are only about 100 codes at the highest level of specificity in the three-digit form. See the appendix of *Code It Right* for a list of the three-digit codes. Many payors, including Medicare, do not accept three-digit codes when higher levels of specificity exist. Never use zeroes as fillers.

Time limit – Set number of days in which a claim can be filed.

Tomograms – A specialized type of x-ray imaging that provides slices through a body structure to obliterate overlying structures. This is commonly performed for studies on the kidneys or the temporomandibular joint.

TPA – Third party administrator. A firm that performs administrative functions for a self-funded plan but assumes no risk.

TPL – The third party payor liable for the cost of an illness or injury, such as auto or homeowner insurer.

TQM – Total Quality Management. The concept that quality is an organic part of a plan's service and a provider's care and can be quantified and constantly improved.

Treatment plan – The plan of care submitted by the provider to the case manager when seeking certification for a member.

Triage – 1) Medical screening of patients to determine priority of treatment based on severity of illness or injury and resources at hand; 2) Charge levied by health care facilities for emergency and other patients.

Triple option – The offering of an HMO, indemnity plan, and PPO by one insurance firm.

UB-92 – The common claim form used by facilities to bill for services.

UCR – Usual, customary, and reasonable. The prevailing fees for services in a given geographical area.

Unbundling – Breaking a single service into its multiple components to increase total billing charges.

Underwriting – Evaluating and determining the financial risk a member or member group will have on an insurer.

Unlisted procedures – Codes in each section of CPT. These codes are used when the overall procedure and outcome of the surgery is not adequately described by an existing CPT code. Use unlisted procedures as a last resort in finding an appropriate CPT code.

Unspecified – A term in ICD-9-CM that indicates more information is necessary to code the term to further specificity. In these cases, the fourth digit of the code is always 9. Fourth digits 0 through 7 identify more specific information of the main term or condition. The fourth-digit number 8 is reserved for identifying other information.

Upcoding – Provider billing for a procedure that reimburses more than the procedure actually performed.

UPIN – Unique Physician Identification Number.

URAC – Utilization Review Accreditation Commission. The accrediting body of case management.

USPHS – United States Public Health Service.

Utilization Review Nurse – A nurse who evaluates cases for appropriateness of care and length of service and can plan discharge and services needed after discharge in home health appointments.

Utilization review – The review of facility use for medical care and services based on diagnosis, site, average length of stay, and other factors.

V codes – Also known as The Supplementary Classification of Factors Influencing Health Status and Contact with Health Services (V01–V82), V codes describe circumstances that influence a patient's health status and identify reasons for medical encounters resulting from circumstances other than a disease or injury classified in the main part of ICD-9-CM.

Volume – 1) The number of services performed; 2) the number of patients; 3) The number of patients in a DRG during a specific time.

Weighting – The practice of assigning more worth to a fee based on the number of times it is charged, "weighting" the RBRVS fees for an area.

Well-baby care – Medical services, immunizations, and regular provider visits considered routine for an infant.

WHO (World Health Organization) – This international agency developed ICD-9-CM to track morbidity and mortality statistics worldwide. It recently updated its coding system with ICD-10, an alphanumeric system with much more room for growth.

Withhold – Percentage of payment to providers held by HMO until cost of referral or services has been determined. If the provider goes over the amount determined appropriate, that amount is kept by the HMO.

Workers compensation – Laws requiring employers to furnish care to employees injured on the job.

Wraparound plan – Insurance or health plan coverage for copays and deductibles not covered under a member's base plan.

Appendix 8: Prefixes & Suffixes

PREFIXES

Prefixes are one half of the medical language equation and are attached to the beginning of words. For example, the prefix "eu-," meaning good or well, combined with the Greek word for death, "thanatos," produces euthanasia — a good death.

a-, an-	without, away from, not
ab-	from, away from, absent
acro-	extremity, top, highest point
ad-	indicates toward, adherence to, or increase
adeno-	relating to a gland
adip-	relating to fat (also adipo-)
aero-	relating to gas or air
all-	meaning another, other, or different
allo-	indicates difference or divergence from the norm
ambi-	both sides; about or around (also amphi-)
an-	without
angi-	relating to a vessel
aniso-	dissimilar, unequal, or asymmetrical
ankylo-	bent, crooked, or two parts growing together
ante-	in front of, before
antero-	before, front, anterior
anti-	in opposition to, against
antro-	relating to a chamber or cavity
arch-	beginning, first, principal (also arche-, archi-)
archo-	relating to the rectum or anus
arterio-	relating to an artery
arthro-	relating to a joint
astro-	star-like or shaped
atelo-	incomplete or imperfect
auto-	relating to the self
axio-	relating to an axis (also axo-)
balano-	relating to the glans penis or glans clitoridis
baro-	relating to weight or heaviness
basi-	relating to the base or foundation (also basio-)
bi-	double, twice, two
blasto-	relating to germs
blenn-	relating to mucus (also blenno-)
blepharo-	relating to the eyelid
brachi-	relating to the arm (also brachio-)
brachy-	short
brady-	meaning slow or prolonged
broncho-	relating to the trachea

cac-	meaning diseased or bad (also caci-, caco-)
cardio-	relating to the heart
carpo-	relating to the wrist
cata-	down from, down, according to
celo-	indicating a tumor or hernia; cavity
cervico-	relating to the neck or neck of an organ
chilo-	relating to the lip (also cheilo-)
chole-	relating to the gallbladder
cleido-	relating to the clavicle
cyst-	relating to the urinary bladder or a cyst (also cysto-)
cyto-	in relation to cell
dacry-	pertaining to the lacrimal glands
dactyl-	relating to the fingers or toes
demi-	half the amount
desmo-	relating to ligaments
deuter-	secondary or second
dextro-	meaning on or to the right
dorsi-	relating to the back (also dorso-)
dys-	painful, bad, disordered, difficult
echo-	reverberating sound
ecto-	external, outside
ectro-	congenital absence of something
endo-	within, internal
entero-	relating to the intestines
epi-	on, upon, in addition to
eu-	well, healthy, good, normal
exo-	outside of, without
fibro-	relating to fibers or fibrous tissue
galacto-	relating to milk
gastro-	relating to the stomach and abdominal region
genito-	relating to reproduction
gono-	relating to the genitals, offspring, origination
gyn-	relating to the female gender
hema-	relating to blood (also hemato-)
hemi-	half
hepato-	relating to the liver
histo-	relating to tissue
homeo-	indicates resemblance or likeness (also homo-)
hydro-	relating to fluid, water, or hydrogen
hyper-	excessive, above, exaggerated
hypo-	below, less than, under
hyster-	relating to either the womb or hysteria (also hystero-)
idio-	distinct or individual characteristics

ileo-	relating to the ileum (part of the small intestine)
ilio-	relating to the pelvis
infra-	meaning inferior to, beneath, under
irid-	relating to the iris
ischio-	relating to the hip
iso-	equal
jejuno-	relating to the jejunum (part of the small intestine)
juxta-	next to, near
karyo-	relating to the nucleus of a cell
kerato-	relating to the cornea or horny tissue
laparo-	flank, loins; operations through the abdominal wall
laryngo-	relating to the larynx
lien-	relating to the spleen
lip-	relating to fat (also lipo-)
lith-	relating to a hard or calcified substance (also litho-)
lumbo-	relating to the loin region
macro-	meaning oversized, large
mal-	bad, poor, ill
melano-	dark or black in color
meningo-	relating to membranes covering the brain and spine
mesio-	towards the middle; secondary (also meso-)
meta-	indicates a change
mis-	bad, improper
my-	relating to muscle (also myo-)
myc-	relating to fungus (also myco-)
myelo-	relating to bone marrow or the spinal cord
narco-	indicates insensate condition or numbness
necro-	indicates death or dead tissue
nephr-	relating to the kidney
noci-	relating to injury or pain
nycto-	relating to darkness or night
odont-	relating to the teeth
oligo-	indicates few or small
omo-	relating to the shoulder
omphalo-	relating to the navel
onco-	relating to a mass, tumor, or swelling
onycho-	relating to the finger- or toenails
oophor-	relating to the ovaries
opistho-	indicates behind or backwards
orchi-	relating to the testicles (also orchido-)
oscheo-	relating to the scrotum
osteo-	having to do with bone
oto-	relating to the ear
pachy-	indicates heavy, large, or thick
pali-	repetition, back again, recurring (also palin-)
panto-	indicates the whole or all
para-	indicates near, similar, beside, or past
patho-	indicates sensitivity, feeling, or suffering
ped-	relating to the foot (also pedi-)
peri-	about, around, or in the vicinity
pero-	indicates being maimed or deformed
phaco-	relating to the lens of the eye
phago-	relating to eating and ingestion
pharyngo-	relating to the pharynx

phlebo-	relating to the vein
phreno-	relating to the diaphragm; head or mind
pimel-	relating to fat
platy-	indicates wide or broad
pleio-	more, additional
pleur-	relating to the side or ribs
pneum-	relating to respiration, air, the lungs
pod-	relating to the feet (also podo-)
poly-	indicates much or many
procto-	relating to the rectum and/or anus
proso-	indicates toward the front, anterior, forward
pseudo-	indicates false or imagined
pulmo-	relating to the lungs and respiration
pyelo-	relating to the pelvis
pygo-	relating to the buttocks or rump
pyle-	relating to an opening/orifice of the portal vein
pyloro-	relating to the pylorus, the stomach opening into the duodenum
pyo-	relating to pus
pyreto-	indicates a fever, heat
rachi-	relating to the spine (also rachio-)
recto-	meaning straight or relating to the rectum
retro-	indicates behind, backward, in a reverse direction
rheo-	indicates a flow or stream of fluid
rhino-	relating to the nose
sacro-	relating to the sacrum, the base of the vertebral column
salpingo-	relating to the fallopian or eustachian tubes
sarco-	relating to flesh
scapho-	indicates deformed condition, shaped like a boat
scapulo-	relating to the shoulder
schisto-	indicates cleft or split; a fissure
scoto-	relating to darkness; visual field gap
sial-	relating to saliva
sinistro-	meaning on or to the left
somato-	relating to the body
spheno-	relating to the sphenoid bone at the base of the skull
sphygmo-	relating to the pulse
splanch-	relating to the intestines; viscera
steato-	relating to fat
stetho-	relating to the chest
stomato-	relating to the mouth
sym-	indicates together with, along with, beside
syn-	indicates being joined together
tachy-	indicates swift or fast
tarso-	relating to the foot; margin of the eyelid
teleo-	indicates complete or perfectly formed
teno-	relating to tendons
terato-	indicates being seriously deformed, esp. a fetus
thalamo-	relating to the thalamus, origin of nerves in the brain
thanato-	relating to death
thoraco-	relating to the chest
thrombo-	relating to blood clots
thymo-	relating to the thymus
toco-	relating to birth
trachelo-	relating to the neck

trichi-	relating to hair; hair-like shape (also tricho-)
tympano-	relating to the eardrum
typhlo-	relating to the cecum; relating to blindness
vaso-	relating to blood vessels
ventro-	relating to the abdomen; anterior surface of the body
vesico-	relating to the bladder
viscero-	relating to the abdominal organs
xeno-	relating to a foreign substance
xero-	indicates a dry condition

SUFFIXES

Suffixes are the other half of the equation. These are attached to the ends of words.

-agra	indicating severe pain
-algia	pain
-ase	denoting an enzyme
-blast	incomplete cellular development
-centesis	puncture
-cephal	having to do with the head
-cle	meaning small or little (also -cule)
-cyte	having to do with cells
-dactyl	having to do with fingers
-desis	binding or fusion
-ectomy	excision, removal
-ferous	produces, causes, or brings about
-fuge	drive out or expel
-genic	indicates production, causation, generation
-gram	drawn, written, and recorded
-graphic	written or drawn
-ia	state of being, condition (abnormal)
-iasis	condition

-itis	inflammation
-lysis	release, free, reduction of
-metry	scientific measurement
-odynia	indicates pain or discomfort
-oid	indicates likeness or resemblance
-ology	study of
-oma	tumor
-orraphy	suturing
-oscopy	to examine
-osis	condition, process
-ostomy	indicates a surgically created artificial opening
-otomy	indicates a cutting
-pagus	indicates fixed or joined together
-pathic	indicates a feeling, diseased condition, or therapy
-penia	indicates a deficiency; less than normal
-pexy	fixation
-philia	inordinate love of or craving for something
-phobia	abnormal fear of or aversion to something
-plasty	indicates surgically formed or molded
-plegia	indicates a stroke or paralysis
-poietic	indicates producing or making
-praxis	indicates activity, action, condition, or use
-rhage	indicates bleeding or other fluid discharge (also -rhagia)
-rhaphy	indicates a suture or seam joining two structures
-rrhagia	indicates an abnormal or excessive fluid discharge
-rrhexis	splitting or breaking
-spasm	contraction
-taxy	arrangement, grouping (also -taxis)
-tomy	indicates a cutting
-trophy	relating to food or nutrition
-tropic	indicates an affinity for or turning toward
-tropism	responding to an external stimulus

Appendix 9: HCFA-1500 Form

The following information is a step-by-step guide through the HCFA-1500 claim form. These guidelines reflect the latest changes. You'll find that we've combined the explanations of fields or "items" with related information to show the importance of those relationships.

HCFA is currently working with the National Claim Committee to revise the HCFA-1500, pursuant to the requirements of the changing century (the millennium), and the regulations imposed by electronic transmission. For this year, and as of October 1, 1998, HCFA requires eight-digit birth dates on the HCFA-1500 for Medicare Part B claims. The items affected are item 3 (the patient's birth date), item 9b (other insured's date of birth), and item 11a (insured's date of birth). The eight-digit birth dates must be reported with a space between the month, day, and year. For example, if the patient's birthdate is April 24, 1936, enter: 04 24 1936. Claims without the eight-digit birthdates will be returned.

Item 1
The information in this item identifies the patient's insurers. You may need to check more than one box. Correctly complete item 9 for information regarding other benefits.

Item 1a
Follow individual payor rules for completing this item. Generally, list the insured's identification (I.D.) number here. Verify that the I.D. number corresponds to the insured listed in item 4. The patient and the insured aren't always the same person. Some payors assign unique I.D. numbers to each enrollee or dependent and require the number of the enrollee or dependent receiving services (the patient) instead of the insured's number in this item.

Items 2 and 5
The patient's name and demographic information are extremely important. Instructions tell you to list the patient's last name first, then first name and middle initial. With electronic claims processing, claims listing the first name first may be delayed.

Another important detail is to check your spelling. Simple transposition of letters or misspelled names can result in denial or suspension of your claim. Also, verify the demographic information about your patient. The patient's address may not be the same as the insured's – a common cause of delayed payments.

Item 3
The patient's date of birth and sex are required by most insurance companies. Insurer's use the birthdate as verification of the patient as well as an indication of Medicare eligibility.

Item 6
This item describing the patient's relationship to the insured verifies eligibility. Remember the patient's relationship to the insured is not always "Self." Complete item 4 before item 6.

Items 4, 7, and 11
Demographic information continues with the item asking for the insured's name. As a rule of thumb for Medicare, the patient and insured are the same. For private payors, some insurers assign a unique number to each enrollee. List the name of the insured if the patient's primary insurance is other than Medicare. Enter "Same" when the insured is the patient. Leave item 4 blank when Medicare is the primary insurance.

Additionally, the subscriber's demographics are important. Assuming that the address of the subscriber and your patient are the same may cost you time and result in an unpaid claim. Supplying all information, including phone numbers with area codes, may avoid delays when an insurance company must contact the insured for additional information. Enter "Same" in item 7 when the insured is the patient.

Keep each patient's insurance information up-to-date. With dual coverage becoming more common, confusion easily arises over which insurer is primary and which is secondary. Understanding the "birthday rule" (explained previously) is critical for commercial payors. Carefully follow your carrier's guidelines for Medicare Secondary Payor (MSP) situations and make it a specific employee's responsibility to verify each patient's insurance data at the time of each office visit.

Items 11a–11d expand on the insured's information. Beginning with the policy or group number, you must also list the insured's birthdate, sex, and employer's name or school name. Data from these fields help the payor determine primary and secondary coverage. For Medicare claims, enter "None" and do not complete items 11a–11c if no insurance is primary to Medicare. Item 11d asks for other health plans; if you check "yes," item 9 must be completed.

Item 8

This field indicates the patient's marital and employment or student status. This information relates to item 6. If you check "spouse" as the relationship to the insured and then mark "single" under patient status, a good edit system will suspend your claim.

Item 9

Item 9 encompasses five fields to identify other insurance. For example, "other" may describe the patient, who has Medicare as primary payor and AARP as secondary, or "other" may be the patient's spouse who is insured through an employer. This information assists in coordinating benefits and determining liability. For Medicare claims, leave item 9 blank if no Medigap benefits are assigned, and enter information only if requested by the beneficiary. Beneficiaries are responsible for filing a supplemental claim if the private insurer does not contract with Medicare for electronic remittance of claim information. However, the trend is for physician offices to assume this responsibility. After receiving the Medicare payment, it is very easy for the billing staff to submit a claim, along with the Explanation of Benefits (EOB), to the supplemental carrier for payment of any coinsurance and deductibles.

Item 10

This multiple choice item determines whether the patient's condition is related to employment or an accident. Note that auto accident has its own line and a field exists for the state in which the accident occurred. Use the two-letter U.S. Postal Service abbreviations. You will find a listing of these abbreviations in appendix B of this book. Item 10 is important to the payor because it indicates liability. Incorrect completion of this item will cause your claim to be suspended or denied.

Item 10d is exclusively for Medicaid (MCD) information.

Items 12 and 13

Item 12 authorizes the release of information, allowing you to provide any medical information required to file the claim. Pay attention to the notation "READ BACK OF FORM BEFORE COMPLETING & SIGNING THIS FORM."

It is the assignment of benefits (item 13) that, in many cases, determines where payment is sent. Maintaining current patient and insured signatures is an extremely important aspect of managing your claims information. While it's ideal to have the patient sign each claim, computer-generated and electronic claims make this an impossible task. Many insurance companies accept the phrase "signature on file," but may request a copy of the signature information. The date indicates that the signature is current.

Items 14 and 15

The remainder of the information on the form defines the patient's medical problem and provides information for treatment provided. Most insurance companies require information on the patient's illness, such as when the symptoms first appeared and if the patient has had the same or similar problems. Medicare does not require that item 15 be completed.

Item 16

This field indicates the days a patient may be unable to work in his or her current occupation. While these dates may not be important to Medicare and private payors, they are very important to a workers compensation claim. Your state workers compensation carrier may require additional forms explaining when the patient can return to work or forms providing disability information. Become familiar with these forms when treating an employment-related injury or disease.

Items 17 and 17a

Medicare requires the referring provider's name and identifier number (NPI). All physicians and suppliers who order or refer Medicare beneficiaries or services must obtain an NPI even though they may never bill Medicare directly. However, related regulations regarding electronic transmission have delayed NPI and HCFA has instructed providers to use their Unique Physician Identification Number (UPIN) until such time as the NPI is implemented. The rule recommending the NPI as the standard healthcare provider identifier was published in the Federal Register on May 7, 1998. Providers will be notified of NPI numbers, and physicians who are not assigned an NPI must contact their Medicare carriers prior to submitting a claim.

Item 18

The dates of admission and discharge are necessary for hospital care. The dates you list must match the hospital's dates because payors often use these records to verify billed services.

Item 19

Use this field to enter additional information, including:

- Eight-digit date the patient was last seen and the National Provider ID (NPI) or UPIN of the patient's attending physician for physical and occupational therapists.

- Eight-digit x-ray date for chiropractor services.

- Drug name and dosage when submitting a claim for not otherwise classified drugs.

- A clear description of "unlisted procedure codes."

- Applicable modifiers when -99 is listed in the line items window.

- The statement "Homebound" when a homebound/institutionalized patient has an EKG tracing or specimen obtained from an independent lab.

Item 20

Complete item 20 when billing diagnostic tests subject to purchase price limitations. Enter "No" if no purchase tests are indicated on the claim. Enter "Yes" and complete item 32 if the diagnostic test was performed outside of the entity billing for the service.

Item 21

Finally, we've arrived at the field for information regarding the physician's services. Item 21 has four slots for diagnostic codes, numbered 1 through 4. There was formerly space for narrative ICD-9-CM (International Classification of Diseases, 9th Edition, Clinical Modification) descriptions, but the current form allows only the numeric codes.

The following are common diagnostic coding problems that are likely to cause payment delays:

- The diagnosis doesn't establish the medical necessity of the treatment. When a problem or illness is acute, your diagnostic code must convey the emergent nature of the patient encounter.

- A patient's chronic diagnosis, which is not the reason for this visit, is incorrectly billed as the primary diagnosis.

- The ICD-9 code is incomplete or inaccurate. Always code to the highest specificity, adding appropriate 4th and 5th digits when available. Never "create" codes not actually found in ICD-9.

- Occasionally, the code does not correspond to the treatment provided, e.g., coding treatment of a femoral fracture as a fracture of the tibia.

- Errors can also occur when italicized ICD-9 codes are used as primary diagnoses. Never use these codes alone or as the primary diagnosis. Code first the etiology of the disease, then its manifestations.

- E codes report external causes of injury or poisoning, including place of occurrence, and are never used alone or as primary diagnoses.

Item 22

This item is for Medicaid resubmissions only. Include the appropriate resubmission code and the original reference number

Item 23

List the prior authorization number in this field. It is required by Medicare, Medicaid, and many managed care organizations.

Medicare requires the 10-digit Clinical Laboratory Improvement Act (CLIA) certification number for laboratory services billed by a physician office laboratory. Claims without the CLIA certification number will be denied, as of January 1, 1999.

Item 24

Be sure to complete these fields accurately, including date(s) of service, place of service, procedure codes and modifiers, charges, days/units, and type of service.

List the actual date of service, not the date you file the claim. If you provided a service for several consecutive days, list the beginning and ending dates, and place the number of days of service in column G.

CPT codes are keyed to place of service (POS), so column B has become even more important. Past HCFA-1500 forms listed HCFA's standard POS codes on the back, but they have been deleted from the current form. Because these codes are required by government payors, we've included them here; but you'll need to check with private payors to determine whether they use these POS codes or have developed their own.

There is a new place of service code for an adult living center, which takes effect January 1, 1999. The new POS (35) is used when billing services rendered at a residential care facility which houses beneficiaries who cannot live alone but do not need around-the-clock skilled medical services. The facility provides room, board, and other personal assistance services. The facility services do not include a medical component.

Place of Service Codes

11	Office	53	Community mental health center
12	Patient's home	54	Intermediate care facility – mentally retarded
21	Inpatient hospital		
22	Outpatient hospital	55	Residential substance abuse treatment facility
23	Emergency room – hospital		
24	Ambulatory surgical center	56	Psychiatric residential treatment center
25	Birthing center		
26	Military treatment facility	60	Mass immunization center
31	Skilled nursing facility	61	Comprehensive inpatient rehabilitation facility
32	Nursing facility		
33	Custodial care facility	62	Comprehensive outpatient rehabilitation facility
34	Hospice		
35	Adult living care facility	65	End stage renal disease treatment facility
41	Ambulance – land		
42	Ambulance – air or water	71	State or local public health clinic
50	Federally Qualified Health Center		
51	Inpatient psychiatric facility	72	Rural health clinic
52	Psychiatric facility – partial hospitalization	81	Independent laboratory
		99	Other unlisted facility

Type of service (TOS) codes also appeared on the back of the previous form, but have been deleted from the current one. Even though this field remains on the form (column C), not all government and private payors require this information. For your convenience in providing information for all payors, the following are HCFA's standard TOS codes:

0	Whole blood or packed red cells	5	Diagnostic laboratory
1	Medical care	6	Radiation therapy
2	Surgery	7	Anesthesia
3	Consultation	8	Assistance at surgery
4	Diagnostic x-ray	9	Other medical service

A	Used DME	N	Kidney donor
B	High risk screening mammography	P	Lump sum purchase of DME
		R	Rental of DME
C	Low risk screening mammography	T	Psychological therapy
		U	Occupational therapy
F	Ambulatory surgical center (facility usage)	V	Pneumococcal vaccine
		W	Physical therapy
I	Installment purchase DME	Y	Second opinion on elective surgery
L	Renal supplies		
M	Monthly capitation payment for dialysis	Z	Third opinion on elective surgery

Column D is the place for procedure codes (CPT and HCPCS). Include any applicable modifiers. As with diagnostic information, the procedure description field has been eliminated. A thorough understanding of CPT and HCPCS coding is a must to fill in these columns.

To establish medical necessity for the services provided, use column E to reference the appropriate diagnoses from item 21 to each procedure. List the diagnoses by item numbers 1, 2, 3, or 4 rather than by ICD-9 code.

Obviously, the charges in column F are important since you're telling the payor how much you want to be paid. Each service or line item should have a separate fee with the total charges noted in item 28. Unless there are unusual circumstances surrounding the service (e.g., additional time and effort) or if the service is reduced, the fees you charge should be consistent on a code-by-code basis. Exceptions are noted by adding a modifier to the affected procedure code.

List days or units in column G. This information is essential for payment of multiple days in the hospital or multiple units of the same code, such as drugs. Enter the anesthesia units for anesthesia procedures.

Column H indicates Early Periodic Screening and Developmental Testing (EPSDT) and family planning.

Column I identifies treatment provided in an emergency department. Remember that emergency services must also be indicated with the appropriate place of service code in column B. Medicare no longer requires this field.

Column J is used for coordination of benefits.

Any special use for column K is determined by individual payors. For Medicare claims, enter the carrier-assigned provider number when the performing physician/supplier belongs to a group practice. When more than one physician/supplier within a group bills on the same form, enter the individual provider number for the corresponding line items.

Item 25

Place your federal tax I.D. number in this field. Indicate whether this is your Social Security number or an employer identification number. Use either your employer or tax I.D. number consistently to avoid confusion on the 1099 forms you receive from third-party payors. Always verify the tax I.D. numbers on your 1099 forms because an error in unreported income may trigger an IRS audit.

Item 26

The patient account number field is purely for your convenience. Many payors list your patient's account number on the EOB which saves you the time it takes to research which "Mrs. Jones's" account should be credited with this payment.

Item 27
This item generally applies to government claims but may apply to other payors with whom you have a contractual agreement. If your office participates with Medicare, this item must always be checked "yes."

Nonparticipating physicians may decide on a claim-by-claim basis whether to accept assignment and check "yes" or "no." Medicare assumes the claim is unassigned if this item is left blank and sends the check to the patient. If a participating physician leaves this blank, it could be viewed as a violation of the participation agreement with Medicare.

Items 28, 29, and 30
Many claims are submitted with multiple pages that can be confusing to payors when only the grand total is listed for all services on the final page. Instead, each page of the claim should list the total charges, amount paid, and balance due for that page. Also, report only the services and procedures actually provided.

The amount paid area (item 29) indicates payment by the patient or by another insurance company. Failure to indicate payment by the primary insurer may result in claims denial or overpayment by the secondary payor.

The balance due (item 30) is the "bottom line" and should always appear on the claim. Many payors consider this field a requirement for claims processing. This item is left blank for Medicare.

Item 31
The physician's signature, stamped signature (if acceptable), or an authorized signature must appear in this item. Most payors return unsigned claims. This signature affirms that the information on the claim is correct. For electronic claims, the HCFA-assigned identifier number serves as the provider's electronic signature.

Item 32
Enter the name and address of the facility if the services were furnished in a hospital, clinic, laboratory, or facility other than the patient's home or physician's office. When the name and address of the facility where the services were furnished are the same as the biller's name and address shown in item 33, enter the word "same."

Providers of services (namely physicians) must identify the supplier's name, address, and NPI when billing for purchased diagnostic tests. When more than one supplier is used, a separate HCFA–1500 should be used to bill for each supplier.

This item is completed whether the supplier performs the work at the physician's office or at another location.

If a QB or QU modifier is billed, indicating the service was rendered in a Health Professional Shortage Area (HPSA), the physical location where the service was rendered must be entered if other than home. However, if the address shown in item 33 is in a HPSA and is the same as where the services were rendered, enter the word "SAME."

If the supplier is a certified mammography screening center, enter the 6-digit FDA approved certification number.

Item 33
The information for this item further identifies your practice to the insurer. Enter the appropriate, payor-specific provider number as well as your group name, address, and phone number. For Medicare claims, enter the provider number, for a performing physician/supplier who is not a member of a group practice. Enter the group number for a performing physician/supplier who is a member of a group practice.

Summary

The HCFA-1500 form is also available in a scannable red-ink version for carriers using Optical Character Recognition (OCR) equipment to process claims. The red ink used to print this form cannot be duplicated by your PC, so do not attempt to print red-ink versions of the HCFA-1500 form from your printer. Carriers are not able to process any form but the official HCFA-1500 red-ink version. If a Medicare carrier is not currently using OCR equipment to process claims, they may accept a facsimile of the HCFA-1500 form generated by dot matrix or laser jet printers, as long as the originals are submitted for payment. Contact your carrier to ask which type of claim form is being accepted for processing.

PLEASE DO NOT STAPLE IN THIS AREA

BAR CODE AREA

(APPROVED OMB-0938-0008)

HEALTH INSURANCE CLAIM FORM

Carrier

[ ] [ ] PICA   PICA [ ] [ ]

| [ ] MEDICARE (Medicare No.) | [ ] MEDICAID (Medicaid No.) | [ ] CHAMPUS (Sponser's SSN) | [ ] CHAMPVA (VA File No.) | [ ] GROUP HEALTH PLAN (SSN or ID) | [ ] FECA BLK LUNG (SSN) | [ ] OTHER (ID) | 1a. INSURED'S I.D. NUMBER (FOR PROGRAM IN ITEM 1) |

2. PATIENT'S NAME (Last Name , First Name, Middle Initial)

3. PATIENT'S BIRTH DATE   SEX
MM DD YY   M [ ]   F [ ]

4. INSURED'S NAME (Last Name, First Name, Middle Initial)

5. PATIENT'S ADDRESS (No., Street)

6. PATIENT RELATIONSHIP TO INSURED
Self [ ]   Spouse [ ]   Child [ ]   Other [ ]

7. INSURED'S ADDRESS (No. Street)

CITY   STATE

8. PATIENT STATUS
Single [ ]   Married [ ]   Other [ ]
Employed [ ]   Full-time Student [ ]   Part-time Student [ ]

CITY   STATE

ZIP CODE   TELEPHONE (Include Area Code) ( )

ZIP CODE   TELEPHONE (Include Area Code) ( )

9. OTHER INSURED'S NAME (Last Name, First Name, Middle Intial)

10. IS PATIENT'S CONDITION RELATED TO:

11. INSURED'S POLICY, GROUP OR FECA NUMBER

a. OTHER INSURED'S POLICY OR GROUP NUMBER

a. EMPLOYMENT? (CURRENT OR PREVIOUS)
[ ] YES   [ ] NO

a. INSURED'S DATE OF BIRTH   SEX
MM DD YY   M [ ]   F [ ]

b. OTHER INSURED'S DATE OF BIRTH   SEX
MM DD YY   M [ ]   F [ ]

b. AUTO ACCIDENT?   PLACE (State)
[ ] YES   [ ] NO

b. EMPLOYER'S NAME OR SCHOOL NAME

c. EMPLOYER'S NAME OR SCHOOL NAME

c. OTHER ACCIDENT?
[ ] YES   [ ] NO

c. INSURANCE PLAN NAME OR PROGRAM NAME

d. INSURANCE PLAN NAME OR PROGRAM NAME

10d. RESERVED FOR LOCAL USE

d. IS THERE ANOTHER HEALTH BENEFIT PLAN?
[ ] YES   [ ] NO   If yes, return to and complete item 9 a-d

READ BACK OF FORM BEFORE COMPLETING & SIGNING THIS FORM

12. PATIENT'S OR AUTHORIZED PERSON'S SIGNATURE I authorize the release of any medical information necessary to process this claim. I also request payment of government benefits either to myself or to the party who accepts assignment below.

SIGNED _____ DATE _____

13. INSURED'S OR AUTHORIZED PERSON'S SIGNATURE I authorize payment of medical benefits to undersigned physician or supplier for services described below.

SIGNED _____

Patient and Insured Information

14. DATE OF CURRENT
MM DD YY
ILLNESS (First symptom) OR INJURY (Accident) OR PREGNANCY (LMP)

15. IF PATIENT HAS HAD SAME OR SIMILAR ILLNESS GIVE FIRST DATE MM DD YY

16. DATES PATIENT UNABLE TO WORK IN CURRENT OCCUPATION
FROM MM DD YY   TO MM DD YY

17. NAME OF REFERRING PHYSICIAN OR OTHER SOURCE

17a. I.D. NUMBER OF REFERRING PHYSICIAN

18. HOSPITALIZATION DATES RELATED TO CURRENT SERVICES
FROM MM DD YY   TO MM DD YY

19. RESERVED FOR LOCAL USE

20. OUTSIDE LAB ? $ CHARGES
[ ] YES   [ ] NO

21. DIAGNOSIS OR NATURE OF ILLNESS OR INJURY (RELATE ITEMS 1, 2, 3 OR 4 TO ITEM 24E BY LINE)

1. |___.___   3. |___.___
2. |___.___   4. |___.___

22. MEDICAID RESUBMISSION
CODE   ORIGINAL REF. NO.

23. PRIOR AUTHORIZATION NUMBER

24. A				B	C	D			E	F	G	H	I	J	K
DATE(S) OF SERVICE				Place of Service	Type of Service	PROCEDURES, SERVICES, OR SUPPLIES (Explain Unusual Circumstances)			DIAGNOSIS CODE	$ CHARGES	DAYS OR UNITS	EPSDT Family Planning			RESERVED FOR LOCAL USE
From		To				CPT/HCPCS	MODIFIER								
MM DD YY		MM DD YY													

25. FEDERAL TAX I.D. NUMBER   SSN [ ]   EIN [ ]

26. PATIENT'S ACCOUNT NO.

27. ACCEPT ASSIGNMENT? (For govt. claims, see back)
[ ] YES   [ ] NO

28. TOTAL CHARGE $

29. AMOUNT PAID $

30. BALANCE DUE $

31. SIGNATURE OF PHYSICIAN OR SUPPLIER INCLUDING DEGREES OR CREDENTIALS (I certify that the statements on the reverse apply to this bill and are made a part thereof.)

SIGNED _____ DATE _____

32. NAME AND ADDRESS OF FACILITY WHERE SERVICES RENDERED (If other than home or office)

33. PHYSICIAN'S, SUPPLIER'S BILLING NAME, ADDRESS, ZIP CODE & PHONE #

PIN #   GRP#

Physician or Supplier Information

Please Print or Type

Approved by AMA Council on Medical Services

FORM HCFA - 1500   (12-90)
FORM OWCP-1500   FORM RRB-1500

Appendix 10: Answers

Chapter 1 — Diagnosis Coding

CODING PRACTICE 1

800.24	Closed fracture of vault of skull with subarachnoid, subdural, and extradural hemorrhage, prolonged (more than 24 hours) loss of consciousness and return to pre-existing conscious level
865.04	Massive parenchymal disruption of spleen without mention of open wound into cavity
867.0	Bladder and urethra injury without mention of open wound into cavity
808.43	Multiple closed pelvic fractures with disruption of pelvic circle
E812.0	Other motor vehicle collision with unmoving motor vehicle, injuring driver of motor vehicle other than motorcycle

When coding multiple injuries, the code for the most severe injury as determined by the attending physician should be sequenced first. The scenario presented does not specify which injury is the most severe. All required surgical intervention. Therefore, the physician should be queried regarding the sequencing of these codes.

CODING PRACTICE 2

Rural Hospital

V30.01	Single liveborn, born in hospital, delivered by cesarean delivery
769	Respiratory distress syndrome in newborn
764.07	"Light-for-dates" without mention of fetal malnutrition, 1,750-1,999 grams

Tertiary Care Hospital

769	Respiratory distress syndrome in newborn
764.07	"Light-for-dates" without mention of fetal malnutrition, 1,750-1,999 grams
774.6	Unspecified fetal and neonatal jaundice

CODING PRACTICE 1

Diagnosis

813.42	Other closed fractures of distal end of radius (alone)
E849.0	Place of occurrence, home
E880.9	Accidental fall on or from other stairs or steps

Procedures

25600-50	Closed treatment of distal radial fracture (eg, Colles or Smith type) or epiphyseal separation, with or without fracture of ulnar styloid; without manipulation — Bilateral Procedure
73110-50	Radiologic examination, wrist; complete, minimum of three views — Bilateral Procedure
73110-50-76	Radiologic examination, wrist; complete, minimum of three views — Bilateral Procedure; Repeat Procedure by Same Physician

CODING PRACTICE 2

Diagnosis

701.9	Unspecified hypertrophic and atrophic condition of skin
709.9	Unspecified disorder of skin and subcutaneous tissue

Procedures

11100	Biopsy of skin, subcutaneous tissue and/or mucous membrane (including simple closure), unless otherwise listed (separate procedure); single lesion
11101	Biopsy of skin, subcutaneous tissue and/or mucous membrane (including simple closure), unless otherwise listed (separate procedure); each separate/additional lesion (List separately in addition to code for primary procedure)
11200-59	Removal of skin tags, multiple fibrocutaneous tags, any area; up to and including 15 lesions — Distinct Procedural Service

This is an outpatient physician service. The lesions on the face are suspected to be basal cell carcinoma but at this point the diagnosis has not been confirmed. Therefore, it would be incorrect to report with a malignant neoplasm code. If possible, the claim should not be filed until pathology reports are returned.

Procedure 11101 has been designated as an add-on procedure and as such does not require a -51 modifier. The skin tags are separate lesions removed from a separate site which is designated with modifier -59.

Chapter 3 — Evaluation and Management Services

ICD9 DIAGNOSIS CODING PRACTICE ANSWERS

These answers are based on the information in the E/M service scenarios and are intended to report the physician services as opposed to the facility services. In some instances it has been noted that additional information should be obtained prior to assigning a diagnosis code. These scenarios were not altered to provide all the information required for reporting the services because coders often are required to obtain additional information. Providing scenarios with all the required information as well as scenarios where the physician should be querried for more specific information allows the coder to learn to identify situations in which more information is required for correct assignment of diagnosis codes.

INTERNAL MEDICINE SCENARIO

443.9	Unspecified peripheral vascular disease
305.1	Nondependent tobacco use disorder

Both the peripheral vascular disease and the tobacco dependence would be reported.

DERMATOLOGY SCENARIO

692.9	Contact dermatitis and other eczema, due to unspecified cause

GYNECOLOGY SCENARIO

789.03	Abdominal pain, right lower quadrant

This is a physician service and at the time of the dictation no specific cause of the right lower quadrant pain had been found. It would be a good idea to query the physician prior to submitting this claim to determine if follow-up examinations during the observation period provided a more specific diagnosis.

GENERAL SURGERY SCENARIO

577.0	Acute pancreatitis
276.5	Volume depletion
799.0	Asphyxia

The ETOH abuse should also be reported but we need to clarify whether the patient is currently dependent on and abusing alcohol in which case the correct code would be 303.90. If the patient has a long past history of alcohol abuse but is no longer dependent a personal history of alcohol abuse would be reported with V11.3. A

third code is available 305.00 for alcohol abuse nondependent and this might also apply depending on the specific circumstances.

CARDIOLOGY SCENARIO

359.8	Other myopathies

UROLOGY SCENARIO

592.1	Calculus of ureter

ONCOLOGY SCENARIO

516.3	Idiopathic fibrosing alveolitis
E933.1	Antineoplastic and immunosuppressive drugs causing adverse effect in therapeutic use
202.88	Other malignant lymphomas of lymph nodes of multiple sites

RHEUMATOLOGY SCENARIO

719.41	Pain in joint, shoulder region

The physician states that the patient has a history of rheumatoid arthritis affecting fingers and wrists. However, the reason for the exam was to evaluate the patient's shoulder pain. The arthralgia of the shoulders was not identified as due to rheumatoid arthritis.

GENERAL SURGERY SCENARIO

578.9	Unspecified, hemorrhage of gastrointestinal tract

Even though the request for consultation related to the complaint of rectal bleeding, it had already been identified that the source of the bleeding was not the rectum because a colonoscopy identified blood in the sigmoid colon. However, because no site or cause for the bleeding was identified on colonoscopy, the nonspecific diagnosis code 578.9 must be reported. The angiograms and the abdominal exploration may provide more specific information; however, at this time it is only known that she has gastrointestinal bleeding.

CARDIOLOGY SCENARIO

427.69	Other premature beats
276.6	Fluid overload
276.8	Hypopotassemia

Even though the patient was admitted for uncontrolled epistaxis, the cardiologist was not treating that condition. The cardiologist only reports diagnosis codes related to the care he has provided.

NEUROSURGERY SCENARIO

722.71	Intervertebral cervical disc disorder with myelopathy, cervical region

MEDICAL SPECIALTIES SCENARIO

493.90   Unspecified asthma, without mention of status asthmaticus

V15.81   Personal history of noncompliance with medical treatment, presenting hazards to health

CARDIOLOGY SCENARIO

427.5   Cardiac arrest

This scenario does not provide any information as to the cause of the cardiac arrest. Therefore, at this point in time only the cardiac arrest code can be reported.

NEONATOLOGY SCENARIO

770.1   Meconium aspiration syndrome

486   Pneumonia, organism unspecified

Two comparative conditions have been designated as the possible cause of the respiratory distress, so both would be reported. Additional work-up will likely provide a more specific diagnosis.

FAMILY PRACTICE SCENARIO

348.9   Unspecified condition of brain

905.0   Late effect of fracture of skull and face bones

V44.0   Tracheostomy status

E929.0   Late effects of motor vehicle accident

The acute injury is no longer the reason for medical care. The residual brain damage which is a late effect of the fracture and intracerebral hemorrhage is the condition currently being treated.

INTERNAL MEDICINE SCENARIO

340   Multiple sclerosis

GERONTOLOGY SCENARIO

707.0   Decubitus ulcer

342.90   Unspecified hemiplegia affecting unspecified side

INTERNAL MEDICINE SCENARIO

486   Pneumonia, organism unspecified

496   Chronic airway obstruction, not elsewhere classified

250.10   Type II (non-insulin dependent type) or unspecified type diabetes mellitus with ketoacidosis, not stated as uncontrolled

FAMILY PRACTICE SCENARIO

465.9   Acute upper respiratory infections of unspecified site

382.9   Unspecified otitis media

369.00   Blindness of both eyes, impairment level not further specified

PEDIATRICS

310.2   Postconcussion syndrome

599.0   Urinary tract infection, site not specified

The reason for the visit was to discuss the child's postconcussion syndrome. The child was examined due to the urinary tract infection but that was not the reason prompting the visit so the postconcussion syndrome would be sequenced first.

UROLOGY SCENARIO

867.0   Bladder and urethra injury without mention of open wound into cavity

INTERNAL MEDICINE SCENARIO

585   Chronic renal failure

420.0   Acute pericarditis in diseases classified elsewhere

250.41   Type I (insulin dependent type) diabetes mellitus with renal manifestations, not stated as uncontrolled

583.81   Nephritis and nephropathy, not specified as acute or chronic, with other specified pathological lesion in kidney, in diseases classified elsewhere

The patient has multiple medical problems; however, the internal medicine services were directed at the acute uremic pericarditis. The underlying disease, 585 chronic renal failure is sequenced first per ICD9 coding rules. Other relevant codes include the IDDM with nephropathy 250.41 and 583.81 and those should also be reported as secondary diagnoses.

MULTIPLE SPECIALTIES SCENARIO

790.92   Abnormal coagulation profile

REHABILITATION MEDICINE OR INTERNAL MEDICINE SCENARIO

V57.89   Other specified rehabilitation procedure

438.11   Aphasia due to cerebrovascular disease

438.20   Hemiplegia affecting unspecified side due to cerebrovascular disease

The patient is in a rehabilitation facility and the reason for the care plan oversight is to evaluate the rehabilitation services. Secondary diagnoses clarify the patient's condition as being due to late effects of a CVA. Normally late effects require both a late effect code and a residual effect code with the residual effect being sequenced first. However, codes in category 438 are combined codes which identify both the residual condition and the late effect.

FAMILY PRACTICE SCENARIO

V70.0   Routine general medical examination at health care facility

MULTIPLE SPECIALITIES SCENARIO

V65.3	Dietary surveillance and counseling
V65.41	Excercise counseling
V17.4	Family history of other cardiovascular diseases

The patient has no current medical problems but has a family history of heart disease which can be affected by diet and exercise. Therefore, this visit would be reported with V-codes describing the counseling services as well as a V-code reporting the family history of heart disease.

PEDIATRICS/FAMILY PRACTICE SCENARIO

V30.00	Single liveborn, born in hospital, delivered without mention of cesarean delivery

Chapter 4 — Anesthesia

CODING PRACTICE 1

Diagnosis

820.8	Closed fracture of unspecified part of neck of femur
250.02	Type II (non-insulin dependent type) or unspecified type diabetes mellitus without mention of complication, uncontrolled
428.0	Congestive heart failure
E849.5	Place of occurrence, street and highway
E885	Accidental fall on same level from slipping, tripping, or stumbling

Anesthesia Procedures

01214-P3	Anesthesia for open procedures involving hip joint; total hip replacement or revision
99100	Anesthesia for patient of extreme age, under one year and over seventy (List separately in addition to code for primary anesthesia procedure)

OR

27236-P3	Open treatment of femoral fracture, proximal end, neck, internal fixation or prosthetic replacement (direct fracture exposure)
99100	Anesthesia for patient of extreme age, under one year and over seventy (List separately in addition to code for primary anesthesia procedure)

CODING PRACTICE 2

Diagnosis

574.10	Calculus of gallbladder with other cholecystitis, without mention of obstruction
278.00	Obesity, unspecified
V64.4	Laparoscopic surgical procedure converted to open procedure

Anesthesia Procedures

47600-P2	Cholecystectomy;

OR

00790-P2	Anesthesia for intraperitoneal procedures in upper abdomen including laparoscopy; not otherwise specified

Obesity, depending on the degree, may warrant a higher physical status modifier.

Chapter 5 — Surgery

CODING PRACTICE 1

Diagnosis

722.10	Displacement of lumbar intervertebral disc without myelopathy

Procedures

63030	Laminotomy (hemilaminectomy), with decompression of nerve root(s), including partial facetectomy, foraminotomy and/or excision of herniated intervertebral disk; one interspace, lumbar
63035	Laminotomy (hemilaminectomy), with decompression of nerve root(s), including partial facetectomy, foraminotomy and/or excision of herniated intervertebral disk; each additional interspace, cervical or lumbar (List separately in addition to code for primary procedure)
22630-51	Arthrodesis, posterior interbody technique, single interspace; lumbar — Multiple Procedures
22632	Arthrodesis, posterior interbody technique, single interspace; each additional interspace (List separately in addition to code for primary procedure)
20937	Autograft for spine surgery only (includes harvesting the graft); morselized (through separate skin or fascial incision)

Procedures 63035 and 22632 are add on procedures and therefore, modifier -51 does not apply. Procedure 20937 is modifier -51 exempt.

CODING PRACTICE 2

Diagnosis Code(s)

996.01	Mechanical complication due to cardiac pacemaker (electrode)
426.13	Other second degree atrioventricular block

Procedure(s)

33212	Insertion or replacement of pacemaker pulse generator only; single chamber, atrial or ventricular
33233-51	Removal of permanent pacemaker pulse generator — Multiple Procedures

Change of a pulse generator battery is actually a change of a pulse generator and should be reported as such. When the pulse generator is changed two codes are required. Report both the removal of the pulse generator and the replacement.

Chapter 6 — Radiology

CODING PRACTICE 1
Day 1
Diagnosis Code(s)
786.51	Precordial pain
272.9	Unspecified disorder of lipoid metabolism
278.00	Obesity, unspecified

Procedure Code(s)

99215   Office or other outpatient visit for the evaluation and management of an established patient, which requires at least two of these three key components: a comprehensive history; a comprehensive examination; medical decision making of high complexity. Counseling and/or coordination of care with other providers or agencies are provided consistent with the nature of the problem(s) and the patient's and/or family's needs. Usually, the presenting problem(s) are of moderate to high severity. Physicians typically spend 40 minutes face-to-face with the patient and/or family.

93015   Cardiovascular stress test using maximal or submaximal treadmill or bicycle exercise, continous electrocardiographic monitoring, and/or pharmacological stress; with physician supervision, with interpretation and report

Day 2
Diagnosis Code(s)

414.01   Coronary atherosclerosis of native coronary artery

Procedure Code(s)

78465   Myocardial perfusion imaging; tomographic (SPECT), multiple studies, at rest and/or stress (exercise and/or pharmacologic) and redistribution and/or rest injection, with or without quantification

78990   Provision of diagnostic radiopharmaceutical(s)

Most cardiologists perform stress ECGs in their offices. Many have the ability to perform more specialized tests like Thallium stress tests as well. Therefore, these codes have been reported as global services. However, if the procedures were done outside the physician's office and the technical component was being reported by the facility, it would be necessary to report only the physician component of these services. Note that there is no code for Thallium stress test in CPT. If the term you are looking for in CPT cannot be found, query the physician about the exact nature of the test. In this case, the correct code is myocardial perfusion imaging; tomographic (SPECT), multiple studies.

CODING PRACTICE 2
Initial Visit
Diagnosis Code(s)

789.05	Abdominal pain, periumbilic
783.2	Abnormal loss of weight
250.00	Type II (non-insulin dependent type) or unspecified type diabetes mellitus without mention of complication, not stated as uncontrolled

Procedure Code(s)

99213   Office or other outpatient visit for the evaluation and management of an established patient, which requires at least two of these three key components: an expanded problem focused history; an expanded problem focused examination; medical decision making of low complexity. Counseling and coordination of care with other providers or agencies are provided consistent with the nature of the problem(s) and the patient's and/or family's needs. Usually, the presenting problem(s) are of low to moderate severity. Physicians typically spend 15 minutes face-to-face with the patient and/or family.

Coding of the E/M services requires some assumptions, i.e. that the patient is seeing her primary care physician and is an established patient. The presenting problems would require at least an expanded problem focused history and exam, but might be at a higher level. In this case, obtain more information before coding the E/M visit.

Duplex Scan
Diagnosis Code(s)

557.1   Chronic vascular insufficiency of intestine

Procedure Code(s)

93975-26   Duplex scan of arterial inflow and venous outflow of abdominal, pelvic, scrotal contents and/or retroperitoneal organs; complete study — Professional Component

Non-invasive vascular diagnostic studies are found in the Medicine Section of CPT. However, the services are frequently performed by radiologists. See the Chapter 8 for further information on these types of studies.

Interventional Radiology
Diagnosis Code(s)

557.1   Chronic vascular insufficiency of intestine

Procedure Code(s)

36245   Selective catheter placement, arterial system; each first order abdominal, pelvic, or lower extremity artery branch, within a vascular family

36245-59   Selective catheter placement, arterial system; each first order abdominal, pelvic, or lower extremity artery branch, within a vascular family — Distinct Procedural Service

75726-26   Angiography, visceral, selective or supraselective, (with or without flush aortogram), radiological supervision and interpretation — Professional Component

75774-26   Angiography, selective, each additional vessel studied after basic examination, radiological supervision and interpretation (List separately in addition to code for primary procedure) — Professional Component

Two first order abdominal (mesenteric and celiac) vessels were studied. Code 36245 is reported twice, with modifier -59 appended to the second procedure to indicate a separate site. Interventional radiology requires two codes, one for catheter placement and another for supervision and interpretation of the angiograms. In this case, the code for angiography of a visceral vessel is reported for the first procedure. Each additional visceral vessel studied after the initial exam is reported with 75774. These procedures are reported with modifier -26 because they were performed as a hospital oupatient service and the hospital will report the technical component. Code 36245, a surgical service, is not reported with a -26 modifier.

Chapter 7 — Laboratory and Pathology

CODING PRACTICE 1

Diagnosis Code(s)

272.0	Pure hypercholesterolemia
412	Old myocardial infarction

Procedure Code(s)

80061	Lipid panel This panel must include the following: Cholesterol, serum, total (82465) Lipoprotein, direct measurement, high density cholesterol (HDL cholesterol) (83718) Triglycerides (84478)
80162	Digoxin

CODING PRACTICE 2

Diagnosis Code(s)

281.0	Pernicious anemia

Procedure Code(s)

85025	Blood count; hemogram and platelet count, automated, and automated complete differential WBC count (CBC)
86340	Intrinsic factor antibodies
82746	Folic acid; serum
82251	Bilirubin; total AND direct
82607	Cyanocobalamin (Vitamin B-12);
82608	Cyanocobalamin (Vitamin B-12); unsaturated binding capacity

Chapter 8 — Medicine

CODING PRACTICE 1

Diagnosis Code(s)

V57.1	Other physical therapy
717.83	Old disruption of anterior cruciate ligament

Procedure Code(s)

97001	Physical therapy evaluation
97110 (x2)	Therapeutic procedure, one or more areas, each 15 minutes; therapeutic exercises to develop strength and endurance, range of motion and flexibility

Physical therapy requiring constant attendance is reported in 15 minute increments so code 97110 would be reported twice. The diagnosis code for physical therapy is a nonspecific service so it is usually a good idea to indicate the condition being treated as well. In this case the patient had an old ACL tear which was repaired surgically so the code for the ACL tear is reported as a secondary diagnosis.

CODING PRACTICE 2

Diagnosis Code(s)

411.81	Coronary occlusion without mycocardial infarction

Procedure Code(s)

92982	Percutaneous transluminal coronary balloon angioplasty; single vessel
93526	Combined right heart catheterization and retrograde left heart catheterization
93545	Injection procedure during cardiac catheterization; for selective coronary angiography (injection of radiopaque material may be by hand)
93556-26	Imaging supervision, interpretation and report for injection procedure(s) during cardiac catheterization; pulmonary angiography, aortography, and/or selective coronary angiography including venous bypass grafts and arterial conduits (whether native or used in bypass) — Professional Component

Coronary angiograms require two procedure codes, one for the injection procedure and one for the supervision and interpretation of the imaging service. The physician should report this service with modifier-26 as the hospital will bill for the technical component. The PTCA is the highest dollar value service so is reported first. The other services are modifier -51 exempt.

Chapter 9 — Inpatient Coding

CODING PRACTICE 1

Diagnosis Code(s)

722.10	Displacement of lumbar intervertebral disc without myelopathy

Procedure Code(s)

80.51	Excision of intervertebral disc
81.08	Lumbar and lumbosacral fusion, posterior technique

In this case the bone graft is not reported separately. The index refers the coder to the term arthrodesis if the procedure when bone grafting is performed with arthrodesis. Unlike CPT coding, ICD-9-CM procedure codes for hemilaminectomy with excision of intervertebral disc and arthrodesis are reported once regardless of the number of levels involved. The code for excision of intervertebral disc contains a 'code also' note for spinal fusion (arthrodesis). The arthrodesis is reported as a secondary procedure.

CODING PRACTICE 2
Diagnosis Code(s)
426.13   Other second degree atrioventricular block
Procedure Code(s)
37.83   Initial insertion of dual-chamber device
37.72   Initial insertion of transvenous leads (electrodes) into atrium and ventricle

Two procedure codes are required when reporting pacemaker placement, one for the generator and one for the electrodes. The procedure will not group to the correct DRG if only the code for the generator placement is reported. Replacement procedures are not reported with the same codes so read operative reports carefully.

Chapter 10 — HCPCS

CODING PRACTICE 1
Diagnosis Code(s)
V25.5   Insertion of implantable subdermal contraceptive
Procedure Code(s)
11975   Insertion, implantable contraceptive capsules
HCPCS Code(s)
A4260   Levonorgestrel (contraceptive) implants system, including implants and supplies

Physicians sometimes make the mistake of reporting both the supply and the implant procedure with code 11975. Generally CPT procedures performed in the physician's office include only the supply of inexpensive routine supplies used by the physician.

Intradermal contraceptive implants should be reported separately with HCPCS code A4260 or CPT supply code 99070.

CODING PRACTICE 2
Diagnosis Code(s)
516.3   Idiopathic fibrosing alveolitis
E933.1   Antineoplastic and immunosuppressive drugs causing adverse effect in therapeutic use
Procedure Code(s)
None
HCPCS Code(s)
E1402   Oxygen concentrator, manufacturer specified maximum flow rate greater than three liters per minute, does not exceed four liters per minute, at 85 percent or greater concentration
A4616 (x50)   Tubing (oxygen), per foot
A4615   Cannula, nasal
E0434   Portable liquid oxygen system, rental; includes portable container, supply reservoir, humidifier, flowmeter, refill adaptor, contents gauge, cannula or mask, and tubing
E0444 (x4)   Portable oxygen contents, liquid, per unit (for use only with portable liquid systems when no stationary gas or liquid system is used; 1 unit = 1 lb)

When a patient requires only temporary oxygen services, the systems are rented. Oxygen concentrators are sometimes used instead of stationary systems. When a concentrator and portable systems are both provided report the portable system as well as the concentrator. Note that oxygen tubing is supplied by the foot. In this case the patient received 50 feet of tubing, so code A4616 would be reported with 50 units indicated on the HCFA.

Index

Continuing Education Module

If you would like to participate in this program that has been prior approved by the American Academy for Procedural Coders for 5 continuing education hours, please send your name, address, telephone number, and a check for $10 to the address below. Medicode will send you a blank test, grade your completed test, and return it to you with a certificate of completion for you to submit to the AAPC.

CEU Testing Unit
Medicode Publications
5225 Wiley Post Way, Suite 500
Salt Lake City, UT 84116

Please allow four weeks for delivery.

- -

Company Name _____

Name _____

Address _____

City _____ State _____ Zip_____

Daytime Telephone number (_____) _____

Continuing Education Module

If you would like to participate in this program that has been prior approved by the American Academy for Procedural Coders for 5 continuing education hours, please send your name, address, telephone number, and a check for $10 to the address below. Medicode will send you a blank test, grade your completed test, and return it to you with a certificate of completion for you to submit to the AAPC.

CEU Testing Unit
Medicode Publications
5225 Wiley Post Way, Suite 500
Salt Lake City, UT 84116

Please allow four weeks for delivery.

- -

Company Name _____

Name _____

Address _____

City _____ State _____ Zip_____

Daytime Telephone number (_____) _____